W9-BJJ-620

Cochlear Implants in Children

Cochlear Implants in Children

Ethics and Choices

JOHN B. CHRISTIANSEN
IRENE W. LEIGH

with contributions from
Patricia Elizabeth Spencer and Jay R. Lucker

Gallaudet University Press
Washington, D.C.

Gallaudet University Press
Washington, DC 20002

© 2002 by Gallaudet University
All rights reserved. Published 2002
Printed in the United States of America

Library of Congress Cataloging-in-Publication Data

Christiansen, John B.
    Cochlear implants in children : ethics and choices / John B.
Christiansen, Irene W. Leigh, with contributions from Patricia
Elizabeth Spencer and Jay R. Lucker.
        p.   cm.
    Includes bibliographical references and index.
    ISBN 1-56368-116-1 (cloth : alk. paper)
    1. Cochlear implants.   2. Hearing impaired children—
Rehabilitation.   3. Medical ethics.   I. Leigh, Irene.   II. Title.
    [DNLM: 1. Cochlear Implants—Child.   2. Decision Making.
3. Ethics, Medical. WV 274 C555c 2001]
    RF305.C485 2001
    618.92'097882—dc21   2001054318

Contents

Preface

During the last few decades of the 20th century, the topic of cochlear implants emerged as perhaps the single most divisive issue among deaf and hard-of-hearing people, educators, parents of deaf children, audiologists, otologists, and others concerned about the welfare and future of deaf people and the deaf community. This topic has become as heated as the centuries-old conflict between oralism and manualism that continues to this day. It is not much of an exaggeration to suggest that the tone of the disagreement approaches that often seen in religious conflicts. The disagreement is particularly intense when the issue concerns implanting children who are too young to decide if they want the implant. The main focus of this book is on pediatric implants and the issues that parents must deal with as they consider a cochlear implant.

We attempt to provide a balanced view of issues that are difficult to deal with in an objective manner. Some opponents of pediatric implants continue to accuse supporters of genocide and child abuse, whereas some proponents of implants have shown little knowledge of, or respect for, the deaf community and its perspectives. We have no illusion that this book will put a stop to all these charges and countercharges. However, we do hope that with knowledge about how children with implants have or have not benefited from them, and information about some of the issues that parents of children with implants have had to deal with, it might be easier to understand the various issues that have emerged and to search for some common ground among those from the different "camps" in the cochlear implant debate.

Both of the authors of this book are deaf, and each has extensive contacts and experience with the deaf community and the hearing world. John B. Christiansen was born in Wisconsin and grew up as a hard-of-hearing child of hearing parents in Utah. He attended public schools, and, during his elementary school years, he occasionally received special instruction from an itinerant speech teacher. For the most part, however, Christiansen dealt with any communication difficulties by sitting in the front row and ignoring anything he could not hear. He managed to make it through the public school system and attended college in Wisconsin, buying his first hearing aid when he was 19. His sensorineural hearing loss became progressively worse over the years, but he never thought about learning to sign and had no idea what an interpreter was while he was in school.

After college, Christiansen attended graduate school in Pennsylvania, Wisconsin, and California, earning a Ph.D. in sociology from the University of California, Riverside, in 1976. Even though one of the residential schools for deaf students in California is located in Riverside, he had little contact with deaf students, or deaf people generally, before coming to Gallaudet in 1977. In fact, he had never even heard of Gallaudet until he was looking for a job in 1976.

Following his appointment as a professor in the Department of Sociology at Gallaudet in 1977, Christiansen quickly learned how to sign. His signing is a hybrid of English and American Sign Language (ASL), a form known as "contact sign." Contact sign is the type of signing that many, perhaps most, people, both deaf and hearing, use at Gallaudet University. His hearing loss has progressed and is currently somewhere in the severe to profound range.

As a sociologist, Christiansen has been interested in issues related to social conflict and conflict resolution, and, with his colleague Sharon Barnartt, wrote a book about the 1988 Deaf President Now protest at Gallaudet University (Christiansen & Barnartt, 1995). Since then, perhaps the most intense social conflict affecting deaf people and the deaf community has centered on pediatric cochlear implants. The primary reason for his interest in writing this book is to see if there might be a way to look more objectively at this contentious issue, and to try to encourage people to identify those areas where they might work together for the benefit of all deaf people, whether they have a cochlear implant or not.

Irene W. Leigh was born in London, England, to refugee parents who had fled Germany immediately prior to World War II. She was diagnosed as deaf on her second birthday. This came as a shock to her parents who had never heard the word "deaf." Her parents were referred to a speech and language therapist who worked to help their daughter develop spoken language. Sign language was never presented as an option.

When Leigh turned 4, her family emigrated to the United States and settled in Chicago, where she attended the A. G. Bell School, a school that encompassed both the local elementary school in its neighborhood as well as an oral day program. This provided her with the opportunity to attend both specialized and mainstreamed classes. She was fully mainstreamed in high school, but always remained anchored to the homeroom, which consisted of deaf students only. Interpreter service was unheard of; Leigh got by with lipreading and listening skills honed through powerful hearing aids. She obtained her training as a teacher of the deaf at Northwestern University and eventually received a master's degree in rehabilitation counseling, a subsequent one in psychology, and her Ph.D. in clinical psychology in 1986, all from New York University. She has always socialized with both deaf and hearing peers, but did not use sign language until her college years, when she began interacting more with deaf people who relied on ASL.

Leigh came to Gallaudet in 1992 from the Lexington Center for Mental Health Services in New York City, where she was assistant director. Currently, she is a professor in the clinical psychology doctoral program in the Department of Psychology. She has published and presented in the areas of parenting, attachment, psychological issues, assessment, and multiculturalism, all related to deafness. Most recently, she has edited a book, *Psychotherapy with Deaf Clients from Diverse Groups* (Leigh, 1999). She is also the parent of two children, one of whom is deaf. Her own personal experience in exploring options for her deaf son have greatly attuned her to what parents go through in making decisions for their deaf child, though she did not have to learn about deafness after her child was diagnosed.

Leigh's exposure to the different ways deaf persons choose to be deaf, whether in the mainstream, with oral peers, as part of deaf culture, or an amalgam of each, has reinforced her interest in understanding how deaf persons experience being deaf, depending on culture, background, and exposure to other deaf models. The topic of cochlear implants represents for her a new way for deaf people to deal with the challenge of being deaf, admittedly a controversial way at present. Her interest in how that process evolves and is influenced by parental decisions, deaf community perceptions, and individual life experiences facilitated her involvement with the research work culminating in this book.

Clearly, both authors come to this book from different professional backgrounds and from different personal experiences of
being deaf. We are part of the deaf and hearing worlds. We have
observed the emergence of cochlear implants on the scene and the
intense reactions of proponents and opponents. We are very much
aware that the entire process of exploring, obtaining, and living
with cochlear implants is heavily colored by hearing and deaf perspectives, as well as medical and cultural perspectives. These are
ripe for investigation by sociology and psychology. Our collaboration is an effort in this direction.

A study of this scope could not have been completed without
the help and support of many people. As will be discussed in the
Introduction, most of the data analyzed in this book come from
two sources: several hundred parents of children with cochlear
implants who responded to a lengthy questionnaire that was distributed by the Gallaudet Research Institute (GRI) in the spring and
summer of 1999, and several dozen parents who talked with us
about their experiences. In a number of cases, parents took time to
do both. We thank these parents for completing the questionnaire,
and for welcoming us into their homes and sharing some of their
family's most intense and emotional experiences with us. We also
thank many of the parents for diligently reviewing the initial transcript of the interview and adding comments that, in some cases,
must have taken several additional hours of their time. Hopefully,
they know how valuable their contribution is to this book. Their
experiences will teach us how the process of pediatric cochlear
implantation, and its aftermath, should be approached by parents,
their children, professionals, cochlear implant centers, and the
deaf community. We are also grateful to the children, adolescents,
and college students who willingly shared with us their experiences with cochlear implants.

Before each interview, parents completed an informed consent
form that had been approved by Gallaudet's Institutional Research
Board allowing us to use the information they shared with us, as well
as their names. Although no one refused to sign the form allowing
us to use the information, some parents did not want their name, or
the name of their child or children, to appear in this book. Most parents, however, indicated that it was fine with them if we used their
names. After much deliberation, we decided not to use the names

of any of the families we talked with to preserve confidentiality. Although some people may be disappointed not to see their name in print, we felt it was more important to ensure that everyone's right to privacy was respected, and we felt it would be confusing to use some, but not all, of the names of the people we interviewed. We have, however, provided identifying information for most of the quotations that are used in the book, usually identifying the source of the quote by gender, the age of the child, and when the child received the cochlear implant. Although the rest of the world might not know who they are, we hope the people who shared these quotations with us will recognize their contribution and accept our thanks.

In addition to the parents, we are grateful for the financial support from the GRI, formerly headed by Brenda Rawlings (now retired) and, before that, by Thomas Allen, currently a dean at Gallaudet. We received considerable support from GRI for 2 years, and the extensive interviewing in various parts of the country would not have been possible without this assistance. We also acknowledge, with thanks, the work of Sally Dunn in GRI who, among other duties, was responsible for administering the funds of the grant.

We are also grateful to Jane Dillehay, the dean of the College of Liberal Arts, Sciences, and Technologies at Gallaudet, and to the former vice president for academic affairs, Roslyn Rosen, who supported sabbatical leaves for both of us during the 1999–2000 academic year so we could devote more time to this project. Rebecca Hogan, Kathleen Annese, Carol Hendrickson, Charlie McKellar, Amanda Hartmann, and Paul Davis did an outstanding job of transcribing the sometimes difficult to understand audiotaped interviews. Some of these transcribers, as well as Jennifer Strunk, David Feldman, Kim Arnold, and Raylene Harris, current or former graduate students at the university, also transcribed the videotaped interviews. Raylene Harris, Jennifer Strunk, Lauren Esposito, and Paul Davis also provided other assistance in securing relevant documents. Raylene Harris ably assisted with the distribution of the questionnaire to Gallaudet faculty, staff, students, and alumni, and Michael J. Gournaris, another graduate student, did an excellent job of compiling and editing the references. Susan Duncan provided us with extensive and thought-provoking comments of the entire manuscript, and Amanda Christiansen patiently taught her father, John Christiansen, how to make duplicate copies of the audiotaped interviews on her stereo equipment. The help of each and everyone is gratefully acknowledged.

Several of our colleagues at Gallaudet warrant special thanks. Senda Benaissa, who currently works for GRI, contributed greatly to the data analysis of both the GRI study and the questionnaires that were distributed to Gallaudet faculty, staff, students, and alumni. In addition, we want to thank Margaret Weigers, a professor in the sociology department, for her assistance in teaching John Christiansen how to use a software program for analyzing the interview data, and for her encouragement and support throughout this project. With over 2,500 pages of interview transcripts, it would have been impossible to systematically analyze these data without Dr. Weigers's assistance. We also thank two people at the Gallaudet University Press: Ivey Pittle Wallace for her valuable comments, good cheer, encouragement, and support over the years, and Deirdre Mullervy for her very helpful editorial assistance. Finally, we want to thank Virginia Gutman, a professor in the Department of Psychology, who provided an abundance of insightful comments on the chapter related to ethical considerations.

One person who needs to be singled out for special thanks is Lisa Holden-Pitt, currently an education research analyst at the United States Department of Education. Dr. Holden-Pitt was primarily responsible for developing the GRI questionnaire that was distributed to parents of children with cochlear implants in the spring of 1999. She also spent countless hours "cleaning" the data after the questionnaires were returned, assisting the authors in developing our parent interview questions, providing an abundance of good advice whenever she was asked, and reading and commenting on drafts of most of the chapters. This book would certainly be quite different, and less complete, without her considerable assistance.

Introduction

The vast majority of parents of deaf children are hearing people who generally have little, if any, contact with deaf people and know next to nothing about deafness before discovering that their child is deaf. Whether they learn of their child's deafness on their own, or whether their child's deafness is diagnosed by an audiologist or pediatrician, many parents are not only shocked and devastated by the news, but they also have few clues about what course of action to take subsequent to this discovery. Many feel the need to "do something," but few have any inkling about what to do when they need to start making decisions about how to socialize and educate their child. This book focuses on some of the issues and questions parents confront when they consider obtaining a cochlear implant for their deaf child.

Rather than simply describe the actions these parents took, we want to draw on some recent social and behavioral science research to interpret why many hearing parents of deaf children continue to find implants attractive. Specifically, we want to know the answers to the following questions: How do parents *perceive their situations?* What are some of the *assumptions* they bring to their decision-making? What are some of the *behavioral patterns* that follow from these decisions? What are some of the *social implications and consequences* of these actions? (Adapted from Anderson, 1999, p. 11; italics added.)

One way to help explain and put into perspective the actions that the parents have taken is to look at some of the assumptions that these parents brought with them to the situation in which they found themselves. That is, how did they (and how do they continue to) define their situation? How one interprets or perceives a situation or circumstance depends in large measure on the assumptions one brings to that situation. Furthermore, the actions one takes depend on one's assumptions about what he or she thinks should be done. And, of course, these actions have intended and unintended consequences or implications. The chain linking situations, assumptions, actions, and consequences is an important one and will be referred to from time to time in this book to organize and help explain our data.

In addition to these questions, we have incorporated some insights from social scientists who have suggested that the traditional anthropological definition of the term "culture" needs to be reconceptualized in a way that can help us better explain why people are more likely to adopt one course of action rather than another. Traditionally, culture has been defined quite broadly as the "way of life" of a people or society that includes norms, values, mores, language, artifacts, and other characteristics. There are few attributes or characteristics of a group or category of people that would appear to exist outside of this global view of culture. We often talk about "deaf culture," for example, and this would include such characteristics as the use of American Sign Language, residential schools for deaf students, and norms governing appropriate interaction between deaf and hearing, and deaf and deaf people. People also discuss "hearing culture" as if that, too, had distinguishing values and norms that can be clearly identified, and are somewhat different from those found in deaf culture.

One difficulty with such interpretations of the term culture is that, by encompassing such a broad range of activities and characteristics, they do not provide us with much help when it comes to using the concept analytically to explain individual actions. There needs to be a better way to link the characteristics of a group or society, which undoubtedly exist and are undoubtedly important, to individual actions.

Instead of a global view of culture that encompasses a society's entire way of life, sociologist Ann Swidler (1986) suggests that a more useful way to conceptualize culture is to see it as a "tool kit," or a collection of resources, from which people are able to select different pieces to construct various "strategies of action" in different situations. Rather than conceptualizing culture as providing us with the "ends" or values that we have learned via the socialization process and that we more or less take for granted, this view of culture focuses more on the "means" by which people pursue various courses of action as they attempt to solve problems of everyday life. One of the advantages of focusing primarily on means rather than ends is that it helps us ask better questions about how people come to make sense of the situations in which they find themselves, and how they act on the basis of their assumptions, exactly the kinds of questions we adapted from Anderson.

In her discussion of culture in action, Swidler focuses on two general situations. In one situation, which she terms "settled lives," culture provides us with a tool kit of skills and knowledge that we use to pursue various activities that are essentially unquestioned and unchallenged. As Swidler notes, when people live settled lives, they "naturally know how to act" (1986, p. 280). Unless something happens to a group or to an individual, most people do pretty much what they have been taught to do, and which they more or less accept as the way things should be done. For example, most parents have not taken a comprehensive course in parenting before becoming a parent. It is likely that most parental skills come either from "on the job training" or from the anticipatory socialization experiences that one had as a child (e.g., trying to remember what your parents did or did not do to or for you when you were young). If nothing happens to question their parental skills, or the course of action they should pursue, parents are likely to stick with the equipment in their cultural tool kit that worked for their own parents and that seems to be working for others.

Not surprisingly, Swidler's other category is "unsettled lives." Although Swidler primarily focuses on unsettled cultural periods, her conceptualization can apply just as well to unsettled periods in a person's (or a family's) life. This occurs because of changing or unforeseen circumstances; people are sometimes involved in constructing new strategies for action that are not simply carbon copies of what they learned during their own socialization experiences.

Where do people look for pieces to add to their new tool kit to develop appropriate strategies for action when their lives become unsettled? Or, more specifically for purposes of this book, what do hearing parents do when they discover their child is deaf and lack even the most basic knowledge of deafness?

Swidler notes that, even during unsettled periods, people are reluctant to abandon strategies for which they already have the cultural equipment. The first reaction people are likely to have when faced with an unfamiliar situation is to fall back on the tools in their cultural kit that have been effective in the past and hope that they will continue to be effective in the future. In this sense, it is "natural" for a hearing parent of a deaf child to think initially in terms of wanting the child to be able to do the kinds of things that hearing parents have taken for granted, like having the child hear and speak without too much conscious training on the part of the parents. Unfortunately, parents soon discover that this assumption is untenable in this situation, and a new course of action is called for. The problem is that there are so many different courses of action available that parents report they often feel overwhelmed with the magnitude of the problem and have little idea about which approach might make more sense. And, given this confusion, it is not surprising that many parents would try to find a "solution" to the problem that does not entail the complete abandonment of strategies with which they are already familiar.

The quest for new strategies of action when faced with the reality of their child's deafness is not an easy journey for parents to undertake. It will be clear from our discussion that much of the attraction that a cochlear implant has for hearing parents of deaf children is that it allows them to use strategies and resources that are already part of their cultural tool kit as they educate and socialize their child.

In addition to information from a number of published books and articles, data discussed in this book are primarily from two sources. Quantitative data were obtained from 439 responses to a 12-page questionnaire entitled "Survey of Parents of Pediatric Cochlear Implantees" that were conducted by the Gallaudet Research Institute (GRI) in the spring and summer of 1999.[1] Most of the qualitative data discussed in the book are from 56 interviews with a total of 82 parents of children with cochlear implants (and, on occasion, the children themselves), and one parent of a deaf child who decided not to get an implant. These interviews were conducted by John Christiansen and Irene Leigh during the summer and fall of 1999. Most of the names of

---

1. A copy of the questionnaire, entitled "Survey of Parents of Pediatric Cochlear Implantees," may be obtained by contacting the Gallaudet Research Institute, Gallaudet University, Washington, DC 20002.

potential interviewees were obtained as a result of the GRI study, noted above, as well as from e-mail discussion groups.[2]

After completing the GRI questionnaire, respondents could indicate if they were willing to participate in a follow-up interview that would focus on some of the issues raised in the questionnaire, as well as a few other related matters. Several hundred survey respondents indicated their interest in such an interview. We subsequently contacted some of these respondents (as well as some of the parents from the e-mail discussion groups who expressed their interest in meeting with us) and arranged to talk with them about their family's experiences with (or without) the implant. We did not attempt to randomly select people to talk with due to the impossibility of covering every part of the United States, although we did try to interview people from different regions of the country to make the sample somewhat representative.[3] Interviews were audiotaped and usually conducted in the respondent's home. Each interview lasted approximately 90 minutes, and respondents were offered $25 for their participation. In one case, an interview was conducted in a shopping center (early in the morning before the crowds arrived), and several interviews were conducted at a hotel in the Los Angeles area where the Cochlear Implant Club International (now called Cochlear Implant Association, Inc.) was holding its biennial convention. In addition, two interviews with parents were conducted at the elementary school their children were attending. All of the audiotapes were transcribed, except for two cases where respondents replied to the interview questions in writing via United States mail or e-mail because an in-person interview could not be arranged. In one case, we also received supplemental information via e-mail

2. One e-mail discussion group is primarily made up of parents of children with cochlear implants. We asked one of the regular contributors to this discussion group to post a short notice that we were interested in talking with parents of children with implants. Some parents willing to share their experiences voluntarily contacted us. A short notice was also posted on another e-mail discussion group primarily made up of adult cochlear implant users or those who are candidates for an implant.

3. We interviewed parents of children with implants in 15 states: Alabama, California, Colorado, Connecticut, Florida, Georgia, Idaho, Illinois, Maryland, New Jersey, New York, Oregon, Pennsylvania, Virginia, and Washington. Irene Leigh also interviewed one family in Australia.

GRI Methodology Used in the 1999 "Survey of Parents of Pediatric Cochlear Implantees"

Each year, for more than 30 years, the GRI has conducted a study called the *Annual Survey of Deaf and Hard-of-Hearing Children and Youth.* According to Brenda Rawlings, a former GRI administrator, "the purpose of the *Annual Survey* is to provide an understanding of the characteristics of this student population and the educational services they receive." Questions about cochlear implant use among deaf children have been included in the survey since the 1992–1993 academic year.

In an effort to obtain more detailed information from parents of children with cochlear implants, a 12-page questionnaire, *Survey of Parents of Pediatric Cochlear Implantees,* was developed and extensively pretested. Brenda Rawlings describes below the methodology used in developing this survey in a GRI report of some of the findings from this study:

The population reported to the *1997–1998 Annual Survey of Deaf and Hard-of-Hearing Children and Youth* was used to select the children to be studied in the [1999] *Survey of Parents of Pediatric Cochlear Implantees. . . .* Of the 48,564 children reported to the *Annual Survey,* 1,739 (4%) were reported to have received a cochlear implant; these children were enrolled in 416 educational programs across the nation. Although some of these children (16%) were reported to no longer be using the implant, all children reported to the [1997–1998] *Annual Survey* as ever having had an implant were included in the study group [for the 1999 survey].

In the spring of 1999, the GRI contacted each of the 416 educational programs that had reported enrolling one or more children with a cochlear implant and provided information about the *Survey of Parents of Pediatric Cochlear Implantees.* The program administrator was asked to forward the questionnaire, along with the GRI cover letter, to the parents of the children identified. If the parent agreed to participate in the study, the parent returned the completed questionnaire directly to the GRI in the postage-paid envelope provided.

Nearly all the administrators agreed to participate in the project and forwarded the survey materials to the children's parents; follow-up phone calls were made to encourage the cooperation of the educational program administrators and to answer any questions they might have about the study.

Beyond the core group of children identified through the *1997-1998 Annual Survey*, GRI recruited the parents of an additional 102 children to participate in the study; these children were identified through various other means. First, a number of program administrators indicated that additional children with cochlear implants had enrolled in their program during the 1998–1999 school year who were not previously reported to the *Annual Survey* and thus were not included in our initial selection of students. When notified of these additional children, the GRI forwarded additional questionnaires and cover letters for the administrator to disseminate to the parents.

Second, researchers became aware of additional children with cochlear implants who were attending educational programs not participating in the *Annual Survey*. These contacts were made through [an] e-mail discussion group . . . and attendance at professional meetings. ([The e-mail discussion group] is a web-based discussion and support group for parents of children with cochlear implants and others who are interested in learning more about pediatric cochlear implants.) GRI shared information about the study, and if the parents indicated an interest in participating in the project, the survey materials were sent to these parents who then returned the completed questionnaires directly to the GRI. In all, 1,841 children with cochlear implants were identified for the project, and completed questionnaires were received from the parents of 439 (24%) children.

because the transcriber could not hear much of the audiotaped interview. Unedited transcripts of the interviews were sent to all the respondents who were asked to make any corrections, and to return those pages on which the corrections or additions were made (a stamped, self-addressed envelope was included with the transcript). In this manner, many of the parents we talked with made extensive and very helpful additions and clarifications to the transcript.

A total of 63 children were the focus of our attention in the 56 interviews we had with the 83 parents we talked with. Seven families we interviewed had two children with cochlear implants. The youngest child in our interview sample was 2 years old, and two young adults were 20 at the time of the interview. Eight of the children were between 2 and 3 years of age, 22 were between 4 and 7 years old, 18 were between 8 and 12, and 15 were 13 years of age or older. Fourteen children, most of whom were in their teenage years (or 1 year beyond), participated in the interview with their parent or parents.

We wanted to interview parents whose child or children had used the implant for at least a year, although we were not able to adhere strictly to this goal (three children had used the implant for 11 months, one for 10 months, one for 9 months, and one for 7 months at the time of the interview). Overall, the average length of time of implant use prior to the interview for all of the children in the families we talked with was approximately 4 years.[4] Most of the children were still using their implant at the time of the interview, although three had stopped using it for one reason or another, and several others were not able to use the implant for a period of time because the implant was not working properly.

In addition to the amount of time that an implant has been used, another important variable in terms of being able to explain and predict implant effectiveness is the age at which a child receives his or her cochlear implant. In our interview sample, there was a considerable range: The youngest child was implanted at 15 months

4. One child in a family that had two children with cochlear implants actually started using the implant 2 days before the interview! Needless to say, little information about how this child was actually benefiting from the implant was available at the time of the interview.

5. As will be discussed in chapter 1, current Food and Drug Administration (FDA) guidelines stipulate that the minimum age for pediatric implantation is 12 or 18 months, depending on the cochlear implant model. In November

and the oldest child was implanted at 17 years.[5] The average age at which the children included in our sample received their implant was a little less than 5 years. This number is a bit misleading, however, since seven of the children and young adults whose parents we interviewed received their implant when they were 10 years of age or older. If these seven are excluded from the calculation, the average age at which the children in our sample received their implant drops to about 4 years. Thus, the "average" or typical child included in our interviews with parents was about 4 or 5 at the time of the implant and had used the implant for about 4 years.

It is important to note that, as we progressed in our interviews, it became apparent that the great majority of parents participating in this study were strong supporters of the cochlear implant. Clearly, sample bias is evident in our interviews. We realize that it is very difficult for parents of children with cochlear implants who are not doing well with the device to voluntarily come forward and recount their experiences and frustrations. Although we were able to find several such parents who were willing to talk with us, the need for more information about this "hidden" group of parents (as well as, of course, the children themselves) continues to be critical.

In addition to these sources of data, we also conducted eight videotaped interviews with current or former Gallaudet students who are using, or have stopped using, a cochlear implant. We also conducted several audiotaped interviews with adolescent cochlear implant users (as noted, a few other adolescent users were interviewed with their parents). In addition, we distributed a four-page questionnaire dealing with cochlear implants to a sample of Gallaudet faculty, staff, students, and alumni.[6]

2000, one implant manufacturer (Cochlear Corporation) received FDA approval for implantation in children as young as 12 months; for other implant companies, the minimum age is 18 months. (See Appendix for names and addresses of cochlear implant companies.) Cochlear implant surgeons do, however, have the flexibility to implant at a younger age than stipulated in FDA guidelines, if they believe it can be medically justified.

6. A copy of this questionnaire may be obtained by contacting John Christiansen at the Department of Sociology, Gallaudet University, Washington, DC 20002. The questionnaire was sent to a random sample of 110 faculty and staff, 120 students, and 125 alumni in April and May 2000. An additional nonrandom sample of approximately 20 Gallaudet summer school students was distributed in May 2000.

Although this book is essentially about parents of children with implants, family considerations, and some of the experiences of the children themselves, we will examine a number of other questions and issues, including:

1. What exactly is a cochlear implant?
2. How long have implants been available for children and adults?
3. What technological developments are likely to occur in the future?
4. What are some of the ethical issues involved in the debate between supporters and opponents of implants?
5. Is there any possibility of a rapprochement among the different factions?
6. Is a child who uses an implant generally able to hear sounds and understand speech, and, if so, how well and under what conditions?
7. What do young deaf people think about cochlear implants?

Cochlear implant history and technology are discussed in part I. The first chapter discusses the history of cochlear implants; an overview of cochlear implant technology is presented in chapter 2. Chapters 1 and 2 provide background information that will enable readers to place the issues discussed in parts II and III of the book in context.

The seven chapters in part II focus specifically on pediatric cochlear implants. Chapter 3 examines how parents discovered their child was deaf or severely hard-of-hearing, how they reacted to this (usually) unexpected news, and some of the actions and attitudes of these parents immediately following this discovery. Where did they go for information? What kinds of recommendations did they get? What did they do with the conflicting information they often received? What type of information sources did they find helpful or unhelpful? How did they initially communicate with their child?

In chapter 4, we discuss how parents arrived at the decision to get an implant for their child. With whom did they talk? What were their reasons for getting an implant? What did they expect the implant to do for their child? How much, if any, contact with deaf persons or the deaf community did they have?

Chapters 5 and 6 cover the implant surgery itself and some of the child's post-implant experiences. Chapter 5 looks at a variety of issues, including how parents selected a cochlear implant center, the child's initial response (during the first year or so) to the implant, problems regarding insurance, and speech/listening therapy and other communication issues. Chapter 6 looks at how the child adjusts to life after getting used to the implant by focusing on the following questions: How much does the child actually hear with the implant? How motivated is the child to use the implant? What type of communication is emphasized, and to what extent does the child continue to require speech and listening therapy? How much time and effort did parents and significant others invest during the post-implant period toward helping the child acquire speech and/or language?

Chapters 7 and 8 focus on educational choices and the overall progress that the child has, or has not, made with the implant. Where do children with implants generally go to school? How satisfied are parents with the education their child is receiving? What special needs or accommodations do children with implants require in the classroom? What special challenges do mainstreamed students with implants face? Looking back, if parents knew at the time the decision was made what they know now, would they still have decided to have their child implanted when they did? If not, what would they have done differently? Chapter 9, the last chapter in part II, is a review of some of the literature on language acquisition among children who have a cochlear implant.

In part III, we take a look at some of the issues that are unresolved or controversial and that continue to generate ongoing debate. Chapter 10 looks specifically at cochlear implants and the deaf community. Why has the deaf community been so opposed to pediatric implants? How has the position of the National Association of the Deaf in the United States, the premier advocacy organization within the deaf community, evolved over the years? How do parents of children with implants view the deaf community? How do faculty, staff, students, and alumni at Gallaudet University, the world's premier liberal arts university for deaf students, look at cochlear implants? How are students with implants perceived at the university? What are the implications of all this information for parents of children with implants?

Closely related to these questions are some ethical considerations that many people have raised over the years and that are addressed in chapter 11. For example, should parents implant a child without the child's consent, or should they wait until the child is old enough to decide? Does implanting a deaf child deny the child "the right to be deaf"? Is cochlear implantation of a deaf child tantamount to "child abuse" or "genocide" against the deaf community, as some allege? How do parents perceive these ethical issues?

In Concluding Thoughts, we summarize our observations and make some recommendations. Also, we make some suggestions about future research needs, because cochlear implants, or their equivalent, are clearly here to stay.

Cochlear Implant History and Technology

CHAPTER

1

History of Cochlear Implants

with Patricia Elizabeth Spencer

By the middle of the 20th century, the medical profession had made great strides in understanding important physiological aspects of hearing, but nevertheless had little to offer people who experienced a profound sensorineural hearing loss (frequently, but inaccurately, called "nerve deafness"). The first attempt to achieve auditory sensation through electrical stimulation probably occurred two centuries ago when Italian Count Alessandro Volta inserted metal rods in his ear canals and connected them to an electric circuit (an unpleasant experience he seldom repeated—"a boom within the head" [Niparko & Wilson, 2000]). However, little occurred between 1800 and the mid-1900s to give profoundly deafened people any indication that their hearing could be even partially restored (Beiter & Shallop, 1998; Blume, 1999; Epstein, 1989; House & Berliner, 1991).

The first modern attempt to electrically stimulate the auditory nerves in the cochlea[1] occurred early in 1957, in Paris, when French otologist Charles Eyries and his colleague A. Djourno implanted an electrode in a man who was eager to have at least a minimal sensation of sound. Under local anesthesia, the electrode

---

1. An explanation of the function of the cochlea, what a cochlear implant does, the surgical procedure, the equipment involved, and other technical matters is found in chapter 2.

was placed on the bony wall that separates the middle ear from the cochlea. After subsequent electrical stimulation, the patient reported hearing a few different sounds and some common words. The effect was not sustained, however, and the implant was eventually explanted (Beiter & Shallop, 1998; Blume, 1999; Nevins & Chute, 1996).

Four years after Eyries and Djourno performed their surgery in France, William House, an otologist in Los Angeles, and his colleague James Doyle made another attempt to electrically stimulate the auditory nerve endings in the cochlea. House and Doyle implanted several adult deaf volunteers in 1961, and one of them received a multichannel cochlear implant.[2] The purpose of this early multichannel implant was to attempt to provide some speech discrimination. This implant "stimulated the cochlea at five different positions along its length, each sensitive to a different range of frequencies" (Blume, 1999, p. 1258). After additional trials, House decided to focus on a single-channel cochlear implant rather than a multichannel one because he felt that single- and multichannel implants could be equally effective (House, 1995). However, virtually all of the cochlear implants today are multichannel models that have, as their goal, the type of speech discrimination that was of interest to House 40 years ago. Ultimately, because of technical problems with the insulating material, House and Doyle's early implants were unsuccessful and had to be removed (House & Berliner, 1991).

Several years after his first effort, House teamed up with Jack Urban, an electrical engineer, and tried again. In 1969 and 1970, House and Urban implanted three adult patients with multichannel devices that were constructed with insulation material that had been perfected in the 1960s for use with heart pacemakers. These cochlear implant surgeries were somewhat more successful than earlier attempts in that the patients experienced a sustained sensation of sound; still, House and Urban focused on developing a

---

2. Cochlear implants are either multichannel or single-channel. Multichannel implants feature a number of electrodes on the electrode array that is inserted into the cochlea, whereas single-channel implants have only one electrode pair. A more detailed discussion of single- and multichannel implants, as well as the difference between an electrode and a channel, is found in in chapter 2.

single-channel implant (House, 1995). Other researchers in the United States, France, and Australia, however, continued to work on the development of a multichannel device. In addition to House and his colleagues, the most important North American contributors to cochlear implant research during the latter part of the 1960s and the early 1970s were F. Blair Simmons and Robert White at Stanford University, Donald Eddington at the University of Utah, and Robin Michelson, Michael Merzenich, and Robert Schindler at the University of California, San Francisco (House & Berliner, 1991; Schindler, 1999). Most of these researchers focused their attention on the development of a multichannel device that could, according to Schindler (1999, pp. 5–6), "provide speech understanding to totally deaf persons."

Reaction from the Scientific Community

In the 1960s and well into the 1970s, there was a considerable amount of skepticism about the efficacy of cochlear implants, and it was very difficult for researchers such as House and Schindler to secure funding for their work. The opposition to implants during this period did not come from people in the deaf community who, like almost everyone else, were largely unaware of developments in the field. Instead, the opposition came from many people in the scientific community, especially those engaged in basic, as opposed to applied, research. As House (1995, p. 4) notes: "There was much skepticism and even outright hostility that we, as clinicians, should be invading the cochlear domain of the neurophysiologists." Schindler (1999, p. 4) remembers that "auditory physiologists and histopathologists dismissed them [cochlear implants] as misguided attempts by surgeons—who know little or nothing about auditory neuroscience—to stimulate nerves that were already dead." Moreover, according to House, many people in the scientific community did not initially support cochlear implants because implants were judged to provide something less than ideal speech discrimination. House and his colleagues argued, however, that whereas cochlear implants were not perfect, an implant did at least provide some sensation of sound for most of those who had received one. Consequently, they suggested, the ongoing work necessary to improve implant performance was worth pursuing (House & Berliner, 1991).

Opposition was also evident in France and Australia, where otologists Claude-Henri Chouard and Graeme Clark faced funding difficulties and hostility from the scientific community. Like Schindler, Simmons, Michelson, and other researchers in the United States, both Clark and Chouard elected to focus on developing multichannel, rather than single-channel, cochlear implants.

Claude-Henri Chouard, a student of Charles Eyries, "dreamt constantly of an electrical system, a James Bond-style gadget which would be able to alleviate the formidable handicap of total deafness" (Chouard, 1978, quoted in Blume, 1999). During the 1970s, Chouard worked to develop a multichannel cochlear implant with Bertin, a small French electronics firm. Beginning in the mid-1970s, early Bertin models were implanted in deaf patients at the rate of about one per month (Blume, 1999).

In Australia, Graeme Clark was also motivated to develop a "bionic ear," largely because of his experiences living with the consequences of his father's deafness (Clark, 1999).[3] As Clark recalls:

> I knew what it was like to have a severely deaf father from a very early age and that affected the dynamics of our family. It affected our relationships with the community and also was particularly evident in the shop. Dad had a chemist shop [pharmacy] and I used to, as a young boy, go and help him quite frequently to serve at the counter, work in the dispensary. I was embarrassed on many occasions when people would come into the shop asking for personal items. Dad would not hear or he would guess at it. He would ask them to raise their voice and, of course, everyone else in the shop could hear. . . . We would have people come home and dad could not participate in the conversation. Mum had to be the ears of the family. . . . Mum had to be the worrier. . . . I was quite confident by the age of 10 [that] I wanted to be an ear, nose, and throat doctor.

3. In the fall of 1999, Patricia Spencer, a professor of social work at Gallaudet University and one of the contributors to this book, spent several months at the University of Melbourne on a Fulbright fellowship. As part of her work, Spencer was able to interview Graeme Clark and several of his colleagues at length about their contributions to the development of a multichannel cochlear implant.

In an interview with Patricia Spencer, Richard Dowell, the director of the Cochlear Implant Clinic at the Royal Victorian Eye and
Ear Hospital in Melbourne (which is affiliated with the University
of Melbourne), expressed his great respect for the early implant
pioneers who underwent experimental surgery: "In the early
stages it was pretty hard on those people. The [first] two . . .
guys were pretty tough—they weren't getting much benefit.
They had to spend long hours connected up to the computer,
and people were playing them things that sounded like squeaks
and buzzes. Meanwhile, the researchers were grilling them about
what it sounded like, asking them to rate sounds with a number.
This sort of thing is quite hard work for the average person, but
those first two guys took it really well. They were just ideally
suited and committed to the whole thing. . . ."

Field Rickards, now professor and head of the Department
of Learning and Educational Development at the University of
Melbourne, was also a member of the department involved in
implantation research when the first two implants were done.
He recalled the spirit of adventure among both the recipients
and the research team during this period. He also noted that
initial results were more positive than had been expected by
some of the scientists involved. In an interview with Patricia
Spencer, Rickards said: "In those early days the dreams were
[just] that [an implant] would be an assistance to lipreading.
When people started to do some open-set[4] understanding of
words without lipreading, it just blew us away. Just blew us all
away!" This result, of course, motivated further work.

---

4. This means that the person being evaluated is asked to repeat a selection
of words and sentences read by an audiologist in a sound-proof room. The person does not know in advance, or at the time of the testing, what speech
sounds or words (including nonsense words and sentences) to expect. Lipreading is not permitted in open-set testing.

By the mid-1960s, Clark had established a thriving surgical practice, but decided to leave that work to focus on developing a way to electrically stimulate the auditory nerve. According to Clark, "speech understanding" for profoundly deaf people "was the essential goal." After a decade of study for a doctorate, and meticulous research and experimentation with animals to determine if electrical stimulation could, in fact, produce the perception of sound, in August of 1978 Clark implanted his first patient, a middle-aged deaf man who had recently lost his hearing in an automobile accident. Two other people were also implanted with a multichannel implant by Clark's team during that year.

In one of his interviews with Patricia Spencer, Graeme Clark recalls that there were two primary sources of opposition from the scientific community in the late 1960s and early 1970s. One was from physiologists who said that, given the structure of the ear, the implant would simply not work. As it became apparent that the implant was effective, at least to some extent, opposition from this quarter lessened somewhat. Opposition from the ear, nose, and throat (ENT) community, however, was somewhat different. Many ENT physicians suggested that implants would damage the cochlea, since they had been taught that nothing should be placed in the inner ear. Opposition from the ENT specialists also diminished a few years later as the potential benefits of a cochlear implant became more apparent.[5]

The problem of funding the early development of cochlear implants was resolved in different ways in different countries. In Australia, when Graeme Clark initially tried to secure funding for his research in the early 1970s, he was turned down by the National Health and Medical Research Council of Australia, the Australian

---

5. Opposition from medical professionals did not disappear completely, however, and continued in some quarters for another few years, at least as far as children were concerned. As House (1995) notes, one "well-known department head and pediatric otolaryngologist," who was interviewed in 1984 regarding pediatric cochlear implants, was quoted in the June 11, 1984, issue of *Medical World News* as follows:"'There is no moral justification for an invasive electrode for children.' Speaking for himself, he says he finds the cochlear implant a costly and 'cruel incentive,' designed to appeal to conscientious parents who may seek any means that will enable their children to hear.'It's a toboggan ride for those parents, and at the end of the ride is only a deep depression and you may hurt the kid.'"

equivalent of the National Institutes of Health (NIH) in the United States. Accordingly, in the early years, Clark was forced to give speeches for minimal fees and to ask organizations like the Lions Club and the Rotary Club for small contributions so he could continue with his basic research program. He and his colleagues participated in local telethons and even "had to go down . . . shaking tins in the streets of Melbourne asking donors to give to the development of a bionic ear." They spent a considerable amount of time soliciting funds from foundations and other sources during the 1970s. It was not until the late 1970s that he finally succeeded in obtaining research funding from the National Health and Medical Research Council and other governmental agencies in Australia.

As part of his effort to secure funding for his research in Australia, Clark received a government grant that included a provision for a detailed survey of the potential market for cochlear implants. This survey was actually done by a company called Telectronics that, at the time, manufactured heart pacemakers. Eventually, this company developed and marketed the Nucleus cochlear implant device. At present, a large proportion of the implants in the United States, and worldwide, are manufactured by Cochlear Limited (Cochlear Corporation in the United States), the name of the Australian company that now manufactures the Nucleus implant.

While Clark was trying to secure private and public funding for his research in Australia, much of the early funding for cochlear implant research in the United States came from NIH, although the Department of Defense was involved to some extent as well. The NIH was involved in sponsoring basic research and in developing clinical research programs (Schindler, 1999).

An Early Technical Challenge

Blair Simmons, Graeme Clark, and others decided early on that in order for speech to be understood by a person using a cochlear implant, it would be necessary to stimulate different areas of the cochlea. This is because different areas of the cochlea respond to sounds of different frequencies. Among those with normal hearing, when a sound is of low frequency, the hair cells in the apex (top) of the snail-shaped cochlea are activated and stimulate the auditory nerve endings located there. Conversely, when a person hears a higher frequency sound, it is because the hair cells in the base of the cochlea are activated. It was reasonable to assume, therefore, that it was necessary for a cochlear implant to stimulate the auditory nerve endings in different areas of the cochlea in order for the implant user to more accurately understand speech, which consists of various frequency components (see chapter 2 for additional information).

One challenge in manufacturing a multichannel cochlear implant that would stimulate the appropriate auditory nerve endings in the cochlea was the problem of how to shape the electrode wire to allow easy insertion into the snail-shaped cochlea. According to Clark (1999):

> First attempts [in Australia] and in San Francisco showed that [the electrode wire] did not seem to want to go into this tightening spiral. One of the challenges I helped resolve was to play around with a shell on the beach the same shape [as the cochlea] with blades of grass and sticks. And I found a fairly obvious thing. If [the electrode wire] is flexible at the tip and increases in stiffness towards the base it will in fact have enough flexibility to take the curves [in the cochlea] but also have enough rigidity at the base to help overcome the friction that it experiences as it goes around.

Bilger Report

One of the first efforts to independently evaluate the efficacy of cochlear implants in the 1970s was undertaken by Robert Bilger of the University of Pittsburgh and sponsored by NIH. The 1977 Bilger report was based on a study of 13 adult subjects, all of whom were using some type of single-channel implant. The Bilger study suggested that, whereas those with implants were bothered by background noise (a problem that is by no means resolved, even today), they nevertheless could hear sounds of different frequencies, could identify environmental sounds, and experienced an improvement in speech- (lip-) reading (Bilger, Black, Hopkinson, Myers, Payne, Stenson, Vega, & Wolf, 1977). The study did not, however, test whether or not implantees could understand speech independent of lipreading, since it was assumed at the time that this was beyond the capability of cochlear implants (Bilger & Black, 1977; House & Berliner, 1991). Schindler (1999, p. 6) notes that the Bilger report "provided substantial scientific evidence for the benefits of cochlear implantation and gave credibility to the emerging technology." Up to this point, professional journals contained few articles about implant effectiveness, and this absence apparently fueled scientists' skepticism about whether or not implants could ever enable users to understand speech sans lipreading. Until the Bilger report provided independent evidence that implants were providing measurable benefit to at least some implant users, there was a vicious circle of sorts: The opposition of the scientific community to implants made it difficult for clinicians and implant advocates to present their findings at professional meetings or publish the results of their research in peer reviewed professional journals. This, in turn, made it difficult for clinicians to obtain funding for their research. The lack of research was then seen by some in the scientific community as evidence that implants must not be performing very well after all.

The First Cochlear Implants in Children

With the publication of the Bilger report in 1977, 20 years after Eyries performed his first implant operation in Paris, cochlear implants emerged from the confines of the relatively small group of clinicians, scientists, and implant recipients who had been involved with implant development and began attracting the attention of a much wider audience. The year 1977 was a watershed in another way as well: In August, the first child received a cochlear implant. Claude-Henri Chouard implanted two young children, one 10 years old and the other 14 years old, in France. Although, at the time, there was some concern expressed among other professionals about implanting children, Chouard hoped to be able to implant children as young as 6 to 8 years of age in the not-too-distant future (Blume, 1999).

As was the case with cochlear implants for adults a few years earlier, in the late 1970s there was considerable disagreement, particularly among neurophysiologists, about the appropriateness of implanting young children (Blume, 1999). The controversies during the 1960s and 1970s concerning adult implantees, although important at the time, fade into relative insignificance compared with the strong disagreements that emerged among those who support or oppose pediatric implants.

One of the reasons for supporting pediatric implants advanced during this time was that it was important to implant children during the "critical period" of language development. It was thought that if profoundly deafened children missed this optimum period, it would be very difficult for them to acquire a spoken language like English or French (see chapter 9). Even though there is still some debate about when this period actually ends, consideration of a critical period for language acquisition continues to act as a catalyst for progressively lowering the approved minimum age for cochlear implants. Indeed, for many of the parents of children with cochlear implants that we interviewed, as well as for many of those who responded to the Gallaudet Research Institute questionnaire, acquisition of spoken language was one of the reasons frequently cited by parents for implanting their young deaf child.

Reaction from Deaf Communities

Opposition to cochlear implants from deaf communities in different countries, as well as from some organizations of parents of deaf children, began in the late 1970s and has continued in varying forms to the present day. For example, in December 1977, in France, a number of deaf people suggested that cochlear implants were not needed, since they were perfectly happy the way they were. Moreover, many deaf people did not appreciate the suggestion that they needed to be able to hear and speak to lead productive lives. Some asked: "Why not bleach the blacks and blacken the whites? When are they going to stop, once and for all, using us as guinea pigs?" (Albinhac, 1978, quoted in Blume, 1999). Arguments such as these have frequently reappeared during the past two decades and will be examined in more detail in part III.

Opposition to cochlear implants expressed by deaf people in Australia arose about the same time as it did in France. According to Graeme Clark (1999), some deaf people in Australia did not appreciate what they perceived to be the negative image of deaf people that was conveyed in some of the fund-raising telethons conducted by Clark and his colleagues during the 1970s. This opposition made it difficult to raise funds via telethons for a while and forced Clark to look elsewhere for funding.

In the United States, opposition to cochlear implants among deaf people appeared a bit later than it did in other countries. Moreover, most of the opposition in America, and elsewhere, has been directed primarily at pediatric implants. According to Lane, Hoffmeister, and Bahan (1996), the first protest from the deaf community against pediatric implants occurred in 1985, when the Greater Los Angeles Association of the Deaf expressed its displeasure.

> In an interview with Patricia Spencer, Phil Harper, until recently the coordinator of the Victorian Council of Deaf People, said that many deaf people were initially angry about the money being spent to develop cochlear implants and "fix up Deaf people" because deaf Australians had so many other needs. For example, when the early telethons were being held to raise funds for cochlear implant research, deaf citizens still had to pay for TTYs[6] and interpreters themselves. There is now more government support for the needs of deaf people in Australia. In addition, as Harper pointed out, there is "more acceptance and recognition of AUSLAN [Australian Sign Language] as a language." However, he expressed ongoing concern that information given to hearing parents about cochlear implants fails to emphasize other options, such as signed communication for deaf children. He commented that "parents need to understand the benefits of both [using and not using implants.] . . . . [Right now] it's too one-track."

6. A TTY (an abbreviation derived from old teletype machines that were used in the early 1960s) makes it possible for deaf people to communicate on the telephone. By using a specially designed modem with a small keyboard, users are able to communicate with anyone who has a similar device.

Developments in the 1980s

The 1980s were characterized by large-scale clinical trials involving both children and adults, the first Cochlear Implant Consensus Conference sponsored by NIH, numerous other professional meetings regarding implant effectiveness, and the entrance of several commercial manufacturers into the field (House & Berliner, 1991). The 1980s also saw the continuation of strong opposition to cochlear implants, particularly pediatric implants, from deaf communities in several nations.

In 1980, the first child to receive a cochlear implant in the United States was implanted at the House Ear Institute in Los Angeles with a 3M/House device (Clark, 1997). By the end of the following year, House and his associates had implanted 12 children under the age of 18, including two preschool age children, with similar devices (House & Berliner, 1991). This 3M/House single-channel implant, along with the multichannel Nucleus device being developed by Graeme Clark and his associates in Australia, were the primary implant devices available around the world during the 1980s (Blume, 1999).

Both of these cochlear implants underwent clinical trials during the early 1980s. In late 1984 the 3M/House model became the first cochlear implant to be approved by the U.S. Food and Drug Administration (FDA) for use in postlingually deaf adults.[7] According to Beiter and Shallop (1998, p. 6), those who received a 3M/House implant "generally gained the benefits of sound detection, environmental sound awareness, and the perception of some speech cues. . . . In general, recipients were unable to recognize or

---

7. "The first device ever approved to replace a human sense," according to House (1995).

8. There are several stages in the process of obtaining FDA approval for new medical devices. Clinical trials begin with an experimental stage in which only freely consenting adults are involved. Safety and effectiveness are prime considerations during this period. After the experimental phase, an application is made to the FDA for "investigational status." According to Nevins and Chute (1996, p. 24), this status "will permit a predetermined number of facilities across the United States to perform similar tests on a designated group of subjects who meet specified criteria for selection." After the investigational stage is completed, results are reported to the FDA and "premarket" approval is sought. Once this is granted, the new device is generally available to anyone deemed eligible to receive it through various designated centers. FDA premarket approval was granted to the 3M/House device in 1984 and the

understand speech without visual cues." About a year after it approved the 3M/House device, the FDA approved Clark's multichannel implant.[8]

In the 1980s, several companies were involved in the development and manufacture of multichannel cochlear implants.[9] One of the models available in the United States, Australia, and elsewhere was the Nucleus 22, originally designed by Clark and his associates at the University of Melbourne. Another model was developed at the University of Utah and marketed by Symbion as the Ineraid. Like all multichannel implants, both models were designed to stimulate the auditory nerve endings along the length of the cochlea, thus helping the user discriminate among sounds of different frequencies. However, reflecting the experimental nature of multichannel implants in the 1980s, these models were structured quite differently. The Nucleus model had an implanted receiver designed to receive electrical signals from the external transmitter, which was connected to it by a magnet. In the Ineraid model, on the other hand, the only part of the implant that was implanted was the wire that extended into the cochlea. There was no implanted internal receiver. Rather, a percutaneous (through the skin) connector was used (Dorman, 1998). Because this system was likely to lead to more infections than the transcutaneous (across the skin) system employed by the Nucleus model, it was not widely used (see chapter 2). In fact, as a practical matter, in order for implants to become more widely used by children, it was necessary to use a magnet that attached the internal receiver to the external transmitter. Not only did this development help reduce infections, but it also made it easier for the user to keep the equipment in place.

Nucleus cochlear implant in 1985. Premarket approval for a number of other cochlear implants and speech processing strategies for children and adults has also been granted by the FDA during the past 15 years. Data collection continues through the premarket phase to monitor the device's performance. The final stage is "full-market" approval. Although additional data collection is not required when a device has full-market approval, there is little practical difference for the consumer between pre- and full-market approval, since the device is readily available in either case (Nevins & Chute, 1996).

9. During this period, another single-channel cochlear implant was developed in Austria. This instrument, dubbed the 3M/Vienna device, was originally manufactured by 3M and later by Med-El. In its latest manifestation, Med-El is one of three manufacturers of multichannel cochlear implants that are available in the United States. (See the Appendix.)

Early cochlear implant models were much larger than those available today, and they frequently consisted of cumbersome externally worn devices that were difficult to keep securely attached to the user's head. Asking a child to sit still or remain inactive so the equipment would stay in place was asking for the impossible.

Another company that was involved in multichannel cochlear implants during this period was the Storz Instrument Company that began manufacturing devices for researchers at the University of California, San Francisco. This company no longer manufactures cochlear implants, but the redesigned University of California, San Francisco, implant is now being developed and marketed by Advanced Bionics as the Clarion cochlear implant (Beiter & Shallop, 1998).

In the early 1980s, some of the research related to multichannel implants focused on improving the externally worn sound (speech) processor. Speech processing strategies are necessary because the range of electrical stimulation available in a cochlear implant is much narrower than the range of sound intensity in the speech signal. Blake Wilson and his colleagues at the Research Triangle Park in North Carolina, and Graeme Clark and his colleagues at the University of Melbourne in Australia, developed strategies for coding speech signals so they could be more effectively processed by the implant user. The work done in the later part of the 1980s by the scientists in North Carolina resulted in what is called a Continuous Interleaved Sampler strategy. This strategy involves stimulating the electrodes implanted in the cochlea sequentially (rather than simultaneously).Wilson and his colleagues at the Research Triangle Institute donated all the results of their NIH-sponsored cochlear implant research, including the development of the Continuous Interleaved Sampler strategy, to the public domain. Consequently, this coding strategy has been employed by many manufacturers of cochlear implants and is used, in one form or another, in many multichannel implants today (Dorman, 1998). (See chapter 2 for additional information.)

The number of people receiving cochlear implants increased steadily around the world during the 1980s. There were only a few hundred implant users at the beginning of the 1980s, but this number rose to approximately 5,000, most of whom were late-deafened adults, by the end of the decade (Mecklenburg & Lehnhardt, 1991). This growth was particularly pronounced after the

FDA gave premarket approval for the single-channel 3M/House device in 1984 and the multichannel Nucleus 22 implant in 1985. Nevertheless, the growth was still less than what many professionals and manufacturers of cochlear implants had anticipated, and, by 1986, the 3M Corporation began to reduce its commitment to the device. The company stopped marketing its single-channel implant in 1987 and elected to put an end to any additional research on an advanced model (Blume, 1999). Cochlear Corporation purchased the rights to the 3M/House cochlear implant, and those who had received this single-channel device before 3M left the field were subsequently serviced by Cochlear.

Although the growth of the adult implant market appears to have been relatively stagnant in the mid-1980s, the demand for implants nevertheless grew, in part because another market for the device continued to develop. That market, of course, was deaf children. A few children had received a cochlear implant prior to the mid-1980s, primarily at the House Ear Institute in Los Angeles, but it was not until clinical trials under the auspices of the FDA began in 1986 that pediatric implants became more widely available. Initially, implants were only available for older children who received little if any benefit from a conventional or a tactile hearing aid.

One of the centers selected by the U.S. FDA for funding was the Cochlear Implant Clinic, associated with the Bionic Ear Institute and the Department of Otolaryngology at the University of Melbourne. The first child implanted there by Graeme Clark and his colleagues (actually a year before the FDA clinical trials began) was a 10-year-old boy who had become deaf about 7 years before receiving his implant. Clark (1997) reports that he and his colleagues were encouraged with the results of their first pediatric implant and, about 6 months later, decided to operate on a 5-year-old boy who had been deaf for 2 years. The fact that both of these early multichannel pediatric implants were seen as relatively successful, at least by Clark and his associates, led them to operate on still younger children, some of whom were deaf from birth. As Clark (1997, p. 16) notes: "Prior to implanting young children it must be appreciated how important it was to obtain good results on older children, and to see a trend for performance to improve at younger ages." Elsewhere in Australia,

William Gibson was also performing implant surgery on children during this period. [10]

Many of the children implanted in other cochlear implant centers in the United States during the FDA clinical trials were also judged to be doing reasonably well with their implant, at least well enough for the FDA to give premarket approval for the Nucleus device for children about 4 years after the clinical trials began.

The question of "doing well enough" or "doing reasonably well" is obviously somewhat subjective, and the lack of a standard protocol for evaluating the effectiveness of either pediatric or adult implants has understandably led to a good deal of disagreement between implant supporters and opponents. This is particularly true for pediatric implants. Although this issue will be discussed more fully later in the book, it is useful to note here that the U.S. FDA clinical trials in the last half of the 1980s were undertaken on 142 children using the Nucleus system, and, according to Clark (1997, p. 22):

> 51% of the children had significant open-set performance with their cochlear prosthesis compared with 6% preoperatively. In addition, 68% of the children could perceive some spectral cues for speech perception with their cochlear prosthesis compared with 23% preoperatively.

Other results of these clinical trials showed similar postoperative improvement. Findings like this, of course, do not answer the question of whether such outcomes (as well as other, more impressive, results in recent years) are of such magnitude, particularly in real-life situations, to warrant a major operation on a young deaf child. Ultimately, such value judgments will always be subjective, at least to some extent, and for many parents it is an extremely difficult decision to make.

In the mid-1980s, another attempt to independently evaluate implant performance was undertaken at the University of Iowa by Bruce Gantz and Richard Tyler. This research determined that multichannel implants generally provided better performance than

10. The Children's Cochlear Implant Centre in Gladesville, New South Wales (a Sydney suburb), under the leadership of surgeon-professor Gibson, has provided at least 200 children with cochlear implants. This program has a strong emphasis on postoperative habilitation (language, speech, and hearing) services for the children and their families.

In his interview with Patricia Spencer, Richard Dowell, the director of the Cochlear Implant Clinic in Melbourne, said that, at the
beginning, only adults with postlingual hearing loss were
implanted. Given the generally positive results from those first
implantations, two congenitally deaf young adults who volunteered for the surgery were subsequently implanted. Dowell said:
"The congenitally deaf young adults were absolutely deaf. They
had never heard before. And, well, it was difficult. They didn't
make much progress (with the implant) at all. So, I would say
that was unsuccessful." Given this lack of success, the cochlear
implant team in Melbourne decided not to do any further
implantations at that time with congenitally deaf adults. Instead,
they chose a teenager who had been born hearing, but lost his
hearing because of meningitis at 18 months of age.This young
man gained minimal benefit from the implant. But, according to
Dowell, he still said that it was of some benefit to him. Because
of this, several more prelingually deaf teenagers were implanted,
and the benefits ranged from none at all to minor benefit with
lipreading. Compared with what postlingually deafened adults
could do with the implants, these were disappointing results.
But a trend was evident: Congenitally deaf young adults received
no benefit from the implant; somewhat younger teenagers could
get some minimal benefit. Then, a 10-year-old was implanted and
"maybe (got) a little bit of speech perception," according to
Dowell. This seemed to imply that younger children would do
better than older children. This idea was reinforced after implantation of a 5-year-old child (deafened from meningitis),who eventually achieved very good speech perception, being able to
perform open-set speech perception tasks.

single-channel implants. However, the findings also showed that,
as far as speech understanding with multichannel implants was concerned, it did not seem to make much difference if there were four
active channels (as in the Ineraid system) or more (such as 8 or 12
channels in the Nucleus system).[11] Dorman (1998) notes that the

11. Readers are reminded to consult chapter 2 for a discussion of the difference between channels and electrodes.

average score for understanding words in sentences among users of these two implant models was approximately 30% for both devices, with a considerable variability in performance among implantees: 0% to 92% correct. Results such as this in the 1980s lent additional support to those who opposed cochlear implants since, it was argued, the results were both unimpressive and unpredictable.

The 1988 NIH Conference

By the time the NIH decided to convene a Consensus Development Conference in 1988, approximately 3,000 adults and children had received a cochlear implant at various centers around the world. Even though many of these users, particularly postlingually deafened adults, were benefiting to some degree from an implant, there were still some questions that needed to be addressed according to the Consensus Development Conference Statement (National Institutes of Health, 1988) issued after the conference was over:

1. Who is a suitable candidate for a cochlear implant?
2. What are some of the advantages and disadvantages of different types (single-channel or multichannel) of implants?
3. How effective are cochlear implants?
4. What special considerations need to be given to children who might be candidates for implants?
5. What are appropriate pre-implantation and post-implantation assessments?
6. What are appropriate habilitation and/or rehabilitation procedures for those who have received cochlear implants?

The conference was also concerned about future research directions and suggested some areas where more information was needed.

As far as the question of who is an appropriate candidate for a cochlear implant is concerned, the Consensus Development Conference Statement (CDCS) suggested that less than 1% of those people in the United States who had a significant hearing impairment were potential candidates for an implant (p. 2). Since there were, according to the consensus statement, roughly 15 million people with such a hearing loss in the United States in the late 1980s, this suggests that only about 150,000 adults and children were considered possible implant candidates by the medical community at the time. And, among these potential candidates, only a very small proportion had actually received an implant. Clearly, the "market" for implants, as defined, was far from saturated in the late 1980s in the United States.

Although the primary focus of this book is on pediatric cochlear implants, it is worth summarizing some of the views of the medical community for both adult and pediatric implants as expressed in the 1988 consensus statement. The consensus statement recognized there were no strict standardized criteria for accepting or rejecting an adult candidate for an implant. However, in general, the appropriate adult candidate for an implant was someone who had no residual hearing and who did not benefit significantly from a conventional hearing aid. The consensus statement also acknowledged that it was difficult to identify a suitable adult candidate for an implant "because it has not been possible, preoperatively, to predict success with a cochlear implant in a specific person" (p. 2).

In an effort to bring more order to the selection procedure for adults, the consensus conference suggested some "stringent criteria" (p. 2) for future potential implantees, specifically:

1. A profound, bilateral, sensorineural hearing loss.
2. An aided (i.e., with a hearing aid) threshold greater than 60 decibels (dB). (This means that, even with a hearing aid, the potential cochlear implant candidate could only hear fairly loud sounds.)
3. Zero percent correct on an open-set speech recognition test.
4. A lack of substantial increase in speechreading (lipreading) even with an appropriately fitted hearing aid.

The consensus statement pointed out that, as multichannel cochlear implants became more common in the 1980s, it also became apparent that there was an "exceptional performance by a small percentage of implantees on open-set tests of speech recognition" (p. 2). It was not clear at the time exactly why this occurred, but during the past decade or so researchers have attempted to isolate those factors that seem to be important for predicting implant success, both in adults and children. There is still no consensus about why some cochlear implant users derive more benefit than others; as will be discussed in chapter 9, some variables have been identified as being somewhat more important than others.

The 1988 consensus statement also suggested that multichannel implants were likely to be more effective, at least in terms of speech recognition, than single-channel implants. However, at the same time, the CDCS pointed out that there were not many medical interventions that had outcomes as varied as those that were apparent with cochlear implantation. Only about 1 in 20 adult implantees could carry on a normal conversation without speechreading, according to the report. The most common outcome was "some improvement in speechreading ability" (p. 4), particularly among those who acquired language skills before losing their hearing and who were currently using a multichannel implant. Despite this, the consensus statement suggested that "a large majority of persons welcome their implant" (p. 4).

As far as pediatric cochlear implants were concerned, the 1988 CDCS noted that, at that time, implants were classified by the FDA as investigational devices and were only available in a limited number of implant centers. The consensus statement suggested that children should be no younger than 24 months before being implanted and that the other criteria be similar to those established for adults: a bilateral sensorineural hearing loss with an aided threshold greater than 60 dB. Furthermore, it was suggested that there be a "minimum of a 6-month trial with appropriate amplification and rehabilitation" (p. 6), including a trial for a tactile hearing aid, before pediatric implantation was to be considered. Also, as with adult implant candidates, it was difficult to predict whether or not a particular child would benefit from the device before implantation. However, in contrast to its report of adult implantees, the CDCS suggested that, as of the late 1980s, it was not possible to determine whether a single-channel or a multichannel implant would be more effective in children, nor what long-term changes due to prosthesis–tissue interactions might occur.

The 1988 consensus statement also noted that "children with implants still must be regarded as hearing-impaired, even with improved detection thresholds in the range of conversational speech. These children will continue to require educational, audiological, and speech and language support services for long periods of time" (p. 6). Furthermore, as far as language development was concerned, the CDCS pointed out that no studies had been done that could separate "the effect of the implant from improvement due to maturation and training" (p. 6). In conclusion, the 1988 NIH consensus statement emphasized again that "implantation does not restore normal hearing" (p. 7) and that, for both adults and children, standardized methods needed to be developed to measure implant effectiveness.

The 1990s and Beyond

During the 1990s, the cochlear implant revolution was in full swing. About 80% of implant recipients were implanted with a multichannel Nucleus implant manufactured by Cochlear Limited of Australia (Mecklenburg & Lehnhardt, 1991). Because the FDA granted premarket approval for the Nucleus 22 channel implant for children in 1990, only a very small proportion of cochlear implant users at the beginning of the 1990s were children under the age of 18. At that time, the youngest person to have received an implant was a little over 2 years of age, and the oldest was 87 (Mecklenburg & Lehnhardt, 1991). By the year 2000, the number of people who had received either a single- or multichannel cochlear implant had increased to over 35,000 around the world. About half of the recipients of cochlear implants today are children under the age of 18.[12]

During the 1990s and beyond hundreds of media (newspapers and magazines, both on-line and in print, and television) stories about cochlear implants have increased public awareness, although

12. According to information from the three largest manufacturers of cochlear implants, by the end of 2000, there were approximately 4,000 Med-El implantees (with only 200, more or less equally divided between adults and children, in the United States), 6,000 Clarion implantees (with about 4,000 in the United States, also fairly equally divided between children and adults), and slightly more than 25,500 Nucleus implantees around the world. Cochlear Limited, the manufacturers of the Nucleus implants, estimated that approximately 60% of the 25,500 worldwide recipients of their implants were adults. Currently, however, the proportion of adults to children receiving the Nucleus implant is approximately 1:1. It is important to keep in mind that these numbers are increasing rapidly, and, by mid-2001, several thousand more children and adults had received a cochlear implant.

the information presented is not always in-depth or even accurate. Many of the "human interest" stories are somewhat dramatic, in that parents or children or adult implant users often report "miraculous" differences in their lives after receiving the implant. Some stories, such as a recent article in the on-line magazine Salon (A. Allen, 2000), have dealt, often superficially, with the controversy between opponents of implants from the deaf community and others who generally support cochlear implants. Other stories have dealt with specific aspects of the controversy, such as the cost of implant surgery versus the cost of keeping a deaf child in a residential school. Whereas the entire cost for the operation may be as much as $40,000 to $50,000, the cost for the latter may run into the hundreds of thousands of dollars if spread over the entire period when a deaf child is attending a residential school. In this regard, one recent story in the *Boston Globe* ("Ear Implants Are Found to Aid Profound Deafness," 1999) cites research done by John Niparko, a cochlear implant surgeon at Johns Hopkins University in Baltimore, as finding "that 80 percent of profoundly deaf children who receive the cochlear implant [before age four and who received four years of training after the surgery] were able to move out of special education and into neighborhood schools." (This issue will be discussed in more detail in Part II; suffice it to say here that even if they are mainstreamed in "neighborhood schools," many children with cochlear implants continue to need a variety of support services.) Another recent article in *Business Week* magazine (Williams, 2000) describes the frustrations one family in Ohio have experienced trying to get their insurance company to pay for the implant operation. Insurance reimbursements continue to be a major headache for many people who have received implants, and this issue will also be discussed in Part II.[13] In addition, the business world is sometimes involved in promoting cochlear implants. Telstra (a telephone company in Australia that contributed to the development of the Nucleus implant), for example, has made a series of advertisements shown on Australian television in which successful chil-

13. In contrast to the United States, in Australia a limited number of cochlear implantations can be covered annually by public medical funds. After this limit is reached, families can use private medical insurance to cover most costs. If they do not have private insurance (because Australia has a government-provided medical program on which many people rely), they are placed on a waiting list until more public funds are available.

dren with implants demonstrate their spoken language skills in highly engaging ways. Overall, it seems that media representations of cochlear implants are far more positive than negative and may not be accurately reflecting the current variability revealed in research studies.

In some areas of the world outside the United States, cochlear implants continue to generate a good deal of favorable publicity. This is certainly the case in Australia. Examples of the high regard in which cochlear implant programs are held in Australia include the "state visits" to the Bionic Ear Institute at the University of Melbourne by the president of China in September 1999 and Queen Elizabeth II of the United Kingdom in the spring of 2000. The visit of the Chinese president may be the more significant of the two because it is associated with marketing of the Nucleus implants in China, training of Chinese surgeons in Australia, and collaboration between Chinese and Australian clinicians and educators working with children and adults with cochlear implants. One reason why Australia continues to be important for the development of cochlear implants and auditory brainstem implants (see chapter 2) is because of the close relationship between the university, industry, and the government in various cooperative research centers "focusing and directing . . . research towards commercial outcomes" (Clark, 1999). It is clear that the extensive involvement of the Australian government in the development of cochlear implants during the past two decades, coupled with the involvement of Cochlear Limited and other Australian-based companies in the manufacture and marketing of implants, has led to a considerable amount of national pride.

The 1995 NIH Conference

In May 1995, NIH held a follow-up to its 1988 consensus conference that focused on cochlear implantation. By the mid-1990s, the world of cochlear implants had undergone some dramatic changes. One obvious change was the increase in the number of people who had received an implant. According to the 1995 Consensus Development Conference Statement (CDCS) (National Institutes of Health, 1995), more than 12,000 children and adults around the world had "attained some degree of sound perception with cochlear implants" (p. 3). In addition, it was apparent that multichannel implants were more efficacious than single-channel ones, and that implant technology had improved significantly during the first half of the 1990s.

During the years since the first conference in 1988, however, some things remained more or less the same. For example, the second consensus statement noted that by the mid-1990s "the vast majority of deaf adults with cochlear implants derive substantial benefit when the implant is used in conjunction with speech-reading" (p. 3). This conclusion was not appreciably different from the one made 7 years earlier. Moreover, the new CDCS suggested that it was still difficult to predict, prior to the surgery, how well an implant user would be able to perform with the implant. There was still a lack of consensus about the definition of a successful implant user, and the auditory performance of individuals with implants continued to be highly variable.

Focusing specifically on children, the 1995 consensus statement suggested that, whereas early detection of hearing loss is important, it was not clear if "implantation at age 2, for example, ultimately results in better auditory performance than implantation at age 3" (p. 7). In addition, as was the case in the earlier consensus statement, it was noted that children (and adults) who are postlingually deafened show superior auditory performance, compared with those who are pre- or perilingually (loss of hearing while learning language) deaf. Those who have a shorter duration between the time deafness occurs and the time of the implant also appear to benefit more than those who experience a greater time differential.

The 1995 consensus statement noted that whereas there were speech perception and speech production improvements in children with implants, the "variability across children is substantial," and "factors such as age of onset, age of implantation, the nature and intensity of (re)habilitation, and mode of communication contribute to this variability" (p. 9). Additionally, the perceptual performance of children increases somewhat with each year post-implantation and "oral-aural communication training appears to result in substantially greater speech intelligibility than manually-based total communication" (p. 10). The consensus statement does suggest, however, that even with an implant, "oral language development in deaf children . . . remains a slow, training-intensive process, and results typically are delayed in comparison with normally hearing peers" (p. 10).

The issue of language development is one that has proven to be extremely contentious among those who have participated in the discussion about the efficacy of pediatric implants. Some suggest that children with implants learn spoken language easier than children raised in a predominantly signing (including signing with voice) environment, whereas others lament the loss of the opportunity to teach language to a deaf child in his or her "natural language of signs." The 1995 consensus statement notes that although there have been numerous studies of the speech perception and speech production of children with implants, less attention has been devoted to the issue of language development per se. A major recommendation of the 1995 meeting was a focus on language development, as opposed to investigations limited to speech perception and production.

It is important to note that the studies of language development summarized in the consensus statement were based primarily on children with single-channel implants. Given more recent findings, it seems reasonably clear that children and adults with multichannel implants generally understand speech better than those with the older single-channel models. More recent research in the latter part of the 1990s suggests that the language and speech production of children with multichannel implants is likely to be superior as well (see chapter 9). Nevertheless, it is still clear that implantation, by itself, is no panacea, at least as far as language development in children is concerned. Our discussion in Part II indicates that children with implants invariably require intensive post-implant speech and auditory-verbal therapy to benefit from the device. Not even the most ardent supporter of pediatric implants would suggest that the surgery, by itself, is sufficient for language and speech development.

Technological Developments

The 1990s also saw technological advances in the electrode array and in various processing strategies used in the implant and its associated software. As noted, the U.S. FDA gave approval to Nucleus (Cochlear Limited of Australia) to market its implant for children from 2 to 17 years of age in 1990 following the clinical trials that began in 1986. In April 1996, the Clarion system was approved for adults after 5 years of clinical trials, and in June 1997 Advanced Bionics, the manufacturer of Clarion, received regulatory approval for pediatric implants. In September 1996, clinical trials for the Nucleus 24 model were authorized, and in 1998 the Nucleus 24 multichannel cochlear implant was approved by the FDA in the United States for use in profoundly deaf children. This new model appeals to those who want the external components of their cochlear implant "hardware" located behind the ear (the Nucleus 24 includes a behind-the-ear [BTE] model that houses the external components).

The third major cochlear implant company, Med-El, is more popular outside the United States than inside, since the current Med-El model is only available in the United States on a limited basis as part of FDA-approved clinical trials. However, if FDA premarket approval is forthcoming in the near future, this Austrian-based company could give consumers another option to consider before deciding which implant model to use. Like Nucleus, both Med-El and Clarion manufacture cochlear implants in which all of the external components are completely behind the ear. (Again, refer to chapter 2 for additional information regarding recent technological advances.)

Changing Criteria for Pediatric Implants

Another recent development deals with the changing criteria for pediatric implants. As Blume (1999, p. 1261) notes: "Gradually, it seems, the criteria on which children are to be admitted to implant programmes are being relaxed. In line with the longstanding view 'the younger the better,' minimum ages are falling from 4 years to 2 years and now (in one German centre) to less than 1 year. Audiometric criteria are also being relaxed, so that some of the children now being given an implant have sufficient residual hearing to have been excluded only two or three years ago." It is thought that many children with some residual hearing could benefit from an implant, since this would provide them with more access to sound than would be the case with a conventional hearing aid. This, in turn, would presumably facilitate the acquisition of spoken language. Over 200 children around the world between the ages of 6 and 18 months have received a Nucleus or Clarion cochlear implant (Luxford, 2000). It was reported at the Sixth International Cochlear

Implant Conference in Miami, Florida, in early 2000, that "children as young as 12 months of age, and children with significant levels of residual hearing, are now candidates to participate in FDA monitored clinical trials for the newest generation of electrodes and implants" ("Synopsis of the 6th International Cochlear Implant Conference, 2000"). As noted earlier, current FDA regulations stipulate that implant candidates should be no younger than 18 months, should have a severe to profound sensorineural hearing loss (for adults) or a profound hearing loss (for children) in both ears, and should have no medical "contraindications."[14] These FDA regulations are not invariably interpreted as hard and fast rules, however, and cochlear implant surgeons can substitute their own judgment if it is deemed medically desirable to do so.

Given these trends, it is certainly likely that more and more implants will be given to children 12 months of age or younger in the near future. This prediction, however inevitable it may be, is nevertheless seen with some degree of concern by Graeme Clark. Clark (1999) said: "I am not sure myself whether it is desirable to operate on [a child] under 12 months." One of Clark's concerns in this regard is the need to take time to be sure an infant's hearing loss is fully assessed.

Deaf Community Reactions

Deaf communities around the world continue to express very strong concerns about cochlear implants, especially for children. One example of such an expression occurred in October 1994, when the International Conference on Cochlear Implantation was held in Melbourne, Australia. Members of the Victorian Council of Deaf People, led by Phil Harper and Chris Dunn, organized a protest demonstration outside the conference on the busiest downtown street of the city. A flyer inviting people to attend the protest was headed, "Say NO to Cochlear Implants." In their literature, and on placards, they claimed that media reports focused on positive expectations from the implants and ignored health risks. They

14. As noted in the Introduction, one cochlear implant model, manufactured by Cochlear Corporation (Nucleus), has been approved by the FDA for implantation in children as young as 12 months.

noted that money being spent on implantation would be better spent on other programs and supports for the deaf community in general. Their press release (October 19, 1994), however, states: "VCOD does not totally oppose the cochlear implant—to some it holds great benefits. For the implant program to be beneficial to the community, it requires a balanced approach to be adopted based on ... unbiased information and involvement of a wide range of people (including Deaf people)."

This protest did not go unnoticed. Scientists, clinicians, and managers working with the cochlear implant program in Melbourne remembered and commented on it in the year 1999. Moreover, this protest was a reflection of the strong positions taken against the implant in the 1990s by other organizations of deaf people, as noted in chapter 10. The policy statement of the Australian Association of the Deaf, for example, strongly rejected what it said were implications that "deaf people are ill or incomplete individuals, ... lonely and unhappy . . . [unable to] communicate effectively with others, . . . desperately searching for a cure for their condition." In sum, the strong disagreement between supporters of implants and those who express serious concerns about them tend to focus on sociocultural arguments, as well as medical ones. Large and "vocal" numbers of deaf people around the world continue to express their view of themselves as a unique linguistic and cultural community, not a group of disabled persons.

There is also an international trend, supported by many organizations of deaf and hard-of-hearing people that have vastly different views on many other issues, to identify hearing loss early in life. About half of the states in the United States, for example, are implementing some kind of hearing screening at birth, and many more states are expected to begin doing this in the near future. This is becoming possible due to the identification of cheaper and reasonably reliable methods for assessing hearing loss without any cooperation from (or harm to) a young infant. This trend, plus the strong belief by many cochlear implant professionals that early implantation (18 months old or younger) provides the greatest potential, is leading toward ever earlier implant surgery. Data are just now becoming available on the progress these children make with implants, and it will be well into the 21st century before the effect of implantation of such young children will be known.

Meanwhile, some of the opposition from people who identify culturally as deaf is changing in both tone and, perhaps to a lesser extent, in substance. One example of this is the withdrawal of the strongly negative 1991 policy statement by the National Association of the Deaf (NAD) and its replacement with another, more balanced, document which, among other things, "recognizes the rights of parents to make informed choices for their deaf and hard-of-hearing children" (see chapter 10). Another is the establishment of a cochlear implant center at the Laurent Clerc National Deaf Education Center (consisting of precollege programs for deaf children) on the Gallaudet University campus. Another example of the change in tone was expressed by John Lovette, a leader in the Australian deaf community. In an interview with Patricia Spencer in 1999, Lovette said that he continues to be more than doubtful about the appropriateness of cochlear implantation for children. However, he believes that using much of the community's energy to fight directly against implants may not be helpful. Rather, the best counterbalance to the cochlear implantation movement may be for deaf people to become more visible and to present hearing parents with models of successful deaf adults who may not use speech for communication, but who are active members of the society in general, as well as the deaf cultural community. Hearing parents of deaf children can only benefit—and may consider cochlear implantation with even more care—when they see that being deaf and not speaking do not interfere with a happy and productive life. As Graeme Clark (1999) noted: "Deaf children are still going to need to be educated. Some people are going to want their children to have an implant and some are going to want their children to have sign language. . . . Sometimes you need to see how to combine these, and [that] is where I think we need to do research."

Another issue that is emerging is the question of what the cochlear implant revolution means for deaf people outside of "First World" countries. Clearly, the vast majority of implantees are currently in the United States, Australia, Canada, Japan, and Western Europe. Few deaf people outside these areas have access to implant centers, surgeons, audiologists, auditory-verbal therapists, and other resources necessary to take advantage of cochlear implant technology. Moreover, the cost of cochlear implants is prohibitive for millions of deaf children and adults around the world. Access to modern technology in the Third World is not, of course, limited to cochlear implants. However, the question of the extent to which implants will become a viable option for deaf people, especially deaf children, around the world is one that will continue to be discussed in the years ahead. We will return to this issue in Concluding Thoughts.

Cochlear Implants: A Technological Overview

Jay R. Lucker

When a child is identified with a severe to profound hearing loss, the family is faced with making many decisions. If auditory access is seen as an option, one decision may be whether or not a cochlear implant is appropriate. This chapter will focus on the technological aspects of cochlear implants.

How We Hear and Hearing Loss

Hearing is a sensory system designed to pick up sound and transmit that sound to our brains where we comprehend what we hear. Sound from the environment is captured by the *pinna* or *auricle* (the external part of the ear). The sound is channeled down the ear canal or *external auditory meatus*, where it strikes the eardrum or *tympanic membrane* (TM). The pinna, external auditory meatus, and outermost (*lateral*) part of the TM make up what is called the *outer ear*.

When sound waves strike the TM causing it to vibrate, the three tiny bones of the middle ear also begin to vibrate. Attached to the innermost (*medial*) portion of the TM is a bone called the *malleus* or hammer. Vibrations of the TM cause the malleus to move. This movement, in turn, causes the next bone, called the *incus* or anvil, to vibrate. The vibration of the incus then causes the third bone, called the *stapes* or stirrup, to move. These three bones are called the *ossicles*. They form a chain, known as the *ossicular chain*, transmitting the vibrations of the TM to the end portion of the stapes bone, which is called the *footplate*. Together, the innermost portion of the TM and the ossicles make up the *middle ear*.

The footplate is an oval-shaped portion of the stapes that fits into an oval-shaped hole (the *oval window*) in the bony wall separating the middle ear from the inner ear. Beyond the oval window is the inner ear that contains the *vestibular system* and the *cochlea*. The vestibular system provides the body with a sense of balance by detecting motion and sending feedback about the body's position in space. The vestibular system is *not* involved in hearing. The cochlea, a fluid-filled, snail-shaped bony structure, contains the sensory receptor structures of the auditory system, and is essential to hearing (see figure 2.1).

The central portion of the cochlea houses the receptor structures and is called the *cochlear duct* or *scala media*. This duct is a fluid-filled, membranous canal. Vibrations in the ossicular chain cause the footplate to move, which creates waves in the fluid of the cochlea, similar to how an oar creates waves in water. As the waves travel down the length of the cochlea, they cause the upper and lower portions of the scala media to move up and down, just as waves from a passing ship may cause a nearby dinghy to bob in the water. Housed in the scala media are the auditory receptor cells that have hair-like structures (*cilia*) protruding from them (that is why they are called *hair cells*). The movement of the fluid in the cochlear duct leads to a bending of the cilia, and this causes the hair cells to release neurochemicals from their bases.

Below the hair cells are the fibers or *neurons* of the auditory nerve known as the *8th cranial nerve* (or just the 8th nerve). These neurons pick up the neurochemicals leading to a neural impulse (which is like a jolt of electricity) that travels down the long fibers or *axons* of the 8th nerve. Together, the cochlea, with its internal structures, and the 8th nerve make up the *inner ear*.

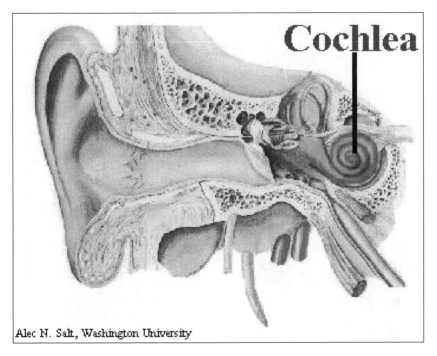

Alec N. Salt, Washington University

FIGURE 2.1
Cross-section of the ear showing the outer, middle, inner ear portions including the auditory (8th) nerve. From "Inner Ear Anatomy," by Alec N. Salt. Available: http://oto.wustl.edu/cochlea/intro1.htm. Reprinted with permission.

The auditory nerve travels from the cochlea through the *brainstem* and projects into the auditory centers of the *cortex* or brain (see figures 2.2 and 2.3).

When we consider hearing loss, we need to consider the part of the auditory system that is not functioning normally. If the problem is in the outer or middle ear, the loss is referred to as a *conductive hearing loss*, and this often can be corrected by medical treatment or surgery (such as insertion of ear tubes to drain fluid in the middle ear). However, if the problem is in the inner ear structures, the loss is called a *sensorineural hearing loss* and is usually permanent. For many people, a sensorineural loss is due to developmental abnormalities of the hair cells, or

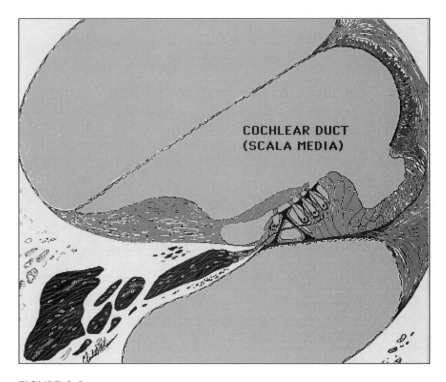

COCHLEAR DUCT
(SCALA MEDIA)

FIGURE 2.2

Cross-section of the cochlea's scala media, including the organ of Corti in which lie the hair cells. From "The Digital Anatomist," by the University of Washington. Available: http://www9.biostr.washington.edu/cgi-bin/DA/ PageMaster?atlas:NeuroSyllabus+ffpathIndex/Syllabus^Chapters/Auditory/ Cochlear^Duct+2. Reprinted with permission.

because of damage to or deterioration of these sensory structures. When sensorineural hearing loss is due to hair cell problems, the normal process of bending these structures, leading to neurochemical release to the auditory nerve, does not take place, and there is consequently little or no access to sound. In short, sound cannot be sent from the inner ear to the brain for interpretation because hair cells for some (or all) frequencies are not available for stimulation. However, in many cases, the auditory nerve itself is undamaged. In such cases, a cochlear implant may be effective. (In cases of less severe sensorineural hearing loss a hearing aid may be appropriate.)

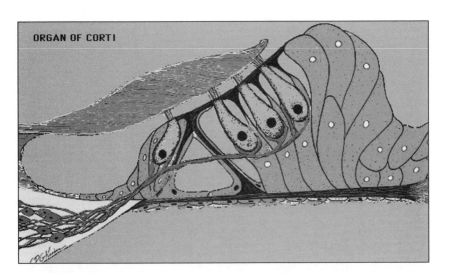

FIGURE 2.3

Close-up of the organ of Corti, including the hair cells and the auditory (8th) nerve fibers. From "The Digital Anatomist," by the University of Washington. Available: http://www9.biostr.washington.edu/cgi-bin/DA/ PageMaster?atlas:NeuroSyllabus+ffpathIndex/Syllabus^Chapters/Auditory/ Organ^of^Corti+2. Reprinted with permission.

Cochlear Implants

Cochlear implants have two distinct components: the internal parts that are surgically implanted, and the external parts that are attached and worn outside the body.

Internal Components

The *internal portion* of the implant includes a series of wires or electrodes that may vary in length with small exposed ends that allow the electrical discharge to be released. This electrode array is housed in material that is both noninvasive to the inner ear structures and that isolates each electrode.

This array is surgically placed in the lower channel (*scala tympani*) of the cochlea of the recipient. The innermost wall of the scala tympani is a bony channel (*modiolus*) through which the auditory nerve fibers or neurons travel. The electrode array is curled or wrapped around the modiolus.

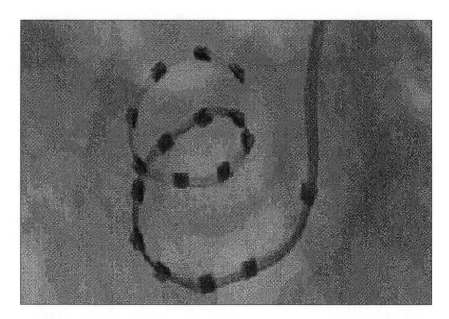

FIGURE 2.4
Actual x-ray photo of the Clarion Hi-Focus electrode in place in cochlea.
Copyright 2001 Advanced Bionics Corporation. Reprinted with permission.

In addition to the electrode array implanted in the scala tympani (*the intracochlear electrodes*), there is at least one *extracochlear* electrode that is placed outside the inner ear in the cavity of the middle ear. This extracochlear electrode serves as a ground. Electricity from the intracochlear electrodes flows to this ground to complete the circuit and create what is known as a *channel*.

Because electricity flows through the electrodes, there needs to be some method for gathering and directing this electrical energy. This is achieved through another internal component, a radio wave receiver. The receiver picks up the electricity that will be delivered to the electrodes along with a program that designates which of the intracochlear electrodes will receive electrical energy, how much energy each electrode will receive, and the order in which the electrodes will be stimulated to discharge. This complexity of programming allows for different electrode stimulation methods provided by cochlear implants (see figures 2.4–2.7).

The internal component of cochlear implants also includes a magnet. This is best understood in relation to the external parts of the device. Its function will be described in the following section.

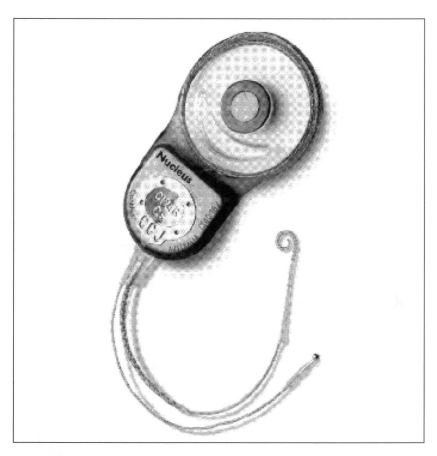

FIGURE 2.5
Internal component of the Nucleus 24 cochlear implant system. Copyright 2001 Cochlear Corporation. Reprinted with permission.

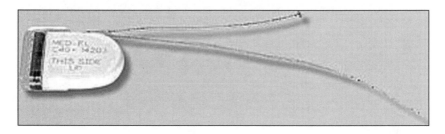

FIGURE 2.6
Internal components of the Combi 40 cochlear implant system. Copyright 2001 Med-El Corporation. Reprinted with permission.

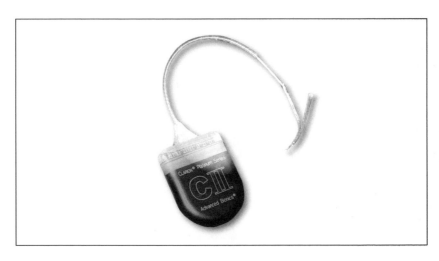

FIGURE 2.7
Internal components of the Clarion cochlear implant system.
Copyright 2001 Advanced Bionics Corporation. Reprinted with
permission.

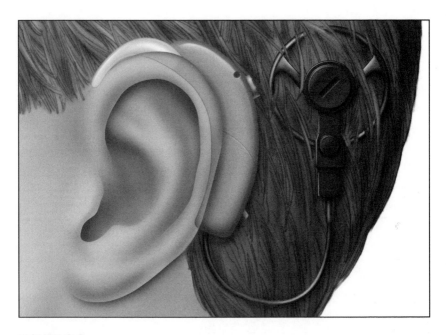

FIGURE 2.8
External portion of a behind-the-ear cochlear implant. Copyright 2001
Cochlear Corporation. Reprinted with permission.

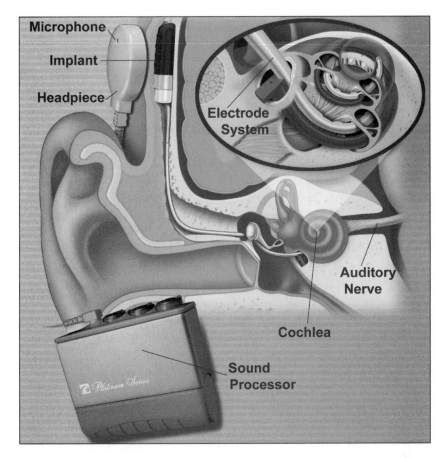

FIGURE 2.9
Cross-section of ear showing cochlear implant with external and internal portions in place. Copyright 2001 Advanced Bionics Corporation. Reprinted with permission.

External Components

The external components of cochlear implants can be divided into two parts. One part includes the sound pick-up (microphone) and speech processing portion, along with the power source or battery. The second part incorporates the program that determines the electrode stimulation strategy, along with the external transmitter that sends this information to the internal receiver. The external transmitter also houses a magnet that attaches the unit to the user's head.

The first part of the external portion of a cochlear implant is, in many ways, similar to state-of-the-art, digital hearing aids. Sounds from the environment are picked up by a microphone that is either worn like the microphone in a behind-the-ear hearing aid or is attached to the external receiver housing that is magnetically attached to the head. The microphone of the cochlear implant sends electrically transformed sound information to the sound analysis system of the implant. This sound analysis system is actually a minicomputer and is usually called the *speech* (or *sound*) *processor*.

After the sound is delivered to the speech processor, it is converted to digital form. This digital information is manipulated by a computer program according to special algorithms called *speech processing strategies* (see below for a brief discussion of some speech processing strategies). Here is where cochlear implants differ from digital hearing aids: Instead of providing amplified intensity to specific aspects of the digitally analyzed information, the speech processor in the cochlear implant converts the digital information into a program that dictates how much electrical energy certain electrodes in the array will receive, and in which order the electrodes will discharge this information. The determination of electrode stimulation is made during a process known as cochlear implant *mapping* that usually begins about 1 month after the surgery is completed. When needed, the implant can be remapped to provide different degrees and modes of electrode stimulation (Nevins & Chute, 1996).

Because of all the computer functions, digital sound processing, electrode programming, and delivery of electricity via radio wave transmission, a great deal of power is needed to operate a cochlear implant. The challenge has been to develop batteries small enough to be included in a cosmetically acceptable device, as well as strong enough to last long and be efficient and economical.

The last components in cochlear implants are the magnets. Recall that the speech or sound processing program and the electricity travel via radio waves from the external transmitter to the internal receiver, and both need to be connected. In some early implant systems, external speech processors were plugged directly into the internal component via a *percutaneous* connection (through the skin). However, problems arose, especially involving risk of infection, and newer approaches using *transcutaneous* coupling (across the skin) were investigated. Eventually, the use of rare earth magnets, noninvasive

Channels and Electrodes: What Is the Difference?

The term *channel* can be confusing when discussing cochlear implants. A channel is often thought of as an electrode; however, this is not exactly the case. A *channel* refers to a *single electrode circuit*. A circuit can best be explained by looking at a basic electrical plug. Most plugs today have two or three prongs. In three-prong plugs, the third or round prong is the ground. The actual electric circuit is made up of the other two (or only two) prongs. Also, one prong is usually fatter or wider than the other. This is often called a *polarized prong.* When a lamp is plugged into the wall outlet, the electricity flows from the wider, polarized prong along the wire to the light bulb, lighting the bulb, then flowing from the light bulb through another wire in the circuit to the thinner prong back into the wall. Now, let's relate this to a cochlear implant to see how a channel works.

Consider the wires inside the wall outlet as the external portion of the cochlear implant and the wall outlet itself as the external radio transmitter. When we place the plug into the wall outlet, this would be like attaching the magnet of the external transmitter to the corresponding magnet of the internal receiver. When the speech processor sends its signal through the wires to the external transmitter, the electricity is transmitted via radio waves to the internal receiver and flows down the appropriate electrode, just as the electricity flows through the polarized prong. To complete the circuit, there has to be a pick up like the thinner prong in the wire of the lamp. In a cochlear implant, the pick up wire is another electrode that is either intracochlear or extracochlear. In contrast to the light bulb, the first or active electrode would end in an exposed tip that would discharge the current in the scala tympani. The current would then flow from this discharge point to the electrode or electrodes picking up the flow (ground electrodes), thus completing the circuit and forming a channel. Thus, a channel in a cochlear implant is composed of at least two electrodes. These electrodes are either both implanted within the cochlea, or implanted so there is one intracochlear electrode and one extracochlear ground electrode implanted in the middle ear space. (It is also possible to have one active or discharging electrode and more than one ground electrode completing the circuit or channel.)

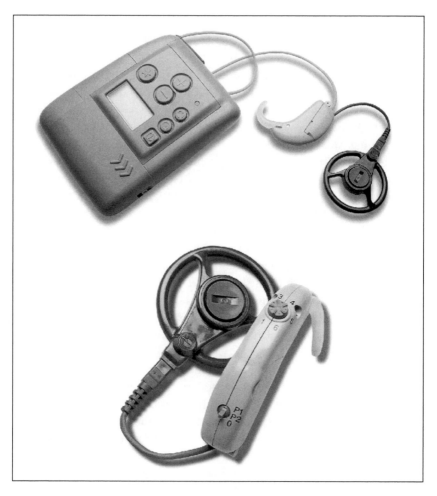

FIGURE 2.10

External components of the Nucleus 24 cochlear implant system. Top: Bodyworn processor showing the speech processor, which also houses batteries, ear-level microphone, and circular headworn external transmitter with magnet. Bottom: Ear-level processor, which houses batteries, microphones, and speech processor, attached to circular headworn external transmitter with magnet. Copyright 2001 Cochlear Corporation. Reprinted with permission.

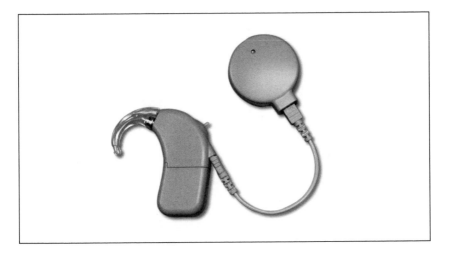

FIGURE 2.11
Ear-level processor of the Clarion cochlear implant system. A bodyworn speech processor would be connected by wire to a headpiece looking the same as the circular headpiece shown attached to the ear-level processor. Copyright 2001 Advanced Bionics Corporation. Reprinted with permission.

to the body, allowed for magnetic coupling of the internal and external portions of the implant. Thus, the external transmitter and internal receiver are connected via magnets that are part of each (see figures 2.8–2.12).[1]

Speech Processing and Electrode Stimulation

Single- vs. Multichannel Systems

When cochlear implants were first investigated and developed, the idea was to provide some degree of sound and speech awareness to persons for whom even the strongest hearing aids at the time could

1. In the past, the internal magnet had to be surgically removed during magnetic resonance imaging (MRI) scans. Today, the use of lower strengths (Tesla rating) of the MRI magnet frequently allows the cochlear implant user to undergo MRIs with the internal magnet in place (Baumgartner, Youssefzadeh, Franz, Steurer, & Gstoettner, 2000; Fishman & Holliday, 2000; Teissl, Kremser,

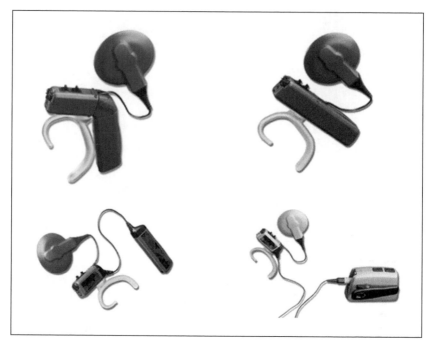

FIGURE 2.12

External components of the Combi 40 cochlear implant system showing the different styles that can be worn with this single unit. Note: The body worn piece in the fourth set is only a special battery pack for longest battery life use with the system. Copyright 2001 Med-El Corporation. Reprinted with permission.

not amplify sound to appropriate levels for such awareness. The goal was to provide electrical stimulation of the auditory nerve, bypassing the nonfunctioning hair cells. Surgeons implanted one or more electrodes into the cochlea and identified which one provided the clearest sensation of sound with the least amount of electrical stim-

---

Hochmair, & Hochmair-Desoyer, 2000). Precautions can be taken after doctors or technicians have been informed that the person undergoing MRI scanning has a cochlear implant. The possibility of "magneticless" coupling to hold the external, hearing aid-like components in place is currently being investigated (Weber, Neuburger, Goldring, Santogrossi, Eng, Koestler, Battmer, & Lenarz, 1999; Weber, Neuburger, Dillo, Battmer, & Lenarz, 2000).

ulation. This electrode was then activated (the others were left inactive), and this single channel of electrical activity (a *single-channel cochlear implant*) provided many users with some awareness of the presence of sound and speech. However, speech understanding was not usually achieved (Osberger, Robbins, Todd, Riley, Kirk, & Carney, 1996).

In contrast to single-channel implants, the development of more sophisticated speech processors and electrode stimulation programs allows for *multiple* channels to be activated and used. In these cases, multiple electrodes are implanted in the cochlea, and, through the mapping process, electrodes are turned on (i.e., activated and coupled with the ground electrode) until more than one channel of stimulation is available.

In addition to the use of multiple channels, the electrodes in most cochlear implants today are varied in length to provide different depths of insertion. A long electrode wire is implanted as far as possible into the innermost or *apical* portion of the cochlea in which lower frequency information is processed and transmitted to the brain. Increasingly shorter electrode lengths are added to the array, and these electrodes are located at the central and *basal* areas of the cochlea where increasingly higher frequencies are processed. In short, a series of electrodes is implanted at different sites in the cochlea, thus providing different frequency information at each site. During the mapping phase, the electrodes can be activated to provide differential frequency information when such information can be obtained from the listener, such as a cooperative adult. In children and recipients who cannot provide this frequency information, estimation is used to determine which electrodes will provide different frequency information.

The general procedures of surgery involve the following: Surgery is performed under general anesthesia, and antibiotics are administered. Since the components are placed within the middle and inner ear near the facial nerve, this nerve must be monitored to ensure that it is not compromised during surgery.

Prior to surgery, the patient is prepped and a portion of hair is shaved from the side of the head on which the implant will be inserted. Then, an incision line is drawn. After the incision is cut, the skin and underlying tissue are moved out of the way, and the mastoid portion of the temporal bone is drilled to provide an insert (well) and tie-down holes for securing the internal receiver housing

---

Surgical Implantation of the Internal Components

Cochlear implants involve a surgical procedure to insert the internal components (Aschendorff, Marangos, & Laszig, 2000; Balkany, Cohen, & Gantz, 1999; Cohen, 2000b; Tucci & Niparko, 2000). The basic goals of this surgery are as follows:

- Inserting the electrode array deeply and atraumatically (i.e., without damage to cochlear structures)

- Placing the internal receiver components carefully against the side of the head to ensure minimal impact from external trauma

- Securing the electrodes and receiver to prevent movement (migration)

- Completing the surgery successfully with minimal danger to adjacent tissue and prevention of infection

- Providing satisfactory cosmetic results (Cohen, 2000b).

---

and allowing for exposure to the bony wall separating the skull from the middle ear space. The electrode array is then inserted into the cochlea. In some cases, a device is used to assist the insertion process; in other cases, the device serves both to assist insertion and hold the electrodes in place permanently. In the latter case, the device is implanted along with the electrodes. Although some of the specific surgical techniques for each cochlear implant are unique, the general procedures are basically the same (Aschendorff et al., 2000; Balkany et al., 1999; Cohen, 2000b; Tucci & Niparko, 2000).

Once insertion is completed, the extracochlear (noninserted, ground) electrode is placed in position. Care is taken to ensure that this electrode does not interfere with the facial nerve, surrounding tissue, or other structures. Then, telemetry is performed to check whether there are any nonfunctional electrodes or electrodes that cannot be used. If any are found, they are identified so they can be permanently disabled during the mapping procedure. This may occur because the surgeon is unable to insert all electrodes, such as in the case of ossification (abnormal calcification or hardening of the soft tissue of the cochlea) caused by meningitis. Once this is completed, the receiver housing is anchored and the surgery is completed.

To ensure proper insertion of the internal components, a postoperative X-ray is usually taken in the operating room. This serves as a baseline for future radiographic studies should electrode movement (migration) be suspected, especially in young children.

Electrode Activation Modes and Speech Processing

When the postoperative healing is completed, the implant recipient is scheduled for activation of the device in what is called *mapping* or programming (Nevins & Chute, 1996; Shapiro, 2000; Zimmerman-Phillips & Murad, 1999). Because of the different ways that electrodes can be paired to create multiple channels, different modes of electrode activation become possible. Additionally, each implant manufacturer has developed different speech processing strategies and electrode activation schemes, although some strategies are similar across devices.

One strategy that is common to all three devices (Clarion [Advanced Bionics], Combi 40 [Med-El], and Nucleus [Cochlear Corporation]) uses one channel stimulated at a time in series. In other words, the channels are stimulated *sequentially*. This mode of stimulation is called *Continuous Interleaved Sampler* (CIS). The CIS strategy provides a very rapid (6,500 pulses per second) rate that can be used by the listener to interpret the incoming auditory information (Shapiro, 2000; Zimmerman-Phillips & Murad, 1999).

In contrast, Advanced Bionics has developed a strategy in which all channels are activated and stimulated at the same time. In this *Simultaneous Analog Stimulation* mode, all channels discharge *simultaneously*, but at different rates and at different places in the cochlea. This provides a digital form of an analog neural stimulation closer to what occurs in the inner ear when sound is processed by a person with normal hearing or a person with a hearing loss using a hearing aid.

In addition to sequential and simultaneous stimulation modes, there are combination forms, such as *Paired Pulsatile Sampler* (pairs of channels are stimulated simultaneously) (Zimmerman-Phillips & Murad, 1999). However, no one mode of electrode stimulation appears to be preferable over the others, and many users have different modes programmed into different memories in their cochlear implant to allow for switching during daily use (Battmer, Haake, Zilberman, & Lenarz, 1999; Osberger & Fisher, 1999).

In addition to the different modes of electrode stimulation, the implant companies use different speech processing strategies. Some strategies look at the general pattern of sound or speech, whereas others look at specific patterns. Often, speech processing strategies try to extract the maximal energy found in the speech signal and deliver that information in the form of specific frequencies of information to electrodes corresponding to those frequencies. Acronyms such as MPEAK, SPEAK, and ACE refer to these types of speech processing strategies.

Some research has been done to compare the effectiveness of different speech processing strategies. In general, the findings show no one strategy to be superior to another, although newer speech processing strategies provide better speech perception and awareness than older strategies (Geers, Brenner, & Davidson, 2000a; Osberger et al., 1996).

In addition to investigating differences between speech processing strategies and modes of electrode stimulation, some research has compared the relative merits of the Nucleus and Clarion devices. One problem with comparing devices is that, as noted, each company has developed different speech processing strategies and electrode activation schemes, and CIS is the only strategy common to both Nucleus and Clarion implant systems. Thus, trying to determine whether one implant system is more effective than another presents many confounding differences. Nevertheless, some of the investigations that have been completed have found that speech perception scores are generally higher for subjects using the Clarion device, compared with the Nucleus implant system (Osberger et al., 1996; Nevins & Chute, 1996; Young, Grohne, Carrasco, & Brown, 1999). Furthermore, both the Nucleus and Clarion devices have been found to provide better speech perceptual performance and expected outcome than hearing aids when matching subjects for similar degrees of hearing loss (Osberger et al., 1996; Svirsky & Meyer, 1999).

Where Are We Headed?

There has clearly been a great deal of progress since the days of single-channel cochlear implants. More sophisticated electrode arrays and placements and more sophisticated speech processing strategies have been developed. Additionally, improvements in electrode development have provided for newer surgical techniques that allow electrode placement much closer to the bony wall of the modiolus. This placement requires less electricity to provide sound awareness, thus improving access to sound and speech. Lastly, the development of improved battery consumption and smaller batteries has allowed for the development of smaller, totally ear-/head-worn devices that are more cosmetically appealing and that may provide for greater mobility with less chance of damage to the body-worn wires and speech processor. Some possible future developments are as follows:

- A totally implantable system with *no* external devices, including a microphone implanted in the ear canal picking up sound much as the eardrum does. This is being investigated by a number of cochlear implant companies and is a realistic possibility for the not-too-distant future. However, problems related to power source, implant size, the body's acceptance of a foreign object, and product failure issues that may lead to additional surgery have to be resolved before totally implanted devices become a reality.
- Significantly more sophisticated speech processing strategies and electrode stimulation modes that provide greater representation of the normal analog speech signal to the listener.
- Greater and more accurate prediction of what is actually being stimulated using electrode discharges. This is currently being investigated through such strategies as *Neural Response Telemetry* (NRT) in some Nucleus devices. NRT provides feedback from the cochlea regarding what is happening with the auditory nerve after electrode stimulation has occurred.

- Better mapping for difficult cases and for young children. NRT may be one answer to this problem.
- Wider use of auditory brainstem implants that function like a cochlear implant, but whose electrodes stimulate the auditory pathways beyond the 8th cranial nerve. A brainstem implant may be appropriate in cases of damage to the 8th nerve when the higher central nervous system pathways are still functioning normally (Otto, Ebinger, & Staller, 2000; Vincent, LeJeune, & Vaneecloo, 2000).

Pediatric Cochlear Implants

3

Pre-Implant Issues

When we met with parents, we asked them to describe the process leading to the realization that their child was deaf. Most of them learned of their child's deafness quite gradually, except, of course, in those cases where the child had an illness, such as meningitis, which caused an immediate loss of hearing. In the absence of early screening for hearing loss, it was difficult for many parents to determine if their child was deaf until the child was at least several months old. In fact, this delayed awareness was the case for almost all of the parents we talked with, since they were not expecting a deaf child and had little familiarity with deafness. Moreover, many of these parents, like most parents, were not sure how much children were "supposed" to hear during the first year of life, or how a hearing infant typically reacts to sound. Only four of the families in our sample became aware of their child's deafness at birth, or shortly thereafter, primarily because early screening happened to be available at the hospital where their child was born, or because they specifically requested it. Of course, not all of the children were deaf at birth, but most of them probably were, even though the parents did not realize this until months later. Of the parents who discussed this issue with us, about a third of them became aware of their child's deafness before the child was 12 months old, and about half learned of their child's hearing loss between 12 and 24 months. Only a small handful learned of their child's deafness after 2 years, and in many of those cases deafness was due to meningitis.

The question of how parents became aware of their child's deafness is one that caused many parents to look back in both wonder and, sometimes, anger, at the delay in getting the "official" word that their child was deaf. Many parents had suspicions months before they were able to get confirmation, either from an electrophysiological procedure such as an auditory brainstem response (ABR) test, a passive test that measures the electrical activity of the brain in response to sound, from the absence of a response from their (presumably alert) child in a hearing test in a sound-proof booth, or from another test (such as a tympanogram that measures the condition of the eardrum and the middle ear, or an otoacoustic emissions test that measures the functioning of the cochlea) (Copmann, 1996).

Several parents said that they initially became suspicious when their child did not react to loud noise. Even though many parents were suspicious several months before a final diagnosis was made, some tried to ignore or otherwise explain away the fact that their assumptions about their child's "normal" hearing ability were being challenged.

> FATHER: It didn't even occur to us that there was a possibility [that she might be deaf]. We just slowly . . . began to realize that [our daughter] wasn't responding to her name.

> MOTHER: [Our] daughter might be confused, because we speak two languages, and so we always thought that [she] was just delayed. . . . We would tap and she still wouldn't look at us . . . and she wouldn't turn, but it never occurred to us that she couldn't hear.

> The father finally recognized that his daughter was probably deaf rather suddenly: One day, I was taking a nap with [my daughter] and it just hit me that I didn't think she was hearing. So I put an alarm clock next to her ear. She didn't wake up, so that's when I realized. . . .
> *Parents of a 3-year-old girl implanted in 1998*[1]

---

1. Unless otherwise noted, ages given for the children at the end of the quotations are as of 1999.

MOTHER: We suspected that there might have been a problem ... when [our son] was maybe 4 or 5 months old. We noticed that he was not consistently responding to sounds. We were able to vacuum in his room when he was asleep, and it wouldn't wake him up. ... So we took him to the pediatrician and asked. The pediatrician snapped his fingers in front of [our son's] face and [our son] blinked.

INTERVIEWER (seeking clarification): Snapped his fingers behind his head?

MOTHER: No, in front of his face.

INTERVIEWER (somewhat incredulous): In front of his face.

MOTHER: In front of his face. ... [The pediatrician] did not think there was a problem with [our son's] hearing. And, not wanting to believe that there was, we continued on [for several more months].

As was the case with several of the parents we talked with, confirmation of their child's deafness came only after the intervention of a third party. The mother of the boy above and her husband served in the military, and while they were overseas their son went to stay with her brother and sister-in-law in another state.

[The brother and sister-in-law] have a son who is a year older than [our son] and they were able to compare his responses, and it was obvious at that time that there was a problem. And they took him to be evaluated in [city], and it was determined that he was deaf.

Mother of a 10-year-old boy implanted at age 6

A number of other parents we talked with reported that others, such as a babysitter or a relative, suspected a hearing loss in their child even before they, the parents, did. Several parents mentioned that an in-law, or one of their own parents, was the first to notice that the child was not hearing. A father said that he and his wife discovered that their son, 13 months old at the time, was deaf after his sister-in-law, a speech therapist, noticed that the child was not developing speech and encouraged the family to have the boy's hearing tested. After her mother-in-law noticed that her grandson did not appear to be hearing well, one mother said:

We took him to our pediatrician at 12 months, I believe, and asked if there was a hearing problem of any kind. And they rang a few bells on either side of his ear and his head turned slightly and they sent us home. That went on about two or three times. . . . It wasn't until he was 19 months old that he was diagnosed by an audiologist. . . . Basically there was no response on the ABR.

Mother of a 5-year-old boy implanted in 1996

Another mother said that her babysitter noticed that the couple's 10-month-old daughter did not respond to the thunder that scared many of the other children in a group she was with. The mother subsequently took her daughter to their pediatrician for advice and, after doing a tympanogram (which does not evaluate the condition of the cochlea), the doctor told the mother: *She hears beautifully, go home.* The mother still had her suspicions, however, and a week later took her husband with her to the next appointment with the pediatrician. The mother recalls that her husband

. . . had a little toy that made a loud noise and he set it off behind [our daughter's] head and the doctor's eyes popped out because she did nothing. . . . We had to wait a month before they had time [for an ABR test].

Mother of a 9-year-old girl implanted in 1994

Many parents did not have to rely on others to tell them that their child might have a hearing loss. In fact, several parents began to suspect this within a few weeks of their child's birth, even though they had no particular reason to suspect that their son or daughter might be deaf.

A number of parents performed the classic banging of pots and pans routine (or even screaming) behind their child to try to determine if their suspicions were true. One mother said that when her daughter was 10 months old, the daughter's grandmother noticed that her grandchild seemed not to hear something that was said to her. In an effort to convince her own mother that her daughter did, in fact, hear, this mother started banging pots and pans together. She soon realized that her daughter did not appear to be hearing anything, and, after getting little support from their pediatrician, was finally able to schedule an appointment with a university audiologist several weeks down the road. The mother recalls:

I made the appointment and then for about four or five days I went around, testing and banging and trying to wake her up and doing all those crazy things. And after about five days I said, I can't do this for another five weeks. I need to know what's going on.

She finally called the audiology department at the local university back and said:

She's not hearing me! I can't wait! Something's wrong. So then they said they would see her the next day and I thought: Okay, this is how this goes, I've learned something important here.
Mother of a 4-year-old girl implanted in 1997

A mother of one deaf child was very eager to determine if her second and third children were deaf. Before the births of her second and third children, she

. . . was banging pots and pans in front of my stomach, and I could sometimes get him [hearing son] to move and I really couldn't get her [third child, a deaf daughter] to move. So, I had this nagging doubt, and she was tested less than 24 hours after her birth, and [there was] no response.
Mother of a 12-year-old girl implanted in 1989 and
a 4-year-old girl implanted at 15 months

One family had more difficulty than most in getting an accurate assessment of their daughter's deafness. In this case, the pediatrician recommended a hearing test when their 2-year-old girl still was not talking. The mother took her daughter to an audiologist for a hearing test in a soundproof booth.

[Our daughter] immediately saw the toys in the back and corners of the booth. She wanted to play and play and play. She kept trying to climb up and reach the toys and I kept trying to get her to sit. The audiologist kept calling her name and calling her name and continued to play the sounds. And when it was over the audiologist said her hearing was normal. She saw no reason for concern. She told me she responded to her name, and I remember saying I don't think she does because at home I call her and call her and call her, but she never turns or anything. This should have been a red flag. I took her advice. I didn't know anything about deafness. I just thought there was no reason for her to be deaf. I had a healthy pregnancy and delivery.

> *Mother of a 5-year-old girl implanted at age 4 and a*
> *3-year-old boy implanted at age 2*

It was not until a year later, when her daughter was about 3 years old, that this mother had her suspicions confirmed by, not surprisingly, a different audiologist, after being told by a third party that she should have her daughter's hearing tested again.

Another mother experienced one of the strangest responses from her pediatrician that we heard after she expressed her concern that her newly adopted daughter might be deaf. Since the daughter had only recently arrived in the United States after a long trip, the doctor thought that the problem was probably due to "jet lag." *Wait a month,* the pediatrician reportedly said, *and we'll check her again.* A month later, the doctor checked again and thought that there was probably nothing wrong with the girl's hearing, but referred the family to an ear, nose, and throat specialist anyway. Getting an appointment for a hearing test required another month and, after several additional months, finally led to an ABR test that confirmed her daughter's deafness. In many other cases, when parents did take their concerns to their pediatrician or other health professional, they were called "neurotic," "overanxious," or "overworried."

Cause of Their Child's Deafness

We asked parents about the cause of their child's deafness in 51 of the families we talked with, and about half of them (25) did not know why their child (or children) became deaf. Among the remaining families, 8 reported that their child became deaf because of meningitis, and 11 reported some type of genetic cause, including one case of Usher's syndrome and one case of Waardenburg's syndrome.[2] In addition to these causes, another 7 families reported

2. Usher's syndrome is an autosomal recessive form of genetic deafness that involves hearing loss and later loss of sight due to retinitis pigmentosa. Waardenburg's syndrome is an autosomal dominant form that is characterized by hypopigmentation that frequently results in a white patch on one's hair, or irises of different colors.

causes such as the illness of the pregnant mother (such as rubella or chicken pox), cytomegalovirus, which can cause hearing loss in infants, and birth complications that occurred during delivery. Some of the parents we talked with expressed interest in learning about the cause of their child's deafness, but most showed only a perfunctory interest or had little interest in the topic at all. As a father of an 11-year-old boy said, *The bottom line is he's deaf so it [the cause] doesn't really matter.*

Many parents felt that there was not a lot they could do about it anyway and were more inclined to focus on the future rather than the past. Some parents initially irrationally blamed themselves for causing their child's deafness, but, in the few cases where this occurred, it was not a long-term obsession. One mother said:

> I spent a good month calling doctors, trying to find out why. Was it because I did something wrong? Maybe I didn't exercise enough. Maybe I exercised too much. Maybe I ate something . . . I drank something. Maybe I took a bath when I shouldn't have . . . I mean just the craziest things. Maybe I woke up too early one day.
>
> *Mother of a 2-year-old girl implanted in early 1999*

After a while, though, and with some appreciated advice from trusted professionals, this mother stopped thinking about possible causes of her child's deafness and decided *to get her the best of care so she can have the best, fullest life possible.*

Reactions

As might be expected, considering their unfamiliarity with deafness, most of the parents of the children we interviewed were shocked and, in many cases, devastated, by the news that their child was deaf. As one parent said: *My first reaction was, I didn't believe it.* A young mother recalled that one of her first questions after learning of her daughter's deafness was, *How can it be? . . . I couldn't believe it because it [deafness] was not in our family anywhere.* Indeed, given the general unfamiliarity with deafness and deaf people that characterizes American society today (see Sacks, 1989), any other reaction would be unexpected. Several parents specifically mentioned that they felt reactions such as these were perfectly natural and normal, given their assumptions about what their child "should be like."

A little more than half of the parents we interviewed used one or more words or phrases, such as the following, to describe the way they initially reacted to their child's deafness: *a huge loss, mad at the world, shocked, depressed, frustrated, a tragedy, sad, scared for what the future would bring, devastated, afraid, confused, a nightmare, the worst thing that had ever happened, in denial,* and *feeling the need to grieve.* Because not all of the parents we talked with actually commented on this issue, the actual number of parents who felt this way is likely considerably more than half. One parent, whose son was diagnosed as deaf more than a decade ago, said:

> Oh, we were really devastated. Our whole life changed that day. We still talk about that. . . . In fact, it brings back emotions to me now. . . . You know, I never even saw a child with hearing aids. That was the first time it hit me.
>
> *Parent of a teenage boy implanted in 1993*

One mother described her feelings of sadness as follows:

> I remember going to the grocery store and a mom was singing to her daughter and I thought, my daughter is never going to be able to do that.
>
> *Mother of a 5-year-old girl implanted in 1998 and a 3-year-old boy implanted in early 1999*

> For the first month I've got this new baby, and I'm singing to him, I'm telling him how much I love him, and I'm doing all this stuff and it was sad to think he might not be hearing any of it.

> I needed to have the [auditory brainstem response] test done to confirm it for me, and once it was confirmed I admit I cried in the parking lot for a good half-hour afterwards.
>
> *Mother of a 2-year-old boy implanted at 19 months*

Another mother said that, when she discovered her young daughter was deaf, *it was very hard to take. I think the worst thing I had to deal with in my life was finding out [that my child was deaf]. It was almost like a part of you dies.* Perhaps the most important reason why so many parents felt this way is because, as one parent said: *The scariest part of it is that you don't know what you're supposed to do next. And no one's telling you; there is no road map.* Another reason many parents were angry or confused was because of what they perceived to be the cavalier treatment on the part of some of the health care professionals they dealt with during the period when they were trying to determine whether their child did, in fact, have a hearing loss. One parent recalled her experience with an audiologist after she learned of her daughter's deafness after a bout with meningitis.

AUDIOLOGIST: Well, one ear is dead, it has nothing, and the other has very little left.

PARENT: What do you mean?

AUDIOLOGIST: I mean, she is deaf. She has lost her hearing.

PARENT: What does that mean?

AUDIOLOGIST: Well, she won't hear any consonants, and she will go to a special school. She can have a life.

PARENT: So, our first experience with anybody explaining hearing loss was pretty, incredibly insensitive.

Parent of a teenager implanted in 1987

Although most parents reacted quite emotionally to the fact that their child was deaf, some of the parents we talked with responded in a way that is perhaps best described as "surprise," along with some degree of sadness to be sure, rather than devastation or depression. This comparatively subdued reaction was characteristic of several of the parents who had more than one deaf child; their reactions were quite different, and somewhat less intense, than those that were apparent after their first child's diagnosis. A few parents actually felt some relief after they learned that their child was deaf. This was often the case when, following an illness such as meningitis, parents were relieved that their child was still alive. Given the alternative, deafness, at that point, seemed almost like a blessing in disguise. When asked about their initial reaction when they discovered that their daughter was deaf, one parent said: *[I had thought that] maybe . . . she was autistic. . . . She . . . didn't smile and didn't look at us. So when they said that she was deaf, I thought, Oh, I can live with this. . . . It was kind of a relief in a way. There was still a lot of sadness, you know, but it was okay.*

Although many parents initially had a difficult time accepting their child's deafness, a number of parents decided, after a short period of grieving, that they had to do something, and not just brood about "what might have been."

One parent said:

> You realize that they can still grow up. They can still get married, and they can still leave the house.
> *Parent of a 6-year-old son implanted at age 5*
> *and an 8-year-old son implanted in 1995*

Another parent said her reaction when she learned that her daughter was deaf many years ago was:

> Boy, we've lost a lot of time. I better get a decision going here . . . where we have to go with [her].
> *Mother of a college-age girl implanted in 1995*

The husband of the mother who frequently sang to her deaf baby during her baby's first month of life and cried in the parking lot after the baby's deafness was confirmed said:

> I'm already thinking about learning sign language or maybe some type of improved audiology, and then I still have these goals for his life, and I'm still going to try to assist him in reaching these goals . . . but my mind is already working on taking a different path to get there.
> *Father of a 2-year-old boy implanted in 1998*

> For me the sorrow or the mourning, I guess is what you would call it, was very short-lived. It lasted just a day or so because there really wasn't anything to do about it. It was just how do we make life better for her?
> *Father of an 8-year-old girl implanted in 1993*

One mother of a 5-year-old boy recalled that after she learned that her son was deaf at 18 months she went from the audiologist's office *to [a bookstore] and bought some books on sign language and was not going to waste any more time. I felt bad that we had waited so long.*

Given the lack of experience virtually all the parents had with deaf people generally or, specifically, with deaf children, many of their initial efforts amounted to "information gathering" more than anything else. And, as conscientious parents gathered information, many of them became more and more confused about what course of action they should take. Part of the reason for this confusion is that many of the people that the parents talked with, including pediatricians, knew little about deafness, deaf people, or about the various methods for raising deaf children. Nevertheless, the most common action taken by parents after they started to look for ways to assist their child was to seek out a pediatric audiologist and have their child fitted for hearing aids. Learning to sign (primarily signing with speech) was also something that many parents did soon after learning of their child's deafness. Apart from this, where did many of the parents we talked with get information about what steps to take after they learned that their child was deaf?

Sources of Information

Everyone we talked with got some advice or recommendation from the physician or audiologist who initially informed them that their son or daughter had a significant hearing loss. In some cases, however, this information was conveyed in a way that was perceived as heartless and cruel. One mother, whose first child, a son, was identified as deaf when he was about 18 months old, recalled that when she was pregnant with her second child she and her husband went to a hospital to learn about the results of their son's hearing evaluation.

> We were frightened, and my husband said I really hope you
> have some good news, you know I hope this is a positive.
> And he [the health professional] said, I don't have any good
> news for you. Your son is profoundly deaf. And you better run
> to Gallaudet and get him into a sign language program
> because that's all you can hope for. Okay, that's how we were
> told. I was really surprised at the lack of information that
> came from [the hospital].
> *Mother of a 14-year-old boy implanted at age 3*

Another mother recalled:

It wasn't like the hospital said, Okay, your child has a profound
hearing loss, you need to give her intervention somehow or
she won't learn language. You can give her intervention visually. You can give her amplification, and give her information
through an auditory means, or you can do a combination. Here
is information about this, here are phone numbers about that.
Here are resources about this, here is a list of names, here is a
list of contact people, here is a list of families and their children, here is where they live. None of that, nothing. We did
basically all the legwork ourselves.

Mother of a 4-year-old girl diagnosed at 2 weeks
and implanted at 18 months

Although many parents expressed some degree of exasperation,
or worse, with their pediatrician or audiologist, some of the parents appreciated the amount of time these health professionals spent
with them, particularly since they were overwhelmed with the
number of choices they would have to begin making. One family
we talked with recalls that their audiologist sat down with them for
2 hours to explain the options after informing the family of the ABR
test results.

Well, the day he was diagnosed . . . they told us that he was
profoundly deaf. . . . They . . . told us all kinds of things that
day, but I don't think a whole lot of it sunk in. We were, you
know, kind of reeling from what we were told, the information we were just given. We were told about hearing aids, and
cued speech,[3] and sign language, and they said there is a
device called the cochlear implant. . . . We were given a list
from [the hospital] of different centers to go to for hearing
therapy and speech therapy within our schooling district and
hospitals in the area, so with that we just made some phone
calls to find out how to get started.

Mother of a 5-year-old boy diagnosed at 1 year
and implanted at age 2

---

3. Cued speech involves the manipulation of hand shapes and hand placements
near a speaker's mouth to produce a visual code representing the phonemes
of spoken language.

Another mother remembers:

We were starving for information. We wanted to learn as
much as we could. And they [the audiologist] gave us the
names of some other people in the community who had
recently had children diagnosed with deafness. And that was
probably, for me, the most useful thing, other parents. We
talked to other parents. And then she [the audiologist] also
gave us . . . a packet of information. . . . I don't remember anything about what was in the packet. . . . I just got on the
phone. Every day I was on the phone. I called Gallaudet. I
called the Clarke School [in Massachusetts]. I called every
national deaf organization that I could find. I called all the
parents. I called the [state school for the deaf]. So we just
kept calling and calling and calling and talking and meeting,
and then we started to meet some people. And then we
started visiting different places that educated deaf children.
Mother of a 5-year-old boy implanted in 1996

A number of parents did benefit from some of the referrals
that were made by those who initially determined that their child
was deaf. About two-thirds of the 51 families that discussed this
topic with us said they were referred to early intervention programs, schools for deaf students, teachers, speech and hearing
clinics, advocacy organizations, and others who had extensive
professional experience with deaf children. Most of the parents
appreciated the information they received from these programs.
In one state, a mother stated the following about her county's
early intervention program:

[They were] wonderful. I mean I walked in and I just . . . cried
and [they] just listened to me and said there are options, you
know, it's not terrible, she's going to be fine, we have lots of
kids and . . . they are fine. So that was the next thing that happened, and I think that was my ray of hope that things were
going to be all right.
Mother of a 4-year-old girl diagnosed at 10 months and
implanted at 19 months

The mother of the teenage boy, noted previously, who had such
a negative experience at the hospital that confirmed her son's deafness, said:

A.G. Bell [Association of the Deaf] was extremely helpful.
They were so wonderful. That's what kept me going, I can
tell you, were the people at A.G. Bell.
Mother of a 14-year-old boy implanted at age 3

In many states, parents were able to take advantage of programs
for infants and toddlers (early intervention programs), and they frequently benefited from programs that sent people to their homes
each week or so. Other parents were able to take their children to
a preschool setting where they socialized with other deaf children.

Not all of the experiences with early intervention programs
were completely positive, however, although many parents did not
realize this until later. Many programs are geared toward a single
"philosophy," be it oral education, total communication (primarily
signing and speaking simultaneously), American Sign Language
(ASL), or some other method. Many parents, however, were not
aware of these options at the beginning and simply accepted whatever was convenient or what happened to be available in the area
where they lived. In retrospect, some parents were pleased with
the choices that were available to them, but others expressed some
frustration with the limited options at their disposal.

We didn't know anything about being deaf. They were the
professionals. And it's not until time has been wasted, and
years have gone by, until you realize that they've been lying.
. . . They don't know everything, and they push whatever
they believe is right, which is wrong.
Parent of a 7-year-old girl implanted in 1996

A number of parents contacted other parents of deaf children,
joined support groups, or participated in on-line discussion groups.
Many also spent a good amount of time reading about deafness and
issues related to raising deaf children. As one parent said in response
to a question about whether she did any reading about deafness
after discovering her daughter was deaf: *Oh, tons, tons! In fact, I
wrote to everybody and got things from Gallaudet University, all
over.* One book that was frequently mentioned by parents as being
particularly helpful was *Choices in Deafness* (1996), edited by Sue
Schwartz.

One problem with reading about deafness and the challenges
of raising a deaf child that was encountered by several parents who
visited their local public library in search of information was the

fact that many of the books were outdated. One parent recalled that when he started searching for information in the mid-1990s, *I found very little in the public library. I think most of our help came from talking to people, because we went right into the family ed program at [a residential school for deaf students] and talking to some of the other parents and meeting some of the other parents and children. I think [that] was probably most helpful, really.* In addition, this man's wife responded *absolutely* when we asked her if she felt that a parent had to be very "proactive" to get the information she felt she needed, because information about what to do was often not readily available. This is a theme that appeared again and again in our interviews: Parents who really wanted to get something accomplished often had to spend a great deal of time talking (and fighting) with pediatricians, audiologists, school systems, insurance companies, and others in positions of authority who had the power to make decisions affecting their child's life.

Some parents, particularly those who discovered their child was deaf relatively recently, turned to the World Wide Web for information.

> I would get on the computer and type in deaf and read everything there was . . . just everything. All the books I pulled out, I read the backs of them and got the biographies [of the authors] and called the people, I mean like I would call [an author] at home.
> *Parent of a 4-year-old girl implanted in 1997*

In addition to these sources of information, many parents turned to their families, friends, business associates, and other acquaintances in an effort to learn more about what their options might be. Of the 51 families we spoke with about this issue, roughly a quarter of them said that they had, in fact, done this. In some cases, family members had some special expertise that was very useful for parents as they made decisions about options. Other families, however, experienced some pressure from in-laws, the child's grandparents, and others to take one course of action or another. One father said:

> My parents were pretty much guiding the way we went. Just because they were so adamant about he's got to talk, he's got to talk, [he will] never make it if he can't talk.
> *Father of a teenager implanted in 1995*

Another family, frustrated at the lack of information available to them when they discovered that their child was deaf in the mid-1990s, started a parent support group.

> Now ... when a child is diagnosed, not always, but often, they get referred to our parent group and we send them ... this package of information that tells them, and we don't prefer one methodology or another. It just tells them what all the options are, and it also has a reference list so people can look at lots of other books and go find some of these things.
>
> *Mother of a 2-year-old son implanted in 1998 and a 6-year-old daughter implanted in 1996*

Hearing Aids

All of the parents we talked with reported that their child used a hearing aid at some point prior to getting a cochlear implant. The vast majority of children used two hearing aids, and most of them began using their aids within a month or two after their parents learned they were deaf. Many of the parents reported that their child used several different types of hearing aids, including aids with FM systems for enhanced amplification, tactile aids, and frequency transposition aids (aids that are designed to transpose high-frequency sounds to lower frequencies). Moreover, a number of children used increasingly powerful aids as their hearing loss became progressively worse in the years before they received their implant.

It is certainly not surprising that all of the children tried a hearing aid before receiving a cochlear implant. Although some very young children may now receive an implant without prior hearing aid use, at the time most of the children of the parents we talked with got their cochlear implant Food and Drug Administration regulations stipulated that implant candidates receive little or no benefit from hearing aids. A 6-month-long hearing aid trial was usually required before implantation could be considered.

Although hearing aid use was universal among the children in our sample, most of the parents we talked with said that their child received minimal or no benefit from the aids. A little more than half of the parents mentioned that their child heard basically nothing with the aid, and the remainder reported varying degrees of benefit. Of those who received at least some benefit from their aid, most of the children had minimal sound awareness and sound discrimination, and were generally only able to hear environmental sounds of one type or another (such as a loud dog barking, banging drums, or a lawn mower). These children were not able to hear enough to clearly understand the speech of another person, and thus were unable to emulate those sounds. Only about a half-dozen parents said that their child received enough benefit from hearing aids to enable them to hear spoken language reasonably clearly before they received their implant. This group of children had significantly more residual hearing when they began using their hearing aid than they did several years after amplification was started, because their hearing loss was progressive.

Some of the data from the Gallaudet Research Institute (GRI) survey helps to round out our picture of hearing aid use among deaf children before they received their implant. All but 5 of the 439 respondents indicated that their child used hearing aids before the implant, and about three-quarters (76%)[4] of the children used their hearing aids all day, every day.

One of the questions on the GRI questionnaire asked parents to characterize their child's hearing with hearing aids, if used normally but without the support of visual cues, before implantation. Under these conditions, only a small percentage (5%) of the parents indicated that their child could understand many or most of a speaker's words spoken at a "conversational loudness level from a distance of 10 feet across a quiet room." Ten percent of the parents reported that their child could hear "a few" words in such a situation, and another 17% of the parents said that their child could hear a few words if the speaker was talking very loudly from a distance of 10 feet in a quiet room. The remaining children (68%) could hear only very loud noises or nothing at all.

In sum, it appears that the following conclusions concerning hearing aid use among deaf children before they received their cochlear implant have considerable empirical support:

1. The vast majority of parents got a hearing aid for their child soon after their child's deafness was confirmed, and almost all of the children used two hearing aids.

4. All percentages have been rounded to the nearest whole number.

2. Most of the children did not receive much benefit from their hearing aids, even the most powerful ones, certainly not enough to consistently hear speech from their parents or from others interacting with them.
3. Most of the children used their hearing aids every day for most of the day, for several months or more, before getting an implant, even if the aids did not seem helpful.

Conflicting Recommendations

In one sense, all the parents we talked with got the same information from those health professionals who informed them of their child's hearing loss: Get hearing aids for your child as soon as possible. In other areas, however, many of the parents reported receiving conflicting recommendations as they were trying to decide what to do after learning of their child's deafness. Of the 26 parents who discussed this issue with us, 15 said they received conflicting advice about which method of communication they should pursue. Perhaps the most significant area in which conflicting advice was received concerned signing or not signing, although some families reported receiving advice about which type of signing, ASL or Signed English, to use. Other families received counsel, whether solicited or not, about cued speech, lipreading, aural habilitation without lipreading, and other communication choices commonly available to parents of deaf children. Unfortunately for many parents, much of the advice received was couched in absolute terms: Our approach (whatever it might be) will lead your child to the promised land of clear communication and the development of good language skills, but beware of competing "brands" that will likely lead straight to disaster.

> The most shocking thing was to see how rigid and almost religious people were in their beliefs about what was the right thing to do. That was really shocking to me.
> *Mother of a 5-year-old boy implanted in 1996*

> We were told that the cochlear implant would never work. We were told that her only method of communication would

be sign, perhaps lipreading if we worked at it real hard. And that she might develop voiced presentation with enough work when she got older, but she would never perceive sound. And I said, If that's true, that's fine. But these experts couldn't convince me that they really knew. This was an opinion not based on any real body of scientific knowledge.

Father of an 8-year-old girl implanted at age 2

In addition to frequently receiving emotional, opinionated advice often couched as facts, parents usually had few reference points with which to judge the likelihood of success or failure of any particular method since, by and large, they were unfamiliar with any of them. This unfamiliarity, coupled with a perceived need to choose "something," led to a great deal of anxiety on the part of many of the families we talked with.

The biggest conflicting information we had gotten [was that] there's this deaf culture that we didn't know about, and there's Signed English people and there's ASL people, and there's hearing aid people and there's nonhearing aid people, and there's talking people and nontalking people, and you know they all are very adamant about their position, and they didn't seem to be very flexible about other people's positions, and all of a sudden we realized we were in the middle of this.

Parent of a 6-year-old girl implanted in 1998

Another mother who lived in a northern state when her first child was diagnosed as deaf, said:

The [city] area is very pro-deaf culture, pro-signing, and I was getting bombarded everywhere. You need to be signing, you need to be signing, and we really feel that we spent the whole early years with [our daughter] trying one thing and then another, [with] the residual hearing going. . . . Here she is diagnosed so young and people think we were so lucky, you don't know how lucky you are to get started so early, and we felt like we were just getting nowhere.

Mother of a 4-year-old daughter implanted in 1998 and a 12-year-old daughter implanted at age 3

I have a distant cousin who did a graduate degree at Gallaudet. She's hearing. . . . The first thing she said to us was,

Don't trust anybody in this business. And she was right on the mark.

Mother of a 4-year-old girl implanted at 18 months

Although many families reported receiving conflicting recommendations about what to do even before they began considering a cochlear implant for their child, a few families' experiences were quite different. For the most part, in these families, it was decided to use one mode of communication because, for one reason or another, that choice seemed "natural" or "obvious." As one parent said after discovering that their young son had became deaf as a consequence of meningitis:

To us, it was like a no-brainer. You had to use some sign language, some kind of communication with your hands.

Parent of a teenage boy implanted in 1993

On the other hand, another couple said, when they discovered that their young daughter was deaf:

I think we were lucky because we weren't confused at the beginning. We knew that, culturally, we couldn't go signing, and we personally did not want her to sign. So we [live] in a hearing world; she's going to earn money and be a citizen of the world, you know, she would have to learn to talk, and people weren't going to wear FM systems for her, and . . . everyone doesn't know how to sign . . . so it was pretty clear to us.

Parents of a 3-year-old girl implanted in 1998

Perhaps one reason for this family's decision was their experience in another country where, according to the mother, *deaf children are put into a separate, kind of shipped away, into a kind of a boarding school . . . they are just not in society. You know, they are shunned, and I just couldn't do that for [our daughter].*

Despite the fact that many parents were bombarded with opinions and advice (or an *overload of helpful suggestions* as one parent of a teenage boy diplomatically put it), most of the parents we interviewed were eventually able to sift through the conflicting claims based on their own research and the experiences they had with their deaf child. In fact, and in contrast with many of the recommendations they received, many parents frequently solved the problem of "what to do" by doing more than one thing. That is, many parents not only signed with their child and encouraged the child's development of sign language (usually Signed English rather than ASL), but they also encouraged the development of their child's spoken language skills, to the extent that this was possible, before getting an implant. Although many of the "helpful suggestions" often appeared to parents to be doctrinaire and ideological, we found many of the parents we talked with to be pragmatic and non-ideological, and focused on the need to communicate with their child in a way that made sense to them.

> We were getting really confused because we wanted to do the right thing, but we made the decision that we needed to do something that was going to be easy for me and easy for [my wife] and was going to be the most parallel with the way we talk to [our daughter] and how she's going to learn. So we decided that we needed to sign exactly the way we talked.

Later, his wife added:

> Because we chose the Signed English, and because we were more comfortable speaking and signing at the same time, we were doing Total Communication, and [our daughter] started learning all the mouth shapes just by watching us. So, she would practically say something without anybody trying to teach her how . . . because she would be signing and make the mouth shape and make a voice and it would come out and we were like, Wow, that's kind of neat!
> *Parents of a 6-year-old girl implanted in 1998*

In sum, perhaps the most important issue facing parents after they learn of their child's deafness is the question of which mode of communication to pursue. For well over 100 years, there has been an intense debate between those who support signing, especially ASL in the United States, as the primary way to communicate with deaf children, and those who support some variant of oralism. The philosophy of oralism discourages the use of signing, and emphasizes the development of spoken language skills and the cultivation of whatever residual hearing is available. Lipreading (or "speechreading") is often emphasized in oral programs. There have been a number of other approaches over the years, such as Total Communication, a philosophy that was particularly popular in the 1970s and 1980s, in which elements of signing and speaking are combined (it is not possible to sign and speak simultaneously in ASL). Nevertheless, the debate, particularly in recent years, is usually framed by ardent supporters in their respective camps as a fairly clear-cut choice between signing or not signing.

Although the debate may be framed this way, it was apparent to us as we interviewed parents of children with cochlear implants across the country that in "real life," in the world where people actually live and make day-to-day choices, the situation is considerably more complex than advocates of one philosophy or the other might realize. Most of the parents we talked with felt that the most important thing was to be able to communicate effectively with their child, and they often did not care, at least initially, how they managed to do this. If signing worked, then they signed. If their child could hear well enough to develop language through speech, then they did that. Of course, most of the parents wanted their child to develop spoken language and that is one of the major reasons why they decided to get an implant. But between the time they learned of their child's deafness and implantation, most of the parents used some variant of signing to communicate with their child.

Signing

Of the 50 families that discussed the issue of pre-implant signing with us, 35 of them signed with their child. About 25 of these signing families consistently signed with voice. This type of signing includes Signing Exact English, which involves signing each word (and often prefixes, suffixes, and verb endings) that is spoken. Signing with voice also includes simultaneous communication, which generally follows English word order, but does not "require" signing each spoken word (in everyday usage, this method is sometimes referred to as Total Communication). Another 10 of the families who signed used some type of supportive signs to back up spoken English. Only three families reported using ASL to some extent before their child received an implant. (All three of these families also said they signed with voice. Since we did not observe their sign communication, it is not known how much "pure" ASL these families actually used before implantation.) Fifteen of the families we talked with about this issue did not sign with their child at all prior to implant surgery.

The most important reason for signing pre-implant cited by our interviewees was to ensure that at least some communication occurred between the parents and their child.

> We wanted sign language. It just felt like the natural, right thing to do right away, because [our son] could immediately have some form of communication right now. . . . Our county. . . . is an oral county, so we had to do a little pulling strings and battling to get the sign language.
> *Mother of a 5-year-old boy implanted in 1996*

One mother, when asked why she emphasized Total Communication before her son received his implant in the late 1980s, replied:

> To give [my son] an open field of communication. That way if he is with people that don't sign he can read their lips and talk back. If he is with the deaf community that does sign, then he [can use] sign language.
> *Mother of a teenage boy implanted in the late 1980s*

Many parents also felt that, without signing, their child would not have been able to develop language at all before getting an implant.

> Even though I am a big fan of cochlear implants, I think cochlear implants are absolutely wonderful, [our daughter] was able to gain a language very young and very fast with her sign language. . . . If you implant at 18 months . . . I still think that sign language would benefit all [deaf] children [before implantation] because that's how we taught [our daughter].
> *Mother of an 8-year-old girl implanted at age 5*

This mother facilitated her daughter's acquisition of sign by learning to sign herself and even hosted small sign language classes so her daughter's friends could learn to sign as well. She also noted that another daughter, who is hearing, learned signs from birth, and, when she was 9 months old, *she couldn't talk ... [but] she had language ... because we signed to her and she could tell us what she needed.* Another family we talked with also stressed the importance of early signing: *We had behavior problems with [our daughter] about not paying attention, [and being] very stubborn. And she would always get upset. She would throw tantrums. If you went ... grocery shopping, she would scream and holler. Once she began signing [and] she had a language, a lot of those behaviors stopped because then she was able to explain well.*

Interestingly enough, according to many of the parents we talked with, cochlear implant centers are not universally opposed to signing. In fact, one parent said that pre-implant signing was encouraged at the implant center where her daughter received her implant.

> [Johns] Hopkins recommended signing, . . . they wanted them to have some signing before they were implanted. And they wanted you to continue on if you were teaching anything new. Plus an oral program [after implantation].
> *Mother of a 3-year-old girl implanted in 1997*

Another mother of a 4-year-old girl also mentioned that supportive signing was emphasized at this implant center, and that an "auditory sandwich" approach, which emphasizes audition, visual clarification through signing, followed by audition, was encouraged, especially after implantation.

Not Signing

Fifteen of the 50 families we talked with about pre-implant signing said they did not sign with their child. One problem faced by several families that initially tried to use some type of sign communication before the implant was the fact that some family members were either unable or unwilling to learn to sign.

> A lot of my family just was not willing to do anything. They weren't even willing to think about it. . . . [One] side of the family showed no interest in learning any sign so [our daughter] had a real language barrier between cousins and the families. . . . They didn't know how to act around her. They weren't relaxed. . . . They weren't willing [to learn to sign] and I couldn't force them to.
> *Mother of a 7-year-old girl implanted at age 4*

Some of the families that did not sign with their child pre-implant said that the major reason why they decided not to was because signing was perceived as being "too easy" for the child. By this they meant that if the child began signing, then he or she would not want to do the "hard work" of learning to listen and develop spoken language.

> We were hesitant to [teach our son to sign] because some of the literature that we read said that if you do teach them signs, then sometimes they will become more acclimated to that and it will be easier for them to rely on using sign than using speech. Because we had decided to use auditory-verbal therapy, we were really concentrating on getting him to use his voice.
>
> *Father of a 2-year-old boy implanted in 1998*

Many of these parents, however, said they would not object if their son or daughter decided to sign later in life.

> Now if [my daughter] wants to sit down when she's 14 and take a sign language class I will sit right down next to her. . . . If that's the route she wants to go, that's fine.
>
> *Mother of a 2-year-old girl implanted at 19 months*

> Signing did help because initially it was a way to communi- cate and [my son] did pick up signs relatively quickly. He signed a lot and that helped alleviate some frustration. . . . But I think it's probably pretty well documented [that] a young child who is developing will gravitate towards whatever is easiest, so once we started signing he signed all the time.
>
> *Father of a 4-year-old boy implanted in 1997*

This father also said that, because his child was not able to hear with hearing aids, it would have been *very difficult* to have gone into an oral program without the benefit of an implant. A number of other parents we talked with were not particularly satisfied with early oral education because that meant asking their child, who often achieved minimal benefit from a hearing aid, to mimic sounds he or she could not hear.

One family we interviewed did not consistently sign with their daughter, now in her early teens, even though they wanted to, because the school where the daughter was a student before (and after) receiving the implant absolutely prohibited signing. Accord- ing to the parents, their daughter experienced little or no language development in this oral school before she was implanted at 6 years of age (and language acquisition was delayed post-implant as well, perhaps because there was little language base on which to build). For family reasons, however, they were unable to take the child out of the school until they moved to a distant state. Before moving, however, they decided to learn to sign anyway, but were forced to lie about it (under threat of expulsion) when challenged by the principal of this oral school.[5] Other families, too, reported that their initial early or parent intervention programs discouraged signing, but that they eventually decided that some type of visual pre-implant communication was desirable.

Several questions on the GRI survey also deal with the question of pre-implant communication. One question asked parents to indicate how their child was communicating "just before" receiving the implant, and another asked how others in the home usually communicated with their child. These data are reported in table 3.1. A third item asked parents to indicate the "general mode of communication" they desired for their child before they considered getting a cochlear implant.

It is clear from table 3.1 that, although pre-implant signing is fairly common among deaf children, it is less frequently used by other people in the child's household. About half of the children used a considerable amount of signing before getting their cochlear implant. A large proportion of "others" in the home also signed pre-implant, although they tended to emphasize speech more than the child did. It is also clear (and tragic) that one-fifth (20%) of the sample reported that their child had either minimal (if any) spoken words or signs, or simply used gestures, before implantation.

The general mode of communication that parents *desired* before they considered a cochlear implant for their child is quite different from what was actually used by the child, or by others in the home, before implantation. Most of the parents in the GRI survey reported that they "definitely wanted" or were "leaning toward" auditory-oral communication (i.e., communication that emphasizes the development of speech and listening skills). In this case, 46% of the parents said they definitely desired, and another 10% said they were leaning toward, auditory-oral communication. Only 7% said they

---

5. This example should not be taken as illustrative of what happens in a "typical" oral school. It is simply one family's experience.

TABLE 3.1
Communication "at Home" Just before Receiving the Implant

Type of Communication	By the Child	By Others
Mainly signing	32%	17%
More signs than spoken words	8%	7%
Signing and speech equally	9%	23%
More speech than signing	3%	8%
Cued speech	3%	4%
All or mainly speech	25%	25%
Minimal or no spoken words or sign	20%	4%

were leaning toward sign or definitely desired sign communication. More than a third (38%) reported that they desired a combination of auditory-oral and sign as the general mode of communication before considering the cochlear implant.

In sum, a significant amount of pre-implant signing occurs in the families we interviewed as well as in the families included in the GRI study. To be sure, most of the signing is done by the child (who may learn many signs in early intervention programs outside the family), but many parents sign as well. This is particularly noteworthy since almost none of the parents knew how to sign before the birth of their deaf child. Parents generally saw the need to do something to facilitate communication with their child after they realized that their child was deaf and that "simply talking" was not sufficient. For many, signing was this something, and, for many, they were clearly pleased that they had used some type of manual (sign) communication with their child prior to the implant. Although many were pleased, they were not necessarily completely satisfied that signing was the best way for their child to communicate. Many, in fact, while noting that early signing did facilitate communication, and did result in the development of a substantial sign vocabulary, also felt that signing did not necessarily lead to the development of "real" (i.e., spoken) language. As the GRI results suggest, many parents preferred that their child develop oral communication skills, even while their child was using some form of sign communication, prior to receiving a cochlear implant. As we will see, this preference for spoken language development is one of the primary reasons why parents decide to get an implant for their child. Another reason may be the parents' limited exposure to signing deaf people who lead full, productive lives.

Speech and "Oral Education"

Many parents, including many of those who signed with their child, used some type of speech therapy or oral/aural habilitation prior to the implant, and we discussed this issue with 36 of the parents we interviewed. There are several closely related methods that fall under the "oral" umbrella, and they all "share one common aspect: they require children to use only spoken language for face-to-face communication" (Gatty, 1996, p. 163). One of these methods is "multisensory," which involves the use of hearing aids to enhance residual hearing, lipreading, and even touch to facilitate communication. This approach can also be called *auditory-oral.* A "unisensory" approach, however, relies only on the development of listening (aural) skills. This is the *auditory-verbal* (A-V) method. The goal of the A-V approach is for "children who are deaf or hard-of-hearing [to] grow up in regular learning and living environments, enabling them to become independent, participating, and contributing citizens in mainstream society" (Estabrooks, 1996, p. 55). This goal is to be achieved by using amplified residual hearing. Most importantly, parents, or the child's caregivers, must work closely with a certified A-V therapist and become the primary models for spoken language in daily (including playtime and "listening game") interactions with their child.

Approximately one-third of the 36 families that we talked with about this issue followed, at least to some extent, the principles of A-V therapy before their child received the implant. A few more parents may have incorporated some A-V principles into their interactions with their child, but it was not always clear in our interviews exactly what type of pre-implant speech therapy or auditory habilitation program parents used, or how long, or how often, it was used. It is important to keep in mind that the "average" or typical child in our sample had been using the implant for about 4 years at the time of the interview. Thus, it is understandable that, in some cases, it was a little difficult for parents to recall the exact nature of the pre-implant speech therapy their child had received.

Although most of the parents were not devoted followers of any one method, at least not before their child was implanted, many of them did want to try some type of speech therapy while their child was using a hearing aid.

MOTHER: We just decided we would take a shot at teaching him to speak, and if that wasn't an option, we had sign language and total communication to fall back on.

FATHER: We thought that he would probably be better off . . . trying to learn to speak so it would be easier to communicate with other people in the world.
Parents of a 5-year-old boy implanted in 1996

[Our daughter] was born into a hearing family. I have two hearing children . . . everyone in my life experience had been hearing. And this [auditory-verbal] seemed like a very natural approach that made a lot of sense to us. I thought it was something that I had the energy to invest the time, and . . . I wanted that relationship with [my daughter]. I was very hesitant to turn her over to a program where they would do it for me.
Mother of a young woman who received her implant in her mid-teens

Another family said they were told that, *if [our son] was going to succeed, he needed to go the oral route.* Since, at the time, the parents were not aware of any other method for educating their child, and since they wanted to do what they could to ensure that their son would, indeed, be successful, they initially opted for an oral approach.

One reason for emphasizing speech and/or A-V therapy before the implant that was cited by several parents dealt with problems the child might have if he or she were to try to learn two languages at the same time. One mother said: *Because the information that I had read and the conferences that we had been to suggested that, [if] we tried to focus on two languages at one time, one or both [languages would be] impaired to a greater degree than if you just focused on one. So, we decided to teach [our daughter] English, to speak first, and then later, if she wants to learn sign, she can.*

Most of the parents who were able to evaluate the efficacy of pre-implant speech and listening therapy were not effusive in their praise, since most of the children could hear very little with their hearing aids. One mother who used the A-V approach both before and after her daughter's implant said that such therapy was

> no fun [before the implant]. . . . [But] now we have fun. But then [my daughter] wasn't getting anything out of it. She would get aggravated, but we would continue to try.
>
> *Mother of a 2-year-old girl implanted in early 1999*

Some parents became frustrated at the lack of progress and transferred their child to a program that emphasized sign communication.

For those families that experienced a good amount of pre-implant success with A-V therapy, or with speech therapy in general, one common denominator was extensive parental involvement. One spouse, usually the mother, devoted hours to the task of helping her child develop speech and listening skills.

One mother who used the A-V approach recalls that, before her daughter's implant,

> We really emphasized the sounds. We did a lot of sound units where we emphasized particular sounds during a particular week. We had units of work set up for us so that we could continue them at home and I worked with her every day, and my husband worked with her every day, so it wasn't just therapy time or school time, it was throughout the day.
>
> *Mother of a teenage girl implanted in 1997*

Another mother said, concerning her commitment to A-V therapy:

> I incorporated daily lessons into our home . . . in an atmosphere of play . . . reinforcing . . . attending to sounds, then progressing to [the idea that] sound has meaning. Then, finally, to speech sounds, just talking to her all the time.
>
> *Mother of a young woman who received her implant at age 16*

Many of the parents used a combination of public and private speech therapy, but those who used the A-V approach often had to pay for it themselves. In some cases, the use of an A-V therapist was an option in the early intervention program that was available to parents. Most of the time, however, for those parents who relied primarily or exclusively on programs that were offered by local early intervention programs, preschools, or regular public schools, generic "speech therapy" was usually all that was on the menu. Moreover, the amount of such therapy varied from less than an hour a week to several hours per week; the variation in the quality of the publicly supported speech therapy was no doubt even greater (see chapter 7). Even for those parents who did emphasize some type of oral communication in the years before their son or daughter received the cochlear implant, most of the time this was not an exclusive approach. As noted, most of the children in the families we talked with were exposed to both signing and speaking in their pre-implant, formative years.

Conclusions

In the introduction to this book, we suggested that by looking at how parents *perceive their situation,* some of the *assumptions* they bring to their decision-making, some of the *behavioral patterns* that follow from these decisions, and some of the *social implications and consequences* of these decisions, we can get a better picture of how parents use the equipment in their cultural "tool kit" to deal with their child's deafness. Much of the discussion in this chapter deals with these issues, and we have no doubt that most of the readers of this book will be able to apply this framework to many of the experiences of the families we discuss in this chapter and elsewhere. Our own interpretation suggests that many parents perceive the situation in which they find themselves in a rather negative way, at least initially. Since the ability to hear is valued in American culture (and elsewhere), the fact that their child does not have this ability is understandably disappointing and demoralizing to many parents. When confronted with this reality, the parents we interviewed generally sought to act on their assumption that the ability to hear (and speak) was something that they should try to encourage in their child. Moreover, the health professionals with whom they came into contact often encouraged hearing and speaking. At the same time, however, parents valued communication, perhaps even more than hearing, per se, and sought ways to overcome communication barriers between themselves and their deaf child or children. This, of course, often included some form of manual communication. In fact, as noted earlier, some parents brought into their decision-making process the assumption that, because their child was deaf, some form of signing was obviously needed to facilitate communication.

Many of the parents we talked with had similar perceptions about their child's deafness and similar assumptions about what would be a desirable outcome. However, since some of the assumptions about pre-implant communication methods differed, the behavior that followed was sometimes different as well. Some parents focused on oral methods, whereas others focused on signing, and some wanted an implant immediately whereas others took several years to make this decision. In the final analysis, though, all the parents (save one) in our sample decided to get a cochlear implant for their child (or children), thus acting on their belief that hearing was an important attribute and that their child should be given this opportunity, if possible (as will be seen, many children participated in the decision themselves if they were old enough).

The social implications and consequences of the decision to implant are far reaching and are still being played out in America and elsewhere. What will the impact of implants be on the educational system, for example? Since mainstreaming in "regular" classrooms is often cited as a goal for children with implants, what effect will this have on residential schools for deaf children, many of which are already experiencing a decrease in enrollment? Do students with implants still need "special services," and, if so, what type and for how long? Is it reasonable to try to educate deaf students with and without cochlear implants in the same school? In the same classroom? What about medical resources? Cochlear implant surgery is quite expensive; is this a good use of medical resources? What about the many thousands of profoundly deaf people around the world, particularly in Third World nations, who will in all likelihood never have a chance to receive an implant? Will their needs be overlooked in the quest for implantation among those deaf people in more affluent nations? These are some of the questions that will be discussed in upcoming chapters.

4

Language Development and the Decision to Get a Cochlear Implant

Language development is probably the most contentious issue among those involved in the discussion concerning pediatric implant effectiveness, and we devote an entire chapter (chapter 9) to this issue later in the book. One of the major reasons why the parents we talked with wanted to get a cochlear implant for their child was because this would presumably provide the child with the auditory information needed to more effectively develop spoken language. Since this is a primary issue for most parents, we asked them how important their perception of their child's language deficiency was in the decision to get an implant.

We discussed this issue with 45 of the families we interviewed (who had a total of 49 children). Table 4.1 summarizes various pre-implant spoken and signed language development categories as articulated by the parents; obviously, some parents described their child's pre-implant language development in more than one way. For example, some parents reported that their child had a good amount of pre-implant sign language development and, at the same time, had little if any pre-implant spoken language development even with hearing aids.

TABLE 4.1

Parent-Identified Pre-Implant Language Development Categories

Language Development as Identified by Parents	Number of Children as Identified by Parents in Each Category*
Little if any spoken or signed language development *before hearing aids* were used	4
Little if any spoken language development before an implant *even with hearing aids*	21
Speech delayed or absent pre-implant	12
Language delayed vis-a-vis peers pre-implant	15
Some to good *sign language development* pre-implant	19
Some to good spoken language development *before hearing loss*	5
Some to good pre-implant spoken language development *with hearing aids* pre-implant	6

* The total number of children referred to in terms of language development is 49. Many children are included in more than one category.

It is important to keep in mind that table 4.1 summarizes the language development categories as identified by the parents we talked with, not by us. When issues related to pre-implant language development were raised, we wanted to allow the parents to describe the type of language or method of communication their child had acquired and was using before implantation. We did not want to ask parents to choose from a predefined list of options. This approach, while allowing parents to expand on the nature of their child's pre-implant language development, does make it difficult to neatly categorize their responses. Moreover, because of the relatively unstructured nature of our interviews, we cannot say that because a given parent did not mention some aspect of pre-implant language development (speech, for example) that it was not important to them. It is also important to remember that we asked parents to talk about something that, for many, happened several years ago in the context of a wide-ranging discussion that also touched on many other issues.

Perhaps the most appropriate way to interpret table 4.1 is to see it as a "group photograph" of pre-implant language acquisition in which the following images seem to be most salient for the parents we talked with: Spoken language was delayed, in terms of actual achievement and in comparative terms with similar-age children, sign language (or, more broadly, some variant of manual communication) was generally valued and encouraged by many parents, and hearing aids often did not provide enough amplification for oral language development.

One of the major reasons why parents were concerned about pre-implant language development was because of a perceived "window of opportunity" that they felt they needed to take advantage of. Many parents thought that if their child did not develop language at an early age, generally within the first 3 years, then subsequent language acquisition would be truncated. (See chapter 9 for a detailed discussion of this issue and other issues related to language development; suffice it to say here that parent perceptions are not always consistent with research findings.)

The mother of a young boy who was implanted shortly before his second birthday said:

> We were told from the beginning that children only have a certain window of time to get spoken language or to get any language.
>
> *Mother of a 4-year-old boy implanted in 1996*

> And not only the introduction of the language, . . . the wiring of the brain in the first 3 years, or some finite amount of time, [will supposedly be complete]. And we wanted to get that language in [our son] within the window that was already half over, because at this point he was already a year and a half old. So we were worried if we didn't do it now it might be too late.
>
> *Father of the same 4-year-old boy*

As noted, an area of language development that was important to the parents we talked with was the fact that language acquisition was often perceived as being delayed vis-à-vis hearing children of the same age. When asked if she felt that her daughter's spoken language development was equal to her friends or peers during the time she was wearing her hearing aid before the implant, the mother of a girl who was implanted at age 4 said:

> [My daughter] seemed a little bit behind. Her signing ability was great, but her talking, she was behind, she really was. That concerned us.
>
> *Mother of a 7-year-old girl implanted in 1996*

This, again, was a common theme among many of the parents with whom we spoke: a reasonably good sign language, but not spoken language, vocabulary prior to the implant. On this point, part of the interview with a mother whose son was implanted in 1988 is revealing.

> INTERVIEWER: At the time you were thinking about getting the implant, was [your son's] language development where you wanted it to be?
>
> MOTHER: No, no. It was not. He had no language.
>
> INTERVIEWER: At the age of 6 [when he was implanted]?
>
> MOTHER: No language. Very little vocabulary.
>
> INTERVIEWER: You mean spoken vocabulary. What about sign vocabulary?
>
> MOTHER: Signing was humongous. It was tremendous. He had it going.
>
> *Mother of a 17-year-old young man*

In an interesting twist on this theme, one family, whose son was hearing until he became ill with meningitis, was able to use sign language to help preserve and build on the spoken language that had been developed before his deafness. The mother of the boy said:

> [Our son] was 2 when he lost his hearing. . . . He had all that receptive language. He was starting to use expressive language. He was starting to put together two and three words. . . . And my husband and I [made] that effort to continue with

language, and used sign language, so he didn't really have that gap in language [after he became deaf]. I mean, he was really lucky. And I think that's why. . . . Because he just got in there right away. He started using signs right away.

Mother of a 13-year-old boy implanted in 1993

Another mother, whose son received his implant in 1997, said that, although her son's spoken language development was quite good while he was using hearing aids, it did require a great deal of work on her part to facilitate this development. When asked if she had to spend more time working with her deaf son on his language acquisition compared with his hearing brother, this mother said: *No question, no question, no question. My hearing son learned language easily.* This mother used pre-implant auditory-verbal (A-V) therapy with her deaf son, and, in large measure because of her time commitment, the method proved to be quite successful (the son is now attending college). As this mother said, concerning A-V therapy:

If the parents don't become active in the therapy and the language acquisition, then it's not a good decision for the kid. It doesn't happen by accident. It happens very, very purposefully all the way through.

Mother of an 18-year-old young man implanted in 1997

Some parents, particularly parents of younger children who were implanted before they were 2 years of age, reported that there was no language development at all in their children, whether spoken or sign. In some other cases, there was no early language acquisition of any kind for several years. As noted in the previous chapter, one-fifth of the parents who responded to the Gallaudet Research Institute (GRI) survey reported no pre-implant language development. In addition to the many other consequences of delayed language acquisition, one of the immediate problems faced by some parents in this regard centered around the difficulty of explaining to their child what an implant was, and why they had to go to the hospital for an operation. As the mother of a young girl who received her implant when she was 4 years old said:

We got a coloring book that told all about the cochlear implant. But [our daughter] didn't have language at that point. [We were not able] to explain [the operation] to her. She knew she was going to the hospital, and she saw pictures of different things. . . . Did she understand that she was getting an implant? No. Did she understand what it was going to mean for her? No.

Nevertheless, this mother is pleased that they went ahead with the surgery since:

> The longer you . . . wait, the harder it is for the child to develop speech. And I think that was important because I want [my daughter] to have the benefit of both worlds, the deaf world and the hearing world.
>
> *Mother of a 7-year-old girl implanted in 1996*

Reaching the Decision to Implant

Access to spoken language was a primary reason why the parents we interviewed wanted to get a cochlear implant for their child. A number of other reasons were also cited by parents as important, although many of these additional factors were related to spoken language acquisition. For example, most of the parents we talked with cited the ability to speak and to communicate with hearing people as an important reason for implantation. Many parents felt that if their child could more easily communicate with the hearing world, this would enable the child to become more independent, and would open up more opportunities and give the child more choices in the future. Safety considerations were also important, and many said that, even if the hoped-for speech did not materialize, enhanced safety was reason enough to get the device.

About half of the 53 parents we discussed this issue with in our interviews said that their child's hearing aids were not providing the type of access to sound that they had envisioned, and that this was an important reason why they decided in favor of implantation. As one mother said:

> He just wasn't getting it with the hearing aids, it just wasn't there. He wasn't picking up the sounds. . . . I wanted him to be a normal kid, you know.
>
> *Mother of a 5-year-old boy implanted in 1996*

A number of parents said that family considerations were important. They felt that if their child had more access to sound that communication with other family members would be enhanced. Several
parents said that, although sign communication was used, at least
to some extent, in the immediate family, signing outside the family was problematic. Not only was this seen as a problem with the
general nonsigning hearing society, but also sign communication
with extended family members was quite rare among the families
we talked with.

In addition to these important factors, some additional reasons
cited by parents included educational concerns and the hope
that the child would have access to music. A sampling of some of
the reasons why parents decided to get an implant for their child
follows below:

The most important [reason for getting an implant] was that
[our son] needed to be able to speak, to communicate. And,
in order for him to be successful in the world, not just in the
deaf community, but in the world, I really felt that he needed
spoken language. . . . I think that a lot of people would . . .
think it offensive if I said that being deaf could very easily be
a limitation. But it can be if you don't handle it properly, and
I want to make sure that he has every tool possible to be successful. . . . The reality is there are certain people out there
who are not going to go out of their way to communicate
with a deaf person. . . . And it may be wrong, but [our son],
in the future, is still going to have to deal with those people.
. . . Our logic was that we wanted to try to give him every
possibility, every advantage that he could have when it comes
time for him to go out into the world and live his own life.
Father of a 4-year-old boy implanted in 1996

Well, I guess, when [my daughter] was about 2 and a half . . .
the early intervention person [asked], Well, what are your
goals for [your daughter], if you could pick whatever you
wanted for her, what would your goals be? And I said I
wanted her to be able to sing and dance and play and everything else that every child does, but she couldn't hear the
music and she can't sing because it's just blocked off to her.
And that was the most important thing to me. . . . I felt that
although I didn't think there was anything wrong with being

deaf, that hearing is such a gift from God, it's such a rich, wonderful thing to be able to experience, that if she has a chance to experience it I didn't want to keep it from her.

Mother of a 6-year-old girl implanted at age 5

That'll be fine if he could hear a car coming, and he's riding his bike. And, you know . . . we just said, Well, what if we didn't do this [get an implant], and then he later looked at us and said, Well why didn't you do that? And so we just felt that it was just another option for him. I mean we never planned on him becoming only oral, because he already was using sign language so well. His language was fine. . . . We just wanted to make . . . his life with other people outside of school and his immediate family a little easier, if we could.

Mother of a 13-year-old boy implanted in the early 1990s

The most important decision that we made together as a family was that we wanted to enhance [my daughter's] ability to communicate. We could tell that the hearing aids were not helping, and I had a concern with the entire family that she wasn't communicating with them at all. And cousins would come over and they would be playing and she kind of was inched out because she didn't understand what was going on. And that concerned me [and] I wanted to give her the ability of hearing all she could hear and learn by that, but she'll always be hearing-impaired, always.

Mother of a 7-year-old girl implanted in 1996

FATHER: It was not a desperate plea to get an implant, because we were desperate to have him speak. We were never like that.

MOTHER: If he could say, I love you, mom, [that would be] wonderful. And if he went like that, that's all I cared about.

FATHER: We wanted to give him the choice and have him make the decision.

MOTHER: I wasn't out to torture my child so I could have a hearing-speaking child.

Parents of a 14-year-old boy implanted in the late 1980s

We know that . . . when he leaves [school], he's going to have to compete with other hearing children, other hearing adults, and we want him to grow up to be independent and be able to make a good living.
Mother of a 16-year-old boy implanted in 1995

A mother, when asked what her main reason was for getting an implant for her daughter, replied:

That she could hear again and be like us. . . . I wanted her to stay here and I was afraid that she would have to go to the school for the deaf someday. . . . I figured if she had some hearing and speech that it would be more likely that she could stay here.
Mother of a 14-year-old girl implanted in 1988

A sign-based method would have the long-term effect of [our daughter] not being able to communicate with the 99.2% of the population that does not sign. That was one of the biggest reasons.
Mother of a 6-year-old girl implanted in 1996 and a
2-year-old boy implanted in 1998

We thought [our daughter] might make use of it, she might learn language auditorily, might help her educationally, might someday help her in her chosen field. We just wanted her to have opportunities and I think her having sign language will also help her. . . . We've always been glad that she knew sign language because should she choose not to [use the implant], then she has her first form of communication that she ever learned.
Mother of an 11-year-old girl implanted in 1996

Data from the GRI study reinforce the importance of language development, especially spoken language acquisition, in the decision-making process. The GRI survey asked parents to identify the "main reason" for deciding to get a cochlear implant for their child. Table 4.2 summarizes these responses. It is clear that spoken language and safety issues are, by far, the most important reasons cited by parents included in this study.

In sum, data from our interviews and from the GRI survey indicate that many parents hoped that their child's chances of acquiring

TABLE 4.2
Main Reason for Deciding to Get a Cochlear Implant

Main Reason Cited by Parents	Percentage of Parents Citing This as Main Reason
Ease in development and use of oral spoken language	52%
Child's safety or environmental awareness	25%
To gain hearing	8%
Child's expressed desire for an implant	6%
Convenience in daily activities	3%
Better future with more opportunities	3%
Concern for child's self-image	1%

spoken language would significantly improve with the implant. Some parents were also concerned that their child was falling behind his or her peers in terms of oral language development, and many were concerned that, even though their child had good sign language skills, this was not "good enough" for optimal functioning in a world dominated by hearing people using a spoken language.

Sources of Implant Information and Advice

In an effort to learn more about cochlear implants, and to determine whether or not an implant might be appropriate for their child, all of the parents we talked with sought out other people for information. These sources of information included other parents of children with cochlear implants; implanted children themselves; adults with implants; health professionals, such as pediatricians, audiologists, speech/language therapists, and various professionals at cochlear implant centers; and deaf people (both those who signed and those who did not). Many parents expressed appreciation for the advice and counsel they received, although the praise was not uniform from all quarters. As noted in the previous chapter, pediatricians were often not perceived as being particularly helpful, and many parents expressed mixed feelings about the information they received from some people in the deaf community who felt that cochlear implants, particularly pediatric implants, were either unnecessary or unethical or both.

We discussed the issue of implant information and advice with all of the 56 families we interviewed. As might be expected, almost none had heard of a cochlear implant at the time they discovered their child was deaf. Most of the parents reported many different sources of information about the implant. A few parents learned about implants in a chance encounter with someone who already knew about them, whereas others were informed by health professionals, such as audiologists or physicians, at a hospital or clinic. Some learned about implants from articles in newspapers or magazines or from books, and several families heard about them in a *60 Minutes* television program that was broadcast in the early 1990s. This program featured a young girl who was obtaining a good deal of benefit from her cochlear implant. Some parents learned about implants from friends, family members, or parents of children with implants at the school where their child was a student. A few parents learned about the device at conferences, such as at Alexander Graham Bell Association of the Deaf conventions. A mother of a 20-year-old daughter said that they learned quite a bit about cochlear implants at an Alexander Graham Bell convention in Utah in 1996. After talking with a number of people at the convention and still not being sure whether or not an implant was appropriate for her daughter, this mother said:

> Finally, I pulled [a doctor] aside and I said, I just need you to tell me, here's [my daughter], here's where she's been, she was born hearing, she's very auditory, very verbal. He just looked at us . . . and said, Do it! Just get it done. And, you know, to this day I appreciate his honesty because everybody's afraid to say . . . . maybe it won't work for you and then you'll blame them.
>
> *Mother of a young woman implanted in 1996*

A parent who attended the same conference said: *We came back from the Alexander Graham Bell conference, which was in July of 1996, and told the program in [city] that we wanted the cochlear implant. After two months of multiple interdisciplinary evaluations [our daughter's] candidacy was approved. She got it at the end of August, and was turned on in September.*

Parents also reported learning about implants at other conferences and seminars, as well as at classes offered by local colleges
and universities. A few parents attended the 1995 National Institutes
of Health Cochlear Implant Consensus Development Conference in
Bethesda, Maryland, to learn more about implants. One parent, who
was living in a western state at the time she and her husband discovered their child was deaf, learned about cochlear implants at a
seminar sponsored by a local hospital in the mid-1990s. Although
they eventually decided to get an implant for their daughter, their
initial exposure to implants was not reassuring. The mother recalled
that *the surgery sounded scary to us, especially when the surgeon
came out and said, Well, I wouldn't implant my 2-year-old.* Parents also attended other seminars and symposiums, some of which
were sponsored by hospitals or cochlear implant centers.

> [The hospital] had a get-together where they had a man come
> in that had a cochlear implant, and he was like their
> spokesperson . . . and how [the implant] was like the miracle
> cure for deafness. . . . He was an older man and he had hear-
> ing and lost it and was implanted to get his hearing back. So,
> and it worked. So, when we saw that we thought, Hey, this is
> it . . . this is going to be the deal where our child will be nor-
> mal, he'll be able to hear, he'll start to pick up, his speech
> will get better . . . just the difference between not hearing and
> here you go. Of course, that didn't work either.
>
> *Father of a 16-year-old boy implanted in 1995*

This parent's last comment highlights the point, expressed by
many parents and discussed in the following chapters, that things
do not always work out as planned.

Several parents learned about cochlear implants from early intervention programs for young children or from outreach programs
from state schools for deaf students. In addition, an important source
of information for parents was the World Wide Web, as well as information that was distributed by cochlear implant companies. Information about implants is available on the web sites of the three major
manufacturers of cochlear implants (see Appendix), and glossy publications produced by implant companies are typically made available to parents by cochlear implant centers when parents begin
exploring implantation as an option for their child.

Some parents had difficulty getting advice, particularly those who were searching for information prior to the advent of on-line discussion groups and Internet web sites. For almost all of the parents we interviewed, parents of other children with cochlear implants, and often their implanted children, provided an important source of information and advice. A sampling of comments from parents on this point follows:

> I think probably what influenced me most was the parents and meeting the children who had implants.
> *Mother of a 7-year-old girl implanted in 1994*

> FATHER: The professionals telling us about the expectations was a lot lower than the real results that we saw in real families.

> MOTHER: I think for me it was later on, when [my daughter] was outside with another boy and [the boy's] dad just called from, it looked like miles away . . . and [the boy] turned around and that was it. I mean, that was the moment for me [and] I really jumped on the bandwagon. But the first time I ever saw a child with the implant I thought, I don't want that.
> *Parents of a 3-year-old girl implanted in 1998*

> We did . . . talk to a family whose daughter had had a cochlear implant done. And I think she was about 6 or 7; by that time she was 10. So her language was perfect. We had a chance to talk to her. . . . And what problems did she have with it, and was it hard? And . . . she seemed to have a mixed feeling, but not a bad mixed feeling. It was like she liked not hearing sometimes.
> *Mother of a 10-year-old implanted at age 7*

A mother said, when she was exploring the possibility of implantation for her oldest daughter in the early 1990s, that:

> Interestingly enough, what happened when we were [visiting an implant center] we met a child [who] happened to be there with her mother . . . and she was the one who really sold us. . . . [The child] is 2 years older [than my daughter], and I heard this child talking, and I said I had no idea this was possible. It's not like today where there are all these children with

implants and you know what it does and doesn't do. . . . This
was the first idea, [the first] clue, that I ever had that this
could be possible.

Mother of a 12-year-old girl implanted in 1989 and
a 4-year-old girl implanted in 1998

We also talked to parents of kids who had received implants
at different ages for different reasons, meningitis, born deaf,
early diagnosed, late diagnosed. . . . All of the parents, without
exception, that we talked to have said they would do it again
in a heartbeat.

Mother of a 2-year-old boy implanted in 1998

We also asked parents how soon they felt their child might be
a candidate for an implant after they had heard about the device's
availability. Interestingly enough, most of the parents we talked with
said that they felt their child was not a candidate, at least not immediately. Some parents said their child had more residual hearing than
was permitted at the time and was benefiting, at least to some
degree, from hearing aids. Others had some doubts about the surgery
itself, or wanted to wait until the technology improved, and others
were unable to consider an implant because, at the time, the minimum age for implantation was 24 months. For a few parents, money
was an issue because some insurance companies balked at paying
for the procedure, especially in the late 1980s before the Food and
Drug Administration gave premarket approval for pediatric implants.
Most of the parents said that the decision to implant was one that
required a good deal of time; implantation was not something many
parents rushed into. In a few cases, one parent wanted the implant
and had to spend some time convincing his or her spouse that this
was, in fact, a good idea for their child.

Input from Deaf People

Many of the parents we talked with had contact with deaf people
before they decided to get an implant for their child. Others said
that, although they did not specifically talk with any deaf people,
pre-implant, they were nevertheless aware of the expressed opposition to cochlear implants by many people in the deaf community.

Some parents were also aware of the National Association of the Deaf 's (NAD's) 1991 position paper. In fact, many parents said that the position paper, which strongly opposed pediatric implants, was included in the information packet that was given to them by the cochlear implant center when they were debating the pros and cons of going ahead with implantation. The positions in the 1991 paper are no longer officially endorsed by the NAD (a new position paper was released in October 2000); but, at the time most of the parents we talked with were considering an implant, this was the "official" NAD position. By default, many people interpreted it as the position of the deaf community, or, more generally, of those whose primary mode of communication is American Sign Language.

Several parents said some deaf people accused them of being "cruel," "barbaric," or guilty of "child abuse" because of their decision to go ahead with the implant. The message that parents should wait until their child was older and give him or her the chance to decide whether or not to get an implant was also emphasized in our interviews. Perhaps not surprisingly, few parents we talked with agreed with this reasoning. Many parents were not pleased with the comments they received from deaf people, and, for some parents, it caused a good amount of anguish. Other parents reported that the views of the deaf community caused them to think long and hard about getting an implant for their child and what this might mean for their child's future identity as a deaf person. It is important to keep in mind that, when many of the parents we talked with had their initial contact with the signing deaf community, they were searching for information about implants (or, more generally, about deafness and deaf people), had little if any previous contact with deaf people, and were worried about what the future might bring. In chapter 10, we discuss, at length, some of the views of the deaf community held by many of the parents we interviewed.

Concerning the question of pre-implant contact with deaf people or the deaf community, the GRI survey asked parents to indicate if they received "direct information" from a variety of deaf people prior to implantation. As shown in table 4.3, about half of the respondents to this question reported receiving some direct information from deaf adults prior to implantation. (Survey respondents were asked to select all sources of information. Thus, the total exceeds 100%.)

TABLE 4.3
Direct Information Received from Deaf Adults Pre-Implant

Direct Information Received	Percentage of Parents Receiving Information from This Source
From deaf adults *opposed to* cochlear implants for deaf children	29%
From deaf adults *supportive of* cochlear implants for deaf children	24%
From deaf adults who neither strongly opposed nor strongly favored cochlear implants for children	16%
From adults (or parents of children) who had discontinued cochlear implant use	6%
No direct information received from deaf adults prior to implantation	54%

General Sources

As far as general sources of information and advice about implants are concerned, the GRI survey asked parents to indicate the *first* person to suggest a cochlear implant as an option for their child. A plurality of the parents (36%) reported that an audiologist, speech/language therapist, or an A-V therapist was the first to make the suggestion, and another 17% said that an otolaryngologist (ENT) specialist made the suggestion. Slightly more than 10% said the first person to make the suggestion was a family member, and slightly less than 10% said that an educator or a teacher first made the suggestion. Reading material was cited by 8% of the parents and other sources—such as pediatricians, television programs, and friends—were cited by a small number of respondents (5% or less in each case).

Another question on the GRI survey asked what sources of information parents used in making the implant decision. Table 4.4 summarizes the responses from parents on this question.

Given the percentages reported in table 4.4, it is clear that many parents used several different sources of information in their decision-making process.

TABLE 4.4

Major Sources of Information Used by Parents in Making the Decision to Implant

Source of Information	Percentage of Parents Using This Source
Audiologist or other speech and hearing clinicians	81%
Other children with cochlear implants	57%
ENT/otolaryngologist	56%
The child himself or herself	43%
Deaf adults	13%
Printed literature	7%

The GRI survey also asked parents how long they considered an implant before deciding to go ahead with the surgery. About a quarter of the respondents said they considered an implant for less than 3 months, another quarter considered implantation for 3 to 6 months before deciding to go ahead, and another quarter spent from 6 months to 1 year thinking about implantation before proceeding. Slightly less than a quarter of the parents spent more than 1 year considering their decision. Related to this question is the issue of how informed the parents felt they were "regarding the various alternatives and assistive communication options available to [their] deaf child" at the time the implant surgery was performed. These other options might include cued speech, digital hearing aids, tactile aids, and American Sign Language. Only 4% of the parents responding to the GRI survey said they were "minimally informed" about these options. Seventeen percent felt they were "fairly well informed," and 78% considered themselves "quite thoroughly informed" about these alternatives at the time they decided to proceed with the surgery. Clearly, most parents felt that they had plenty of time to become aware of the options available for their children and to decide that a cochlear implant was what was desired.

Child's Participation in the Decision-Making Process

One of the important issues raised by many critics of pediatric cochlear implants, including many deaf people, is that parents should wait until the child is old enough to participate in the decision-making process before obtaining an implant. Consequently, we wanted to ascertain the extent to which parents involved their children in the decision-making process.

We discussed this issue with most of the parents we talked with and, interestingly enough, about half of them said they did involve their child, at least to some extent, in the process. Of course, if the child was only 18 or 24 months old at the time of implantation, there was no child involvement in the decision-making process. However, even among children as young as 4 or 5, many parents made a conscious effort to determine if their child was interested in the implant, even if the child did not clearly understand what was involved. (Issues related to surgery will be discussed in the next chapter.) Among older children, most of the time the decision to get an implant was the child's decision. In only one case did we interview a family where an older child (13 years old) was implanted even though he did not want the device. This issue will be examined in more detail in chapter 11.

Conclusions

In summary, few of the parents we talked with knew about cochlear implants when their child was diagnosed as deaf; most of them got information about implants from many different sources, especially other parents and children with implants, and most of the parents considered the cochlear implant option for 1 year or less before making a decision to go ahead with the surgery. This is not to say that the decision was an easy one; indeed, for almost all of the parents we talked with, the decision was anything but easy, even though parents clearly wanted their son or daughter to acquire spoken language, if possible. The decision-making process was, by and large, a draining and stressful experience for many parents that was, in many cases, even more difficult because of the vocal opposition of many deaf people to pediatric implantation.

In addition to the sources of information discussed in this chapter, parents also received information from the cochlear implant center where they elected to have the surgery. As noted, some parents initially decided to have the surgery after talking with health professionals, many of whom were associated with implant centers. In the following chapter, we will examine the relationship that parents had with the implant center, issues related to surgery, and some of the short-term post-implant outcomes.

5

The Cochlear Implant Center, Surgery, and Short-Term Post-Implant Outcomes

The parents we interviewed reported choosing surgeons in many different hospitals for the cochlear implant procedure.[1] We asked parents what kind of advice and information they received from the implant center, if they felt they were an integral part of the decision-making process, if they felt there was some "pressure" from people at the implant center to go ahead with the surgery despite any misgivings they might have had, and how informed they were about the risks involved in cochlear implant surgery. Several questions on the Gallaudet Research Institute (GRI) survey also dealt with these and other issues related to the implant center.

Following a referral from their pediatrician, or from another physician or health care professional, some of the parents we talked with shopped around for an implant center. Most, however, simply selected a center near their home because it was the

---

1. These included hospitals in the following states: Alabama, California, Colorado, Florida, Illinois, Indiana, Iowa, Maryland, New York, North Carolina, Oregon, Pennsylvania, Tennessee, Utah, Virginia, and Washington. (One family had the surgery performed in Australia.)

only one available or because they had developed a good relationship with some members of the staff. Several families, particularly in the western part of the country, traveled a
considerable distance for their child to get an implant because
there were no implant facilities in their vicinity. The need for
post-implant follow-up habilitation activities, including mapping
and speech therapy, added to the travel burden for a number of
these families.

The entire process from referral to surgery is fairly time-con-
suming, and usually involves an initial consultation at the implant
center followed by audiological, psychological, and surgical assessments. Some of these activities may be combined in a single visit
to the hospital; but, at a minimum, several months are typically
required for the process to run its course. In addition, as will be
seen, many parents we talked with had to spend a great deal of
time struggling with their insurance carrier or their HMO to get permission to go ahead with the surgery. This was especially true in
the late 1980s and early 1990s when pediatric cochlear implants
were much less common than they are today.

Most of the parents we interviewed said that one of the things
their implant center stressed was that positive results were by no
means guaranteed and that there was considerable variability in the
amount of success enjoyed by children after an implant, as
reflected in current research literature (see chapter 9). Most of the
parents also said that both the pros and cons of implantation were
presented by the implant center and that they did not perceive
themselves to be pressured to go along with the wishes of the center. Parents knew the decision was up to them. Moreover, most of
the parents said that implants were not presented by the implant
center as a "cure" for deafness. Many parents also said that the
implant center made them aware of the position of many people
in the deaf community regarding pediatric implants. The following are some of the comments from parents on these issues:

> FATHER: [The implant center] would give us options and give us
> literature and then say, You make up your own mind. And I
> appreciated that . . . because I think we are intelligent, edu-
> cated people, and were able to make an informed decision,
> but they wouldn't give us any real guidance at all. . . . Handing
> my child over to a surgeon was probably one of the hardest

things I ever had to do. And I don't know that they could have increased that doubt any more.

INTERVIEWER: So you don't feel ... [the implant center] was forcing anything on you?

FATHER: No, not at all. I mean, it [was] totally the opposite. . . . They . . . really wouldn't give us any guidance, even when we asked them . . . it was frustrating.

MOTHER: I think they realized that it's a decision that you need to make as a parent . . . it's not a decision that anyone can make for you.

Parents of a 2-year-old boy implanted in 1998

They [the cochlear implant center] made me no promises. [As] a matter of fact, I really thought, Well, why didn't they try to get me a little more excited about this thing? . . . But they guaranteed me nothing. They did not bring my hopes up at all, . . . they said she will never hear like a normal person. The implant is not a cure. It . . . doesn't restore hearing. When it's off she is still deaf. She is still going to be deaf. And you don't know how her spoken language will be, or how she's going to do with it.

Mother of a 2-year-old girl implanted in early 1999

[At] our cochlear implant center, one of their requirements as you go through the evaluation process is that you read the papers of the NAD, the American Academy of Audiology, and the Cochlear Implant Club International, so you get the whole spectrum of opinion by doing that.

Mother of a 6-year-old girl implanted in 1996 and
a 2-year-old boy implanted in 1998

The mother of a young boy who was implanted in 1996 said that, in the packet of information she received from the cochlear implant center:

MOTHER: There were two or three articles written by the deaf community; there was information from Cochlear, the company. They gave us names of other parents of children who had the implant, and we were able to meet other children who had the implant and to meet the parents and talk to them.

INTERVIEWER: So [the implant center] encouraged you to talk with deaf people who were not in favor of implants?

MOTHER: They did. They really did. Whether they were in favor or not. They encouraged us to look at everything, they really did.
Mother of a 4-year-old boy implanted in 1996

At another point in the interview, however, the following exchange took place:

INTERVIEWER: Do you think the [implant center] was advertising their successes too much and not giving you a really objective picture of what to expect?

MOTHER AND FATHER (together): Yes.

INTERVIEWER: I wonder if their emphasis on the success stories is making it more difficult for parents whose kids are not quite at that level.

MOTHER: Oh, absolutely.

FATHER: Absolutely, that's what we felt. . . . Because of [the implant center] talking about the success stories, we came very close to saying we made the wrong decision . . . I do not think *we* made the wrong decision, but I sure wish we had a little bit more information at the very beginning. I think we still would have gone with the implant, but I think we would have made a few more right moves along the way.

INTERVIEWER: Do you think the [implant center] has changed its approach a little bit . . . their approach to parents?

MOTHER: Yes . . . they've definitely modified [their approach] because I met another mother whose son was trying to be in the candidacy program to get the implant and they wouldn't accept him because he didn't have enough communication.
Parents of the same 4-year-old boy

Although most of the parents said that the implant center they dealt with was even-handed in its approach, and that they felt comfortable with the process, a few parents perceived some pressure or encouragement from the implant center to get the device for their child.

> Mother: The medical community acted like, almost, we almost felt as though we would be neglecting him if we didn't follow through on the cochlear implant. It was really presented to us as a gift from God: Why wouldn't you do this for your child? Do you know how horrible it is to be deaf? We were given absolutely no negative information about it at all except for the fact that he would need surgery and general anesthesia.
>
> Interviewer: This was at the [implant center]?
>
> Mother: Yes.
>
> *Mother of an unimplanted boy*

I'm going to say that [the implant center] was the one who handed out the literature, both sides of it, so that we would be able to read and make the decision on our own. But they were like our parents, they were wanting to get it done, pretty much. You really wanted to think that they were looking towards his welfare, but. . . .

> *Father of a 16-year-old boy implanted in 1995*

> Interviewer: Did you feel that they were pushing you to get the implant? Or do you feel that they were just giving information, making it possible for you to make the decision?
>
> Mother: I think they were doing that. Obviously they were pro-implant. I mean they . . . had seen the results of the implant.
>
> *Mother of a 10-year-old boy implanted in 1995*

Related to parent involvement, one question in the GRI survey asked parents if they felt they were "a vital and valued member of [their] child's CI [cochlear implant] team." Parents were asked to consider "the period from before the implant surgery through the habilitation and educational adjustment after the

TABLE 5.1
Professionals Affiliated with the Cochlear Implant Center Involved in Preparing for and Facilitating Child's Use of the Implant

Professionals at the Cochlear Implant Center	Percent of Parents Citing Professional Involvement
Audiologist	95%
Surgeon	86%
Speech pathologist	75%
Psychologist	35%
Teacher of the deaf	34%
Educational consultant	20%
Social worker	10%
Other professionals	3%

surgery" as they answered this question. Of the parents responding to this question, 96% said they either agreed or strongly agreed that they were in fact a vital and valued member of their child's cochlear implant team. Moreover, more than two-thirds of the parents reported that they were well acquainted, or very well acquainted, with the members of their child's cochlear implant team. Parents were also asked to identify the professionals affiliated with their child's cochlear implant center "who were involved in preparing for and facilitating [their] child's use of the cochlear implant." Table 5.1 summarizes the responses to this question.

The results reported in table 5.1 are certainly not surprising, since surgeons, audiologists, and speech therapists are the people responsible for implanting and mapping the device, and for making sure that the child benefits from it as much as possible.

The GRI survey also asked if the parents were satisfied with the counseling they received from their child's implant team before the surgery. Almost 90% reported that they were either satisfied (24%) or very satisfied (65%) with the counseling they received.

Surgery-Related Issues

Almost all of the parents we talked with said they felt they were well aware of the potential risks of the surgery. Perhaps the most common concern was related to possible damage to the facial nerve, which lies close to the cochlea. If this nerve was damaged, some type of facial paralysis could occur. In addition, parents were generally aware of some of the limitations that would be imposed on their child because of the surgery, particularly the fact that a magnetic resonance imaging (MRI) of the head would not be an option in the future unless the implanted magnet were to be removed. Most of the parents understood that the surgery might not be completely successful. But, because they wanted to do what they could to enable their child to be able to hear as much as possible, parents said again and again that they felt the risks were acceptable.

> FATHER: We realized that we were putting him in an operation, and if it wasn't successful he might lose everything. But, we just thought that the results could far outweigh the risk.
>
> INTERVIEWER: What did the hospital tell you about the pros and cons of the implant?
>
> FATHER: Well, they explained what could happen if something went wrong . . . during the operation. . . . And they told us about all [the plastic] playground equipment, about static electricity [that could damage the programs in the speech processor], they went over all that. And we took the steps . . . we gave away all his toys that were plastic and might cause some static. . . . The hospital didn't hide anything, they tried to tell us everything that might happen or could happen.
> *Father of a 7-year-old boy implanted in 1997*

The GRI survey also dealt with the question of risk. One question asked: "When the implant surgery (initially) was performed, were you rather unfamiliar, somewhat unfamiliar, or very familiar with various POSSIBLE negative outcomes of receiving a CI [cochlear implant]?" Responses to this question are summarized in table 5.2. It should be noted that the various categories in the first column of table 5.2 were not explained (i.e., were not operationally defined) on the questionnaire. Rather, each respondent was left

TABLE 5.2
Awareness of Possible Negative Outcomes of Implantation

Type of Possible Negative Outcome	Percent "Rather Unfamiliar" with This Outcome	Percent "Somewhat Familiar" with This Outcome	Percent "Very Familiar" with This Outcome
Auditory or audiological	5%	30%	64%
Medical or health-related	3%	26%	69%
Social	11%	38%	49%
Psychological	13%	39%	45%
Language-related	8%	36%	53%

to his or her own interpretation of what a negative auditory, social, psychological, or other outcome might be.

The vast majority of parents who responded to the GRI survey also reported that they were somewhat familiar or very familiar with each of these items as possible positive outcomes of receiving a cochlear implant. In general, parents reported that they were more aware of possible positive outcomes than they were of possible negative outcomes.

Although parents generally felt that the surgery was highly desirable, this is not the same thing as saying that it was invariably seen as necessary.

The mother of a young boy was asked if she saw implant surgery as elective surgery:

> Oh yeah, yeah, yeah, yeah, yeah. . . . I mean we never felt that it was something we had to do. And that was probably part of the reason why it was a hard thing to decide, because here you are putting your kid under the knife, and is it something you really need to do? I mean it was really hard.
>
> *Mother of a 13-year-old boy implanted in 1996*

Very few of the parents we talked with felt that implant surgery was absolutely necessary for their child to lead a productive and satisfying life. Rather, most parents, after considerable thought and discussion, felt that, given their experiences, their assumptions about the role of hearing in the modern world, their family situation, and the opportunities they hoped would be available for their child, the surgery, however traumatic and nerve-wracking it might be, was at least worth trying.

The mother of a young boy recalled her pre-implant anxieties in the days leading up to the surgery:

> The whole week [before] . . . I really went through a whole reconsideration, like, he's perfect the way he is, why would we cut into his head? He's doing fine with sign language. What are we doing? We're changing him. It was really terrifying.
>
> *Mother of a 5-year-old boy implanted in 1996*

Another mother, whose child was implanted in 1996, said, concerning the surgery:

> We're setting [our daughter] up for her life having a medical need. . . . I realize . . . we're doing that, . . . but we thought even [when] she becomes an adult if she doesn't want [the implant] she can have it taken out.
>
> *Mother of an 11-year-old girl implanted in 1996*

An important issue for many of the families we talked with was how they prepared their child for the implant surgery. Some families visited the implant center prior to the surgery, some said they used coloring books or other books provided by the implant center or from another source, and some used a variety of other creative methods to prepare for the surgery.

> FATHER: We told [our son] all about what was going to happen. We took him down to the hospital [and they had] dolls and everything down there. They showed him all the gowns that would be used by the doctors and what he would wear. . . . That was explained to him before the operation.

> MOTHER: [Our son] still has the coloring books the hospital gave him about the operation and implant and he still reads them occasionally. He knew he would have the same device his school friend . . . had, so that was great to him.

> FATHER: [Our son] had very little language at the time [of the implant]. I want to say he understood . . . we were doing

something. But I can't exactly say that he knew exactly what
was going to happen. I mean he didn't know down to the
last detail what was going on. He just knew we were doing
something and it was going to involve an operation because
that was explained to him pretty clearly, I thought.

Parents of a 7-year-old boy implanted in 1997

One of the more ingenious methods of preparing their child for
the implant surgery is described by the parents of a young boy:

FATHER: We tried to tell [our 7-year-old son] what was going to
happen and we introduced him to another kid that had a
cochlear implant and he was terrified. And . . . then we got
him what they call a kid's kit from the Cochlear Corporation. And it was a little book which, of course, he wasn't
able to read, but it had pretty pictures of a kid getting a
cochlear implant. And it came with a little toy cochlear
implant with a processor and headset and Velcro to attach it
to whatever the kid's favorite little doll was. [Our son's]
favorite thing was a 6-foot-long stuffed snake. . . . We brought
this snake into the hospital for his speech therapy and we
took the snake into the audiology booth and tested the
snake's hearing and I, I am not kidding, we tested, we gave
. . . the snake a hearing test. . . . He was supposed to rattle his
tail when he heard sound, and he didn't hear anything! And
so we reached the conclusion that his ears were broken, like
[our son's], and then we went and took the snake to the
doctor . . . in the clinic there, and we said, Okay, here's his
audiogram, and of course there's nothing. His ears are broken. Can you do anything for him? Can you fix them? And
the doctor looked at this and looked at the snake and took
out his little otoscope and he said, No, there's nothing we
can do. The only thing that might help him to hear is if he
gets a cochlear implant. And [our son] was like, Oh, no!
And then we told [him] they could do it right away. But his
snake was going to have to stay in the hospital to get this
done. He was going to have to [stay] overnight. Actually he
had to stay over the weekend because speech therapy was
. . . Tuesday. And Tuesday came and we went back to the
clinic and the snake was waiting for us there with his head
all bandaged up. And the doctor took his little bandage scis-

sors and cut the bandage off. And there was the snake's new cochlear implant. . . . We took the snake back to the booth and, lo and behold, the snake could hear.

MOTHER: Then. . . .

FATHER: . . . our son decided he . . .

MOTHER AND FATHER (together): . . . wanted a cochlear implant!
Parents of an 11-year-old boy implanted in 1995

A few of the children in the families we interviewed experienced some complications with the surgery. One of the more serious complications occurred in a girl who was implanted in 1992. Part of the interview with the mother is as follows:

INTERVIEWER: Did you feel pretty apprehensive at the operation?

MOTHER: For the surgery, yeah, . . . and her facial nerve was damaged for probably . . . 8 or 9 weeks. It was horrible, it was just really bad.

INTERVIEWER: What happened?

MOTHER: Her eye wouldn't shut and [her face] drooped down so when she smiled only [one] side went up.

INTERVIEWER: So, what did they say about that? Did they say, Don't worry, it will go away, or what did they say?

MOTHER: No, they were worried. . . . They thought it would be permanent. They did some tests on the nerves, I don't know what you call it . . . and they thought it would be permanent.

INTERVIEWER: Did they tell you at the beginning this was a risk?

MOTHER: They did, but the doctor said, It's never happened to me.

INTERVIEWER: Did it clear up gradually?

MOTHER: Yeah, just kind of quickly [after about 2 months].
Mother of a 10-year-old girl implanted at age 3

A mother of a son who was deafened by meningitis when he was 2 years old said she felt that the implant center was not completely honest with her when he was implanted in 1990. She said that after the surgery started:

> [My son] was in for about 2 hours when the doctor came out and said, We could only put in one channel. And I said, Why? He said, Because the cochlea was ossified. I said, Didn't you see that on the X-ray? And he said, Yes, but I thought that sometimes it's not solid, sometimes it's not hard, a lot of times, most of the time, it's soft . . . but his is just like bone in [the cochlea].

Later in the interview, the mother was asked if she had known that only one electrode could be implanted if she would still have gone ahead with the surgery.

> MOTHER: I would not have gone through with it because . . . it's a big surgery to put him through. . . . You know, at least with 7, 15, 21 [electrodes] you have a chance of 1 or 2 or 3 working. But with one, you only have one chance.

> INTERVIEWER: Do you feel like the doctor was honest with you about that, or do you think he was not?

> MOTHER: I feel, really, that he was so eager to do it that he wasn't honest with me.
> *Mother of a teenager implanted in 1990*

Most of the other complications or unexpected outcomes cited by parents were fairly minor and usually disappeared in a day or two. Some of the children experienced nausea, and in one or two cases postsurgical problems appeared to be exacerbated because, in this era of managed care, the hospital was in a rush to discharge the patient. Some parents were not completely prepared for what would happen after the surgery or what their child would look like.

> The scar, the actual incision, is so much bigger, there is so much more hair that went, than I ever imagined.
> *Mother of a 9-year-old girl implanted in 1994*

Most parents, however, were surprised at how quickly their child bounced back after the surgery. Some children were outside playing the next day and others returned to school within a few days after the surgery.

Most of the parents said that the surgery went smoothly and that all of the electrodes were successfully inserted in the cochlea. In the GRI survey, 95% of the respondents said that the electrodes were successfully inserted. Over time, however, some of the electrodes may stop working, either because they fail internally or because unpredictable interference among them can make it difficult for the user to interpret sound. About a fifth of the respondents in the GRI study said that some of the inserted electrodes were inactive, either through hardware failure or voluntary shut off. Another 10% said they were not sure whether or not any electrodes were inactive.

One issue that many people, including parents of children with implants as well as adult implant users, have concerns about is the question of re-implantation. That is, do the internal components have to be replaced periodically, or is it expected that they will remain implanted in the cochlea for the implantee's entire life? In general, the expectation, both from the implant center's perspective and from the patient or the patient's family, is that the internal components will not need to be replaced even though new developments in implant technology continue to be made. Rather, it is expected that any changes that occur will take place in the external components, particularly the speech (sound) processor. Indeed, many of the parents we talked with hoped that their child would be able to take advantage of new speech processing technology, including behind-the-ear (BTE) models that would make the implant more cosmetically appealing. Many parents said they hoped to purchase this new technology even if their insurance carrier refused to pay for it.

Concerning this issue, the GRI survey asked parents if their child's "device (internal or processing components)" ever had to be "upgraded or replaced." Virtually all of the respondents said that some upgrading or replacement was necessary. The vast majority of these responses focused on upgrading the external components, or even replacing cords that had been broken or lost, rather than replacing the internal equipment. Since parents were also asked to describe the circumstances of each upgrading or replacement, it is possible to estimate the number of devices that had to be replaced internally. There were 438 responses to the GRI survey that indicated a specific type of implant received by their child.[2] From the comments made by parents, it is apparent that at least 25 (approximately 6%) of these implants had to be replaced internally one time. This is a conservative number since we only counted those comments in which there was clear, unambiguous evidence that it was the internal component that had to be replaced (e.g., comments such as "implant failed, internal failure" or "internally failed, was replaced as outpatient"). If there was any doubt about whether it was an internal or an external piece that needed to be replaced, we assumed that it was an external part. Thus, because of the ambiguity of a number of comments from parents on the GRI survey, it is likely that at least several additional devices needed to be internally replaced. In any case, this is somewhat more than the 1–2% device failure/ replacement rate commonly cited by implant companies, although it is less than the 10% replacement rate cited by one of the parents we talked with whose son was implanted three times.

INTERVIEWER: What percentage of devices fail, do you have any idea?

FATHER: The doctor in [city] who did the third implant said the literature you get from Cochlear and Clarion say they're 99%; he said actually it's like 90%. . . . So that's one in ten [that] will fail.

Father of a young boy implanted three times

The GRI survey also asked parents if the device had to be replaced or upgraded more than once. Again, using a very conservative estimate, it is apparent that at least nine (2%) respondents

2. Devices manufactured by Cochlear Corporation (Nucleus) were used by 358 children, implants manufactured by Advanced Bionics (Clarion) were used by 70 children, and implants from other companies (3M/House and Med El) were used by 10 children. One respondent did not specify the type of implant used. Most of the parents of the children we talked with also used Nucleus devices (Nucleus 22 or the newer Nucleus 24 model), which have been available for a considerably longer period of time than Clarion. Among the families we interviewed, the ratio of Nucleus to Clarion users was about 5:1; no implants made by other manufacturers were used by the children in the families we talked with. For many families included in both the GRI study and in our interviews, the Nucleus device was the only one generally available when their child was implanted. When a choice was available, many parents spent a considerable amount of time weighing the pros and cons (both cosmetic and technological) of each model.

needed to replace the internal device twice and at least one (less than 1%) needed to replace the internal unit three times.[3]

Another issue related to implant surgery that is of concern to parents is the question of which ear to implant. Not only must parents decide what type of implant to get for their child, they must frequently decide where to put it. In a few cases, the cochlear implant surgeon made the decision about which ear to implant, but in most of the families we discussed this with it was the parents who made the final choice.

Deciding which ear to implant is still far from an exact science, and the parents we talked with described a variety of reasons why they decided to have the implant surgery on one ear or the other. Many parents said they decided to implant their child's "worst" ear (in terms of decibel loss) so that, if the implant did not work as expected, then the "best" ear would be available for later implantation (or for continued hearing aid use). In recent years, it appears that parents and implant centers have been more willing to implant the "better" ear since the likelihood of implant success, at least to some extent, has increased, and because it may be desirable to implant the ear that has a better history (or memory) of auditory stimulation.

In some cases, major or minor medical reasons governed the choice. For example, in one family, meningitis led to more ossification of the cochlea in one ear, which necessitated implantation in the other ear, whereas in another family a pre-existing scar near one ear made it appealing to have the surgeon "use" the same scar for the implant surgery. In another family, X-rays of the cochlea in both ears revealed that the facial nerve was too close to the cochlea in one ear, and the surgeon wanted to avoid possible complications in that ear. A minor skull fracture on one side of the head resulting from a fall led to implant surgery on the opposite side of the head for a child in one family, and, in another, it was determined that, on one side, the mastoid bone in the skull was not thick enough to support the internal transmitter.

---

3. On this point, a recent article in the Health section of *The Washington Post* (Colburn, 2000) entitled "Wired for Sound," includes a sidebar with the heading: "Cochlear Implants at a Glance." The following appears as a caveat in the sidebar: "In about 5 percent of cases, reimplantation is necessary because the original device fails." No source is given for this information, but it is interesting that the percentage is very close to what is reported in the GRI study.

Although medical problems and issues were important for some of the families, much of the time they were not the major factors in determining which ear received the implant. Rather, social factors, including concerns about expected speech and language development, frequently entered into the picture.

A few parents said that they decided to have the implant on the right ear because they thought this might facilitate language and speech development, which is centered in the left hemisphere of the brain. Others decided on the right ear because of athletic concerns (such as a child batting right-handed in baseball or softball and having the implant on the right ear, away from the pitcher), or because it was thought that, in the future, if their child were to be driving a car, an implant on the right ear would be more practical for hearing other people in the vehicle. Another parent decided to have an implant on her child's right ear for a very practical reason: *I usually am using my right hand and carrying [my son] around on my left and I thought that his right ear is going to be most available to me.*

Cochlear implant centers now sometimes perform a promontory stimulation test to determine if implantation in one ear might be more desirable than the other. In this test, an electrode is inserted through the eardrum onto the promontory of the cochlea. Then, tests are performed to determine how the auditory nerve responds to an electrical signal. Presumably, if the response is significantly better in one ear, this might be an important reason to do the implant in that ear. But, there is still no one, single, overriding criterion that is used for determining which ear to implant, and parents and surgeons continue to use a combination of aesthetic, practical, and medical reasons when making the decision.

Insurance Issues

A cochlear implant operation is quite expensive, and implantees and their families encounter additional expenses for postsurgical habilitation procedures, including frequent mapping (programming) of the sound processor and speech/auditory-verbal therapy sessions. At the present time in the United States, the cost for the surgery (including the cost of the device itself) is at least $40,000. Since few families have the resources to pay for implant surgery themselves, the question of how to pay for the device is one that is of great importance to parents and others contemplating implantation. Clearly, it was of concern to virtually all of the parents we talked with in our interviews.

It appears that about 1 of every 5 or 6 families we interviewed had significant problems getting their insurance carrier to pay for the cochlear implant for their child. Of the 52 families we discussed this with, 10 of them said that their insurance company or other medical provider refused to pay anything at all for the operation or for postsurgical mapping and habilitation (3 families), or would only pay after one or both parents spent a considerable amount of time on the phone, writing letters, making threats, or some combination of all three of these activities. Moreover, even when some of these recalcitrant insurance carriers finally did pay, they often did not cover the entire cost. In fact, several families we talked with said they have paid a great deal of money themselves for the surgery or postsurgery mapping and habilitation (primarily speech and listening therapy) expenses.

As far as the surgery/hospitalization is concerned, it appears that, in about 42 of the families we interviewed, their insurance company (or Medicaid or another public program) eventually paid 90–100% of the costs. In another 4 families, the insurance paid approximately 75–80% of the surgical/hospitalization expenses. Not all of the parents we talked with mentioned specific percentages, and, as noted, some of the insurance companies delayed paying for a considerable amount of time.

We heard some very interesting stories about insurance-related problems from many of the parents we interviewed. One mother said, *We went [to the hospital] that day for the surgery not knowing if they were going to pay for it or not. [And] we were prepared to take a loan out to pay for it. But the doctor's secretary came down into the waiting room and told us that she got the word that they were paying for it.* Another family got their insurance company to pay for everything, but, the father said, *then they promptly rewrote the insurance contract so that they would never have to pay for another. . . . In the paragraph where it says hearing aids are excluded . . . the new version [says] that hearing aids and cochlear implants are excluded.*

Perhaps the most important reason why a number of insurance companies delayed paying for the procedure was because it was new and because no one had asked them to pay for it before. In a few cases, insurance companies delayed paying for the implant either because the device had not yet been approved by the Food and Drug Administration (FDA) for use in children or because the child was too young to be implanted according to the FDA guidelines (under 18 or 24 months, depending on when the surgery took place). Thus, it is understandable that, in some cases, a considerable amount of time was needed to secure approval for the procedure. To facilitate this process, the major cochlear implant companies, as well as many cochlear implant centers, now have specific offices or positions assigned to handle insurance-related problems and to secure payment from insurance carriers.

As noted, three families we met, in different parts of the country, were unable to secure any support from their insurance carrier for the implant. In all three cases, however, another agency or person, or even an entire community, stepped in and offered to pay for part or all of the cost of the surgery and hospitalization. The first family had to pay for the surgery themselves, whereas the local Lion's Club paid for the speech processor. The mother of the second family recounts her experience as follows:

> When they did the implant the doctor explained to me that it was a $24,000 surgery [about a decade ago]. . . . I didn't have the $24,000. I said, If you will take my money every month, I will sign whatever it takes, and I will pay you. . . . I didn't have a husband, I didn't have nobody. It was just me and [my daughter] . . . and . . . my son. . . . And I said, If you're willing to let me sign . . . I will pay you a little bit every month. He said there was no problem with that. So I signed the papers. I was responsible for everything that went on at the hospital. After 2, 3, months, I think I made one payment, and the doctor . . . told me that I didn't have to pay [any] more because someone anonymously— I was not allowed to know the name—paid it off.

In the third family, the entire community came together to raise money for the implant surgery:

> MOTHER: I called a lady in . . . a small town nearby who had done fund-raisers before and she told me how to go about it. . . . I asked some people in the community to be the administrators, to be the fund-raising committee, and any money that

was brought in, they were to be in charge of it. . . . From that, the church organized fund-raisers. The baseball team, the parents of the ball team that [my son] played on, they organized a softball game between a [city] TV station and a local industrial park softball team. And they played, and charged admission into the ballpark. . . . The local pizza place donated pizzas for them to sell by the slice. Hamburger joints here in town donated hamburgers to be sold at the concession stand. Everything that night, the money was for [my son].

Interviewer: How much did they raise, do you remember?

Mother: Yes, I do. Forty thousand dollars . . . in 2 weeks.

Not all of the money was raised at the softball game, but additional community activities, including a carwash, food sales, and extensive media exposure, resulted in funds that are still being used (and anonymously replenished) today, more than a decade after the surgery.

Post-Implant Expenses

As far as post-implant habilitation expenses are concerned, it is safe to say that, in general, insurance carriers were much less enthusiastic about paying for postsurgery habilitation costs, especially for ongoing speech or auditory therapy, than they were about paying for the surgery. This reluctance caused considerable consternation among a number of parents we talked with. These parents questioned why their insurance would cover the equipment itself, but not the programming and training that would allow their child to benefit from it.

Slightly less than half (between 20 and 25) of the 52 families we talked with about insurance-related issues said or implied that their insurance carrier paid for post-implant mapping and speech/auditory therapy in full (or close to it). In about the same number of cases, insurance companies paid for some, but not all, of the mapping or habilitation expenses. In general, insurance companies appear to be more willing to pay for mapping than for speech and auditory therapy, perhaps because they see the latter as a long-term commitment. Moreover, a number of parents said that their insurance company would only pay for speech and auditory therapy expenses after a deductible had been met, or would only pay a maximum of several hundred dollars a year; anything beyond that was the parent's responsibility. In any case, it is clear that many of the families we talked with had to pay for much of the post-implant speech and/or auditory-verbal therapy their child received (outside of school) themselves.

> [The insurance company] put a limitation on the amount of speech therapy a cochlear recipient can have. It's not adequate to get through the year at all. And we come out-of-pocket literally in the thousands of dollars for speech therapy for our children.
>
> *Father of a 10-year-old girl implanted at age 4 and*
> *an 8-year-old boy implanted in 1996*

Another family said that, after the surgery, they started paying for speech therapy themselves. However, they soon noticed that their insurance policy stipulated that a maximum of 2 months of therapy would be covered. They subsequently got the company to pay, and, as the mother of the implanted child said, *once they started it I wouldn't let them stop. I said, You can't deny benefits based on services for a disability.* The father argued: *Are you telling me that you're going to pay for a prosthesis [the implant], but you won't pay for the training . . . to learn to use it? . . . Is that your position? And, ultimately, the insurance company that we dealt with didn't really have any experts who knew anything about it, and we went out and hired our own, and they filed reports, and they said, All right, we'll try it for a year and see if she improves.* Not surprisingly, the parents subsequently reported to the insurance company that progress was being made, and payments from the company have continued. Other parents also reported more success in getting their insurance company to pay for post-implant needs when the therapy is called "prosthetic device training" rather than "speech therapy."

As noted, another post-implant issue that is of importance to many of the families we interviewed is paying for upgrading the external speech processor. Most of the children currently use a body-worn processor that is about the size of a deck of cards. The alternative is a BTE processor that is more cosmetically attractive,

TABLE 5.3
Post-Implant Medical Insurance Services

Medical Insurance Service	Percent of Parents Reporting Full Coverage	Percent of Parents Reporting Partial Coverage	Percent of Parents Reporting No Coverage
Implant reprogramming or remapping	58%	29%	13%
Post-implant speech production therapy	41%	34%	25%
Post-implant auditory hablitation training	42%	32%	26%

especially for teenagers, as well as more functional, particularly in sporting events. We asked parents if they have had any upgrades, or if any were anticipated, and, if so, if their insurance company would pay for it. In only a few cases did the insurance company pay for an upgrade or did parents expect them to. Rather, almost invariably, parents expected to have to pay for this significant cost themselves if it was not available from the cochlear implant company at the time their child had the surgery.[4]

The GRI survey asked parents to indicate whether their medical insurance provided full, partial, or no coverage for reprogramming/remapping, post-implant speech production therapy, post-implant auditory habilitation training, or for any other insurance-covered accommodations or services. Table 5.3 summarizes the responses to these questions.

4. Because of rapid changes in cochlear implant technology, some implant companies offer coupons, or other discounts, for new processors that are not ready for distribution at the time a person actually has implant surgery. In addition, if both BTE and a body-worn sound/speech processors are available at the time of the surgery, the implantee may be given both of them as part of the cost of the operation. Each sound/speech processing device must be programmed separately, however.

In addition to these services, a few parents reported that their insurance carrier also paid for such things as batteries, new cables or wires, and summer speech therapy. These findings closely mirror the findings in our interviews in that insurance companies are more willing to pay for mapping expenses than for speech or auditory therapy, and that many families incur significant out-of-pocket post-implant expenses.

The GRI questionnaire also asked parents how long, after the initial "hook up," their medical insurance covered "CI habilitation services such as speech perception training and speech production therapy." A little more than two-fifths of the respondents (43%) said that this benefit was provided for 6 months or less, whereas a little more than one-quarter (27%) said that nothing at all had been covered. Only about 30% of the respondents had habilitation services paid for, in whole or in part, by their insurance carrier for more than 6 months.

Short-Term Post-Implant Outcomes

About a month after the surgery, implant patients need to return to the cochlear implant center to have their implant activated. This involves magnetically attaching the external microphone or transmitter to the internal receiver and programming or mapping the speech (or sound) processor so the implanted electrodes will be able to do the job they are designed to do: stimulate the auditory nerve endings in the cochlea and thereby enable the user to perceive sound. For virtually all of the families we talked with this was a very exciting time; the initial mapping session was the first time they would be able to see if the equipment actually worked as they hoped it might. Of course, many families realized that nothing dramatic might occur since the cochlear implant center had cautioned them against being too optimistic about what their child might be able to initially hear with the implant.

As discussed in detail in chapter 2, mapping is a complex process that involves establishing appropriate levels of sound for each of the implanted electrodes and making sure that the electrodes "work together" to enable the user to perceive sounds as clearly as possible. Under ideal conditions, the implantee is able to inform the audiologist doing the mapping when the sounds (including pure tones at different decibel levels and frequencies) are too soft, too loud, or just right. Of course, there are other ways, such as closed- or open-set word tests or even simple conversations, to determine the extent to which the mapping for the cochlear implant is appropriate.

For a child, it is often difficult to achieve a good initial cochlear implant map because it is sometimes hard for the audiologist to know exactly what the child, especially a very young child, can hear. Many of the parents we talked with said that, although it was clear their child heard *something* at the first mapping session it was not always clear exactly how much was heard. Consequently, it was often necessary for them to return to the implant center quite frequently during the first 6 months or so to "fine-tune" the map.

We asked parents about their child's first reaction at the initial mapping session. The vast majority of parents said that their child did in fact respond in some way to sound at the first mapping session; only three families said that there was no response at all. The most common initial reaction was crying, and about half of the parents said that their child appeared to be scared or frightened when sounds were first heard with their newly activated implant. A couple of parents said that their child was *overwhelmed* at the initial activation, whereas another parent said that their child signed *weird* when asked to describe what the sound was like. Not all of the children necessarily cried because they were frightened, however; as one parent said, her child cried and, at the same time, apparently *loved it*. About a quarter of the families we talked with said that the initial mapping session was uneventful; there was no dramatic scene at all, although it was clear that their child did perceive at least some sounds with the implant. And about another quarter said that their child was surprised or excited, or even laughing, at their first mapping session after hearing sound with the implant.

Many parents reported that their child heard new sounds very soon after the implant was activated that had not been heard with the hearing aids. Frequent mention was made of hearing doorbells, microwave timers, running water, telephones ringing, birds chirping, distant sirens, and other everyday sounds for the first time with the implant within a day (or less) to a month or two of use.

> I took [my son] into the bathroom [halfway through the first mapping session] and he ... reached up and flushed the toilet and he jumped, he was scared. . . . And then I went and I

flushed the toilet again [and] he was scared. And then he
looked up and it was almost like he was afraid of the handle
on the toilet, [but] he finally grabbed it and pulled. And it
made the same noise and he jumped. Then he grabbed it
again and pulled it and he started laughing. And I couldn't get
him out of there.

Father of an 11-year-old boy implanted in the mid-1990s

What follows is a short sampling of some other "first-day"
reactions to implant activation:

I think it was a bit scary, too, because when she got home
[the first day] she didn't like the garage door opener when it
opened. She cried, said not to open it. But she liked to run
water and put my high heels on and click my high heels.

Mother of a 7-year-old girl implanted at age 4

On the drive home after the [initial] mapping I was sitting in
the back seat and could hear the music and the music was
beautiful and I was just going off, This is so awesome, this is
so beautiful, and I could carry on a conversation with my mom
and she was sitting in the front and I didn't have to read lips.

Young woman implanted in 1996 at age 17

I was driving on the freeway [after the first mapping ses-
sion] and [my daughter] started screaming in the back seat
. . . [because] the magnet had fallen off. She was upset
[and] I put it back on. She laughed and laughed and
laughed; she loved it. From the . . . very first moment she
was so upset to have lost it.

Mother of an 8-year-old girl implanted at age 2

When I came in with him, and they turned it on, and gave
him his first sound, he started saying, I hear that, I hear that.
And that day he heard me tell him that I loved him for the
first time. And he turned around and he told me back what I
had said. . . . The first day it was turned on he understood that.

Mother of a teenager implanted in the late 1980s

Many of the parents we talked with said that the stated or
unstated policy of the cochlear implant center where the activation occurred was to start slow and try not to overburden the

child with too much sound all at once. This often involved activating only some of the electrodes at the first mapping session and, even for those electrodes that were activated, setting threshold levels that would allow the child to become gradually acclimated to the new sounds. Although parents sometimes expressed frustration with this policy, since they wanted to see more dramatic, immediate, results, they also understood that it would take time for their child to adjust to the implant.

One of the first things that many parents tried to do was to get their child to respond to his or her name.

> After 3 days, when I said [her name] she could turn around. . . . And within a week she would turn her back to us and we would say [brother's name] . . . and she would say, [brother's name], you said [brother's name].
>
> *Mother of an 8-year-old girl implanted in 1996*

A few families said that after a while they noticed that their child was able to respond to sounds in another room. Sometimes this occurred within a few months or even sooner, but sometimes it took several years to reach this plateau.

> We started with noisemakers [after a month or so]. You know, we would make noise and he would turn one way or the other, and then we started getting further and further away. And I would say within the first 2 months we could go to the bedroom and we would play a game. He would sit in here and listen and we would go to the bedroom and shake it and he would come running in, and my [deaf] mother was like, she was shocked to see that.
>
> *Mother of a 2-year-old boy implanted in 1998*

It often took some time for the child to get used to new voices.

> [My daughter's] first reaction, and actually for a long time [after that] was, I'm waiting for it to be a real voice. It's not a real voice yet. To her, I think, the sound that she had gotten from her hearing aids was real voice sound, and this wasn't a real voice yet. And that's what her reaction was.
>
> *Mother of an 11-year-old girl implanted in 1996*

Almost invariably the progression was from hearing something to making an identification of the sound to, months, or sometimes even years, later, understanding speech. Moreover, this progression usually did not happen naturally. Rather, parents repeatedly acknowledged that hours and hours of work, including regular speech and auditory therapy after the surgery, was necessary for their child to benefit from the implant. As one mother said: *Detection of sound doesn't mean comprehension. So we still had a lot of work to do [after the first day].*

Part of the development of speech discrimination involves the ability to hear high-frequency consonants that the child was usually unable to hear with a hearing aid. For some families, this development came rather quickly after implantation, whereas for others it was delayed for months or even longer.

The difference we see [that] the implant makes are things like, he never heard the 's' sound or 'ts' before and now he not only hears them but he is producing them. And that is a big difference. He now hears up into the 6000 hertz [cycles per second] frequency range whereas before he was only up to 2000 hertz, and he hears better at lower decibels, too.

Father of a 2-year-old boy implanted in 1998

MOTHER: One night [2 months after the implant was activated] we turned off all the lights and I was whispering a few words and [my daughter] was receiving everything I was saying.

INTERVIEWER: She was repeating everything?

MOTHER: Everything.

Mother of a 3-year-old girl implanted in 1998

[My daughter] could hear nothing for, I would say, for 3 weeks; we went back four times for mappings. This is unheard of . . . they couldn't figure out where she was. . . . She didn't hear tones, she heard nothing. Three or 4 weeks later she thought she discerned a beeping. . . . We've gone from . . . understanding speech and understanding stuff [with a hearing aid] to hearing beeping. . . . I mean, I was just beside myself; she had many, many mappings. . . . [My daughter] was all over the map, literally, in her mapping. Now she is doing quite well with the implant but it required 6 months to a year to differentiate between tones and, ultimately, understand speech. Now she is functioning better than she did with the hearing aids.

Mother of a college-age young woman implanted in 1995

My speech got so bad [after the implant]. I felt totally cut off from everyone. But I never reached the point that I thought it wouldn't get better. I never got to the point where I was really concerned. I said, I'll just give it 3 more weeks . . . then I said, just 4 more weeks. Also, I remember my experience with the transonic [hearing aid] and how difficult it was to adapt to that. It was horrible the first 2 to 3 months, just like the implant, then it got better.

The same college-age young woman implanted in 1995

Not all of the children initially liked wearing their implant, perhaps because they did not like the sounds they were hearing or were otherwise uncomfortable with the device. Consequently, sometimes parents had to resort to bribery to encourage their son or daughter to continue to use the implant. As one mother said: *It took a lot of months of bribery and stickers and just [trying] to motivate [my son] to wear [the implant].* Another mother had to resort to similar tactics to get her daughter to use her implant, which she hated at first. In this case, the carrot was a Barbie doll. Others said that it took some getting used to and that a break was frequently needed. Even the young woman who found music so awesome on the first day said: *Sometimes I just don't like to study with my implant on. I just take it off because it's so extremely quiet. I still . . . like doing that. It's nice to have the freedom to be able to take it off and not have to hear anything.* On the other hand, one child liked her implant so well, she insisted on sleeping with the external equipment attached.

Conclusions

There seems to be no one dominant type of post-implant outcome among the families we interviewed. Most young children heard some sounds, especially environmental sounds, more or less right away, whereas a few did not hear anything at all for several months. The most common description that parents offered of their child's progress with the implant was that it was quite slow and gradual, and that considerable post-implant habilitation was needed. It frequently required 6 months or more before the child was able to respond to his or her name, clearly distinguish among voices, and understand at least some speech. After time, though, most of the families we talked with said that their implanted child could clearly hear much more with the implant than they could with a hearing aid.

A lingering problem mentioned by many parents is the fact that it is often difficult for their child to hear in noisy situations, and it is hard for them to interact with strangers, with those whose voices they are not familiar with. Although these limitations are evident during the first 6 months after implantation, they tend to linger, in some cases for years, in many of the families we talked with. Clearly, few implanted children have "normal hearing" with the implant, and most of them continue to rely on lipreading to a considerable extent for communication.

6

Adjusting to Life After the Implant

Parents of children with cochlear implants, as well as the children themselves, typically face several issues after the implant surgery. These include the time commitment parents need to make for their child to benefit as much as possible from a cochlear implant, and the mode or type of communication the children typically use after implantation.[1] Some of the most important post-implant experiences of children with implants occur at school. Because education is so important, the following chapter will focus exclusively on that issue.

Time Commitment

Before implantation, virtually all of the parents we talked with were very much aware of the fact that it was unlikely that their child would demonstrably benefit from the implant immediately after the

1. "Children," of course, in this chapter and elsewhere, is somewhat of a misnomer; it is simply a category of convenience that includes a number of adolescents and young adults who are no longer children.

device was activated. Rather, parents realized that they would probably have to put in a great deal of time to ensure that their child
derived as much benefit as possible from the implant.

> [A speech therapist we see] . . . makes an analogy that receiving
> the implant is like receiving a load of building supplies on a
> lot. And in a couple of years you might have a beautiful new
> house on that lot if you do the work. But, if you don't do the
> work, you'll just have a load of building supplies on that lot. . . .
> Every moment with [our daughter] is a language opportunity.
> *Mother of a 4-year-old girl implanted at 18 months*

A number of other parents we talked with commented on the
amount of time they expected to have to put in with their child
for implantation to "work." A sampling of some of the comments
from parents on this point follows:

> The implant is 5 percent. The 95 percent is what you do
> after the implant. . . . And we were very willing to make the
> commitment, and excited to make the commitment.
> *Family of a 5-year-old girl implanted in the mid-1990s*

> [My daughter] is not the only one who was implanted. I might
> not actually have something in my head, but it was a commit-
> ment. And it was a commitment to know that for this to suc-
> ceed with [her] that I had just as much work to do as she did.
> And [the implant center was] very realistic about that. Don't
> expect it to change overnight. Don't expect her to be turned on
> and . . . to speak the next day. It's not going to happen that way.
> *Parent of a 7-year-old girl implanted in 1996*

> You'd never know how he would do. And that's the hardest
> thing about deciding to do this is because they cannot tell you
> what the outcome will be. That was really hard, . . . and . . . if
> any parent asks me, I tell them the same thing. I say, Look, they
> cannot . . . promise that this is what's going to happen with your
> child. So you have to know that going in. Don't think it's going
> to be like this miracle cure of your kid, . . . you still have to
> work. . . . You're not going to turn it on and he's going to hear
> like a normal hearing person. That's not going to happen.
> *Mother of a teenager implanted in the early 1990s*

We also asked parents if the amount of time they have actually devoted to the post-implant habilitation needs of their child was about what they expected. There was a good amount of variability in the responses to this question. A few parents said that they were surprised to find that, because the implant worked so well, they did not have to spend a great deal of time educating and socializing their implanted child, at least not any more time than they had to spend with their child's hearing siblings (or what they thought their friends were spending with their hearing children). A more common response was that they did indeed have to put in a great deal of time, and that learning to use the implant is, as one parent whose daughter has used her implant consistently for 7 years, said, *still a work in progress*. Several mothers we talked with said that they left their job outside the home to devote themselves full-time to their newly implanted child. (We did not find any fathers who did this, although at least one dad did get a second job after his wife left her job outside the home.) Although many parents could not afford this option, they nevertheless did end up spending as much time, if not more, with their child as the implant center had said they would have to spend.

Many parents said they incorporated constant language reinforcement into their everyday activities, something one mother called *natural learning*. They frequently modeled language for their child, used signing to clarify language concepts, made a conscious effort to speak clearly and maintain eye contact, corrected their child's speech, if necessary (although most parents said they tried not to intimidate their child too much while doing this), sang songs, played games and read books to their child (and had their child read to them), and devised a variety of creative methods for reinforcing language, speech perception, and speech development. Some parents used an "auditory sandwich" approach to language reinforcement. As noted earlier, this involves presenting language orally, reinforcing it visually, and then presenting it again orally. One parent we talked with who used this approach used signs to represent language visually, while another used Cued Speech, which the child had been using before implantation, to accomplish the same goal. Many parents labeled furniture and other objects around the home, for example, and one family created a "visual calendar" in which the activities for the month were displayed so that the child could easily associate a picture on the calendar with a planned family activity. Other families spent time helping their child listen to a variety of sounds around the house, such as a microwave oven, the doorbell, or a telephone ringing. Some parents had to work hard just to ensure that their child continued to use the device. Some of the comments from parents regarding the amount of work they had to put in after their child received the implant are as follows:

> Interestingly enough, since he's had his implant we've spent less hard time because it's easier for him to listen. He overhears and it's more natural, like it is for my 3-year-old. When we had his hearing aids, it was a lot of work to get him to hear things and understand. Now what happens is I can talk to him much more like I do my 3-year-old. . . . The first year was definitely just as hard. But now I've noticed a huge change this third year . . . that he's had it. Things are really just much more natural, and if I use something he doesn't understand he tells me right away like, What does that mean, I don't understand? Whereas before I wasn't sure that was the case; I would have to be sure he heard me. . . . We support him in every way that I possibly can. I make a point of really working with people who work with him. I talk to everybody. I tell them what they can do to help him in a situation. . . . I will make a point of saying he doesn't hear you, you might need to talk to him. I'll do that if it's my mother, or my mother-in-law, or if it's the neighbor, I'll say, He doesn't understand you, you might want to tell him again.
>
> *Mother of a 7-year-old implanted in 1996*

> I would have hoped we [would be] further along at this point than we are. . . . I think it's probably a lot more [work] than I expected, but I don't think that would have changed anything. I mean, you do what you need to do for your children.
>
> *Father of a 4-year-old boy implanted in 1996*

> FATHER: Every moment with [my daughter] is a language opportunity. And when she asks for food, when . . . she's hungry, when she wants to go somewhere, we . . . talk to her in a way that incorporates what we learned from [the therapist]. So it wasn't a lot of work in that you turn to page 19 of the manual and you do these exercises, but it was work.

MOTHER: It was special work, it wasn't medically unpleasant
work. . . . It was just being thoughtful. It was just how best to
teach your child. . . . That's kind of the foundation of the auditory-verbal philosophy, just making language a part of life,
and language is everywhere.
Parents of a 4-year-old girl implanted at 18 months

The mother of a young girl, when asked to compare raising an
implanted child with a hearing child, replied:

You really just have to be more aware. I guess that's probably
where it's different. People with hearing kids don't have to
think much about what they tell somebody, whereas I have to
think a lot more about what I am telling [my daughter] and
saying to her than somebody else would have to do. So, in
that regard, yes, it is more work and I try to keep it as everyday as I can, and . . . I don't want to make this a forced thing.
It should come as natural as possible to me, and that's what I
try to do because I don't want to stress myself out, and I don't
want her stressed out because then you don't get anywhere.
Mother of a 3-year-old girl implanted in 1997

It's less than what I would have had to do if he had not had
the implant. . . . The implant made life easier for everyone.
Mother of a 10-year-old boy implanted in 1995

[First year] post-implant, you know, having to work so hard
with him, and my friends and their children just la de da . . .
and here I am. I'm going to speech therapy twice a week, a
teacher of the deaf is coming in twice a week, I'm going to
[the implant center], two hours away, once a week. And all
day long at home I'm saying, Can you hear that? . . . Why do I
have to do this? . . . Why does he have to go through this? . . .
Also doing sign language twice a week at a local center. . . .
I would just work with him all day. . . . If we were at home [I]
was constantly trying to engage him to listen and look at me.
Mother of a 5-year-old boy implanted at age 2

We invited children over. We created a summer playgroup in
the backyard so that [our daughter] would be surrounded by
other children . . . we wanted her exposed to other kids. . . .

We got [a] speech viewer program for our own home computer. . . . We bought a lot of toys and activities that were sound
rich. I bought her a drum set. . . . When I would come home
from work I would sit down for anywhere from a half-hour to
an hour everyday. . . . And I would just read the book and go
over the book and point to the pictures.

Father of an 8-year-old girl implanted in 1993

One night he was in the hallway and I was making dinner and he
was starting to make sounds in his throat, 'kkkkk,' like a 'k,' but it was
just guttural kind of 'kkkk' nonsense. I dropped everything and I ran
over to him and I started doing it. I said . . . cookie, car, and I started
to make all these sounds that I could think of that started with a 'k,' a
hard 'k' or a 'c' so that he could hear that that's the sound that you
make when you say those words. And within a week or so he
started using the 'k' with those words. . . . This, I believe, was after
six months of use.

Mother of a 5-year-old boy implanted in the mid-1990s

[Deaf kids] are not really designed to hear. Face it, they can't
hear. God did not design them to hear. And we're trying to
force them into the hearing world. . . . It's tough to raise a
hearing-impaired kid. . . . But it's getting better.

Observation of a father of a child with a
cochlear implant

Communication Issues

Almost all of the families we talked with utilize extensive speech
and auditory therapy, including auditory-verbal (A-V) therapy, with
their child. In addition, many of the families said they incorporate some form of signing into their daily post-implant interaction
with their child. As is apparent in a few of the comments noted previously, many of the things that parents do at home, or in other
settings with their child, are activities originally suggested by their
therapists or by others at the implant center. For some parents, the
type of speech and auditory therapy they use is similar to what was
used when their child was using hearing aids before implantation.
For most of these families, it is generally felt that post-implant

therapy is more productive because the child is able to hear and understand more sounds with the implant than with a hearing aid.

Even though many children continue to use speech therapists in school, many parents said they are not satisfied with this arrangement, either because the quality is not what they envisioned or because of time constraints. Consequently, if they can afford to pay for it, many parents also send their child to a private therapist, either after school or during the summer or both.[2] Although a few children participate in group speech therapy, some parents do not like this approach because they feel other children in the class are not always appropriate language models for their child. Most of the parents we talked with also utilized the speech and auditory training services of the implant center, at least during the first year after the implant was activated.[3] Some parents, however, live too far from a cochlear implant center to go every week or every other week, and the speech and auditory training they are able to get is limited by what is available in the community where they live. Although some parents engage the services of a teacher of the deaf in addition to speech and/or auditory therapists, and have their child attend various therapy sessions for several hours each week, most of the parents we talked with limit their child's "formal" therapy to about two hour-long sessions each week. For most families, this is

2. In the GRI study, 52% of the parents who responded said they paid for some speech communication training at their own expense. Slightly more than one-third of these parents paid for this training for one year, another 20% paid for up to two years, and the rest (about 45%) paid for 2 to 16 years of speech communication training at their own expense. Some of this training undoubtedly occurred before implantation, just as it did for a number of families in our interview sample.

3. One of the major cochlear implant centers in the mid-Atlantic region, The Listening Center at Johns Hopkins University in Baltimore, provides parents inquiring about an implant for their child with a comprehensive packet of information. Presumably, most other implant centers do much the same thing (at least most of the parents we talked with reported that they received a good amount of information from their implant center). Included in this packet is a list of "requirements" for parents. And, included among these requirements, is a commitment to "direct rehabilitation services," including individual therapy sessions, for their child at Johns Hopkins for at least a year after implantation. In addition to rehabilitation services at the implant center itself, centers often assist parents in obtaining educational support and services for their newly implanted child. In the GRI study, 62% of the respondents indicated that their implant center provided "moderate" or "generous" assistance in this regard.

in addition to whatever speech and auditory training their child receives at school. Two hours is about all the structured training outside of school that their child is willing to tolerate each week. For some families, this involves a long commute after school, which is often burdensome not only for the parent but also for the child.

There are several different types of speech and/or auditory therapy available for parents. Many of the parents we talked with did not specify which type was used with their child, and some did not know. A good number, however, used A-V therapy or auditory-oral therapy. At least a dozen of the families we talked with used a trained A-V therapist for their implanted child's auditory therapy. A few additional comments from parents regarding speech and/or auditory therapy are presented below.

I was always in [my daughter's] therapy. . . . Besides the speech, language therapy we also had the teacher of the deaf working with her three times a week. At that time it was only 3 hours a week. Now she has 10 hours a week.

Mother of a 7-year-old girl implanted in 1994

We couldn't have done anything without the speech therapy with the cochlear implant.

Mother of an 8-year-old girl implanted in 1996

INTERVIEWER: Did they tell you when you were thinking about the implant how much work you would have to put in to make sure that the implant was successful?

MOTHER (in postinterview written comments): This is an important question. I found a lot of families think you turn it on and instantly you have a hearing child. A good school and therapy are crucial.

Mother of a 3-year-old boy implanted at age 2 and
a 5-year-old girl implanted at age 4

The Gallaudet Research Institute (GRI) study included several items related to speech communication or speech production therapy. On one of the questions, four of every five parents rated the speech training their child received as either "very helpful" (39%) or "indispensably helpful" (41%). The GRI survey also asked parents how often specific speech-language production training activities with their child occurred at home. In response, about three-quarters

(76%) said such activities occurred "frequently" or "occasionally." Less than a quarter (22%) said they rarely or almost never occurred. Moreover, most parents (81%) also said they were satisfied or very satisfied with their child's progress to date in the development of spoken language skills.

Regarding auditory training their child has received since the implant was activated, the vast majority of parents responding to the GRI study said that they found auditory training to be either very helpful or indispensable for their child. Respondents were also specifically asked how many years of A-V therapy their child had received before and after receiving the implant. Although approximately 75% of the parents said that their child had received at least some A-V therapy before and after implantation, it is impossible to say what proportion of these respondents actually received A-V therapy from a certified A-V therapist.

We also discussed with parents a variety of other post-implant communication issues, including the mode or type of communication commonly used by their child and within the family. Most of the 55 families we discussed this issue with said that the quality of their child's speech had improved, sometimes dramatically so, since receiving the implant, although most parents emphasized repeatedly that this took a long time and a lot of hard work on everyone's part. More than half of the parents we talked with now rate their child's quality of speech as quite good, although it may not be as clear as the speech of their child's hearing peers. Some parents said that their child is now able to converse, if somewhat awkwardly, with strangers. Communication with other family members, including grandparents, was also mentioned by many of the parents we talked with as something that improved, albeit slowly, after implantation. In summary, whereas some parents were clearly disappointed with the results so far, most felt that their child's speech had clearly improved over the years.

Although speech is important, signing by no means stopped after implantation for most of the families we talked with; more than half of the children still rely on some type of post-implant sign communication. Many children rely on interpreters in school or places of worship, many use signing to communicate with their deaf (non-implanted) friends, some still sign with their parents, and so on. If other forms of visual communication, including Cued Speech and lipreading, are included, then a large majority of children use some combination of visual communication methods and styles post-implant. Very few rely only on listening skills coupled with speech. Nor are the parents we talked with necessarily disappointed with this result. As will be discussed in more detail in chapter 8, parents are generally pleased with their child's progress with the implant.

In this regard, it is worth mentioning the "Communication Methodology Position Statement" that The Listening Center at Johns Hopkins University routinely distributes to parents who are contemplating a cochlear implant for their child. This position statement is included in the packet of information that is given to parents. The statements says:

> The Listening Center supports that the use of a visually non-ambiguous system of communication be used to develop conceptual and linguistic skills from the time of confirmed diagnosis of profound hearing loss through the time of cochlear implantation. The visual system should NOT be terminated immediately following activation of the cochlear implant. . . . While a visual system of communication is strongly encouraged for communication development, it is also essential to maintain focus on developing any residual hearing a child may have prior to cochlear implantation.

In a similar vein, Marschark (1998, p. 47) observes: "Despite occasional claims to the contrary, there is no evidence at all to suggest that the early use of manual communication (signs or gestures) by deaf children hampers their development of skills in spoken language or in any other area."

What follows is a sampling of comments from parents concerning post-implant communication issues:

> My mom and dad, who do not know sign language, sat down and . . . could communicate [orally] with my daughter [in the last 6 months]. . . . [My daughter] could talk to them and they could understand everything she said. . . . And this is after three years . . . and a lot of hard work, a lot of work that went into [this] on [her] part, and the family, and sacrifices and everything else. But we would never dream of doing anything else. . . . I can never see her not being dependent on an interpreter. If she's in a big auditorium with

people, or even if she's sitting in the front row . . . I think, to catch all of it, that she's gonna need sign language.

Mother of an 8-year-old girl implanted at age 5

In response to a question about whether she thought some signing was compatible with having an implant, one mother replied:

Oh, I think signing is necessary. I think she should always sign forever, and I think her signing vocabulary should get bigger and bigger. So, yeah, I think it's necessary.

Mother of an 8-year-old girl implanted at age 7

We were really just like the movie, *Mr. Holland's Opus*, where . . . the dad is screaming at the mom, you know, What does he want?, the mom is screaming at the dad, I don't know!, and the kid is screaming. I mean, that was us for two years. That's when we decided to sign to [our son] instead of having a noisy dinner.

Mother of a 4-year-old boy implanted in 1997

After it became clear that her child was not getting a lot of benefit from the implant after two years of hard work, one mother said:

MOTHER: We just saw him farther and farther behind, but now I see him catching up closer and closer.

FATHER: And we really feel like that changed the day we made the decision that he needed language and we weren't getting spoken language through to him, so we were going to get sign language through to him and we did.

Parents of a 4-year-old boy implanted in 1996

Cued Speech was only used by four of the families we talked with (and is used to some extent by about 13% of the families in the GRI study post-implant). One father had this to say about Cued Speech:

When [my daughter] was 2 we began using Cued Speech regularly in our home. At this point I must insert a parenthetical comment. The decision by [Gallaudet University] to give up Cued Speech instruction was appalling. This is an incredibly effective communication system. It is especially effective when learning to use a cochlear implant. If this decision . . . was made for "political" reasons, it was shameful! . . . Cued Speech provided [my daughter] a visual representation of the "familiar" sounds at the same time she was receiving this new stimulation. . . . Your vocabulary is at our fingertips (pun intended).

Father of a 12-year-old girl implanted at age 9

Hearing and Understanding With the Implant

We asked most of the parents we talked with how much their child could actually hear with the implant. Could they distinguish among different voices, for example, or converse on the telephone? Only six of the 63 children represented in our family interviews had used the implant for less than one year (and three of the six had used it for 11 months at the time of the interview). As noted in the introduction to this book, the "average" or typical child in our sample had used the implant for about 4 years at the time we conducted our interviews. Among the families we interviewed, the longest any child had used the implant was approximately 12 years (one child was implanted in 1987 and three children were implanted in 1988, although one of the latter stopped using the device several years ago). Thus, the observations from parents about how much their child can actually hear with the implant, or distinguish among and understand different voices, cover a considerable range of years. Nevertheless, it is apparent from our data that there is no simple relationship between the number of years of implant use and the amount of benefit the child is receiving from the device. Some of the children who have used the implant for years still have difficulty using the telephone, for example, and virtually all of them prefer to use closed captions on television. None, as far as we can tell, can listen to the radio (except for music) without difficulty. Almost everyone has at least some difficulty hearing in relatively noisy environments, such as restaurants, automobiles, or movie theaters. Moreover, as will be seen in the following chapter, many children who have had their implant for years still need services, such as FM amplification systems or open captions, or even a sign language interpreter, in the classroom. On the other hand, some of the children who have only recently been implanted are doing so well in different communication situations that their parents claim they are doing nothing very different than they would be doing if the child had normal hearing from birth. Perhaps as these younger children, whose implants include more recent technological advances, grow up they will demonstrate greater success (i.e., improved functional hearing) with the implant than some of the older children who have implants with less advanced components.

Most of the children in the families we met progressed fairly slowly in the sense that fairly loud environmental sounds were heard and recognized first, followed by the ability to distinguish among common sounds in the home, recognizing voices, particularly parents' voices, and then distinguishing among them. This was frequently followed by learning to reproduce speech sounds appropriately, perceiving the differences among consonants and vowels, conversing with people with or without lipreading, learning what sounds to "tune out" in an increasingly noisy world, and so on. These were not hard and fast stages that the children went through, however. A few children in the families we interviewed still do not perceive much more than environmental sounds with the implant even after several years of using it, and some children could hear much more than environmental sounds very shortly after the implant was activated. In general, however, it required at least a year or two, sometimes more, before the children were able to derive enough benefit from their cochlear implant to communicate effectively with members of their family or with close friends. Part of the reason for the gradual progress is because the speech (sound) processor is usually programmed quite low at the beginning to give children a chance to adapt slowly to the new sounds. Other factors may include the quality and amount of post-implant speech and auditory therapy, how often the implant is actually used, the number of electrodes that are functioning properly, and even the number of hair cells remaining in the cochlea (this may indicate that at least some auditory nerve endings are probably still functioning). The simple fact is that predicting whether an individual child or adult will be a successful implant user is still an inexact science, although research continues to suggest that some factors, such as those noted previously, are commonly associated with positive outcomes (see chapter 9). Some comments from parents on this issue are as follows:

With some people, once he . . . becomes familiar with . . . your voice he is able to work on a higher level. When he . . . initially meets somebody he has a little problem focusing on their speech pattern and [the] clarity in their voice. But once he gets that, he's able to be more successful. So he needs familiarity with . . . a voice to really work well with his implant.

Parent of a teenage boy implanted in the late 1980s

Two years after implantation, these parents noted:

FATHER: One thing that a lot of children have trouble with is the 's' sound and the 'sh' sound, which [my son] is starting to get very well. So those are probably the more recent things. Whether that's a matter of him listening or the school doing exercises or a matter of his mappings getting more fine-tuned and turned up, I don't know, but it's really getting good.

MOTHER: If it's something he doesn't . . . like [he says], I don't think so, mom. Like, normally, [if] your 4-year-old says that to you, you would be, like, Don't talk that way to me! We don't care because it's just fine, just talk to us! . . . But it's been 2 years, 2 solid years of 3 days a week therapy.

Parents of a 4-year-old boy implanted in 1997

Three years after implantation, one mother said:

From a little girl who had no speech, she could say Mom, mom, and she could not hear, to a little girl who can be across my home and I can say, [Daughter], it's time for dinner. And she comes in and says, What's for dinner? She can hear me from far away.

Mother of an 8-year-old girl implanted in 1996

Six years after implantation, a parent said:

I don't think his discrimination is very good still. . . . He says that it's all just noise to him . . . so that's why he doesn't like it.

Parent of a teenager implanted in 1993

He is much more relaxed socially, and in group conversations he acts a little bit more appropriately as far as not just busting in with his voice. . . . I don't think he had one decent small group conversation before the implant....He doesn't perform like a hearing person now. He can't do everything I can do, but he's able to hear without speechreading sometimes, and he's more comfortable with himself. He told me that the quality of sound is so much better. So it's not everything he had hoped for, but there are some nice results.... He said it's like a VCR that has a tracking device. And he said with the hearing aid it's like the tracking is off, but with the implant it's like the tracking is locked in. It's much more [of a] clear signal. So he has to fill in a little bit less.... Music still doesn't sound all that great to him. Speech, voices, those are sounding much better to him, and that's from someone who has been deaf his whole life.

Mother of teenager implanted in 1997

She had some real high points that first year [with the implant] ... the dinging of the microwave when she popped popcorn. I walked into the house one time and her ear is right up to the microwave listening to the popcorn. And then when it dinged she said, I always wondered how you knew that the dinner or the thing was done.... There were some real high points that year [including hearing birds and crickets]. The low points were the lack of speech discrimination, that just wasn't coming like we thought.... She started to listen to music for the first time ... she never listened to music ever. And then she started going to dance clubs with her implant, and she said, This is great! ... So, as a teenager, this really set into her social life that now she can enjoy going out with hearing friends and truly enjoy the same things they are enjoying on the same level.

Mother of a young college student implanted in 1995

A father of a young girl who has had her implant for six years had this to say about the amount of hearing his daughter has:

One of the things I like is we go bicycle riding together, she and I. And she can get 20, 30 feet in front of me. And I can yell, Stop, slow down, wait!, and she does it. So I mean [at a] distance she still hears.... What we're experimenting with now [is] we're ... having people she knows, like her teacher from school or grandpa or her babysitter, ... call her a couple of times and just talk on the phone, any subject. She gets 50 percent.

Father of an 8-year-old girl implanted in 1993

We asked almost all of the parents we met if their child was able to understand the dialogue on television without captions, if he or she was able to converse on the phone, and if music was enjoyed or appreciated. As noted, most if not all of the children still preferred having captions turned on when they watched television. As far as the telephone is concerned, it is apparent that this is not an easy device for people with implants, children or adults, to master. Part of the problem, of course, is that lipreading is impossible with the phone, and many of the children whose families we talked with, like many implant users in general, rely to some extent on lip- (speech) reading. Another problem is that people on the other end of the line may not speak clearly or loudly enough, or they may have an accent with which the implant user is unfamiliar. It appears, though, that perhaps the major hurdle that the children in our sample faced with respect to telephone use was primarily psychological rather than audiological. Many parents we talked with said that their child needed to spend a good amount of time, frequently several years, developing enough confidence to tackle this intimidating and ubiquitous aspect of modern culture. Many children began by trying to identify their parents' voices on the phone, and then graduating to grandparents and other relatives and friends, including other children with implants, whom they knew. After the implantees' fear of the phone was reduced, some of them were more eager to try to talk with strangers on the phone. Few, however, currently feel confident enough to use the telephone indiscriminately, although some parents said that their child seems to be able to communicate more successfully when he or she uses a speakerphone than when a handheld model is used. Some children use a plug-in adapter that comes with the cochlear implant when they try to converse on the phone, whereas others simply hold the telephone close to the microphone on the external portion of the implant.

As far as music is concerned, there was a large amount of variability—some enjoyed it and were able to develop their musical skills post-implant, but many have not learned to appreciate music in the years since they received their implant. A few children who tried learning an instrument after implantation seemed to have difficulty distinguishing among the different notes in a musical arrangement. A few others, however, were able to learn to play, and enjoy, a musical instrument. In general, there is no simple linear relationship between years of implant use and music appreciation. In addition, it appears that music is not a particularly important part of the lives of most of the children whose families we talked with.

One question on the GRI survey asked: "Since receiving the CI, has your child ever taken vocal or instrumental music lessons regularly?" In response, only 15% of the parents said yes (and about five of every six of these parents said the music instruction experience was a positive and enjoyable one for their child). The most common instrument studied by the implanted children was the piano (6%); another 3% said their child participated in choir or in another type of vocal music program. As was the case among the children in the families we interviewed, music does not seem to be a major part of the lives of many children in the GRI study.

Some observations from the parents we talked with concerning music and telephones are presented below:

> [My daughter] gets music at school, but not with the mainstream. She goes into the deaf classroom and has music there where it's signed.
>
> *Parent of an 8-year-old girl implanted in 1996*

A mother of a young daughter who has used her implant for about three years said:

> She loves music. Without the cochlear implant she would have never been able to enjoy music. She loves to play the piano. She picks up the violin. She picks up the guitar, and she just loves to hear . . . music; and she loves to make music.
>
> *Mother of a 7-year-old girl implanted at age 4*

> I play the piano. I'm in my seventh year playing the piano. I played the flute. I've been in the band; I've been in chorus; I'm really involved musically in my life.
>
> *Teenager implanted in 1987*

A mother said her daughter, who was implanted in the early 1990s, was just now starting to use the phone

> . . . with other hearing-impaired kids. . . . Which is very interesting because . . . they're both going, What? What?
>
> *Mother of a 10-year-old girl implanted at age 3*

It's been really one of probably the best and most happy things for me . . . to be able to talk with my daughter on the phone which I never could [before implantation]. And I think for me that took a lot of getting used to. And, actually, [she] didn't do it right away; she was really afraid, I think.

Mother of a young woman implanted in 1996

Another mother said her son was now starting to use the phone:

He just held [the phone] right up to his microphone and said, Hi, mom, this is [me], what time will you be home? And I said, Is your dad right there? And he says, No, my dad's not here.

INTERVIEWER: That was the first time he used the phone?

MOTHER: First time, he just decided to call me . . . I was thrilled. I almost started to cry. I didn't believe him, I thought, Your dad was there and you're playing a trick on me. Oh, I was thrilled.

Mother of a teenager implanted in 1993

A young college student said that initially he refused to talk on the phone, but his speech therapist encouraged him. He quoted her as saying:

We'll say nursery rhymes on the phone. You will have the words in front of you, and I'll say them and you will repeat them back to me. . . . It took me a very long time to learn how to use the phone to recognize her voice spontaneously. . . . It's only been very recently that I could talk on the phone with anybody.

Young man implanted at age 12

A father of a young girl had this to say regarding his daughter's use of the phone when he and his wife called from out of town:

We had a complete conversation about what did you do at school and what have you been doing, and she was telling us about all the things she was doing and what was going on at school. And we were asking her lots of questions and she could understand them and answered them all. We were just, you know, even though we live this every day, we were still amazed that at this young age of only 5 years . . ., and having [the implant] three years, that she can already talk on the phone that well.

Father of a 6-year-old girl implanted in 1996

We discussed the issue of post-implant hearing aid use with 39 families (and got information about 41 implanted children). Only six of the children in these families continue to use a hearing aid in their nonimplanted ear. Seventeen children tried it for a while, even if only for a few days, and stopped, primarily because they received little or no benefit from the aid. Another 18 children never tried using an aid at all after implantation. Although most of the comments from parents regarding this issue were relatively brief, one comment from the mother of a child who has stopped using the implant reminds us of the need to exercise caution when deciding which ear to implant.

> INTERVIEWER: You still . . . use a hearing aid in your right ear, right?

> MOTHER: We've tried it . . . it's been a while. It was when he was going through that stage where he didn't want his implant at all, he wanted the hearing aids. So I pulled out his hearing aids and let him wear his . . . aid. And he couldn't because they implanted his good ear; he has very, very, very little hearing, residual hearing in his other ear. So, you know, he couldn't hear anything hardly.

Child's Current Feelings About the Implant

We also asked parents if their child ever wanted to stop using the implant, their perception of their child's current feelings about the implant, and their assessment of their child's sense of self-confidence or self-esteem before and after implantation. In addition, we asked the parents if they had noticed any changes in their child's pattern of social interaction post-implant. In quite a few instances, we were able to ask the child as well.

Of the 63 children in our parent sample, five are no longer using the implant consistently (or at all). The vast majority of the parents we talked with said that their child either never wants to take it off during the day or only wants a brief respite from the sounds they pay attention to most of the time. Some of the children did not immediately like the implant, and some are still struggling with it even though they have not stopped using it, but most have gotten accustomed to it, and appear to enjoy using it, over the years. One boy even got a buzz hair-cut so everyone would notice his scar and his implant, and about a half-dozen parents said their child occasionally even wants to sleep with his or her implant on! (Since the batteries need to be recharged, and since this is not likely to be comfortable in any case, parents generally discouraged this practice.) A small number of children only wear the implant at school, and one uses it only when she wants to hear some-thing special such as music. In addition, a number of parents and chil-dren said that, for cosmetic reasons, they were looking forward to using a behind-the-ear implant model.

As far as issues related to self-esteem, self-confidence, and social interaction are concerned, it is important to note that we did not discuss this issue with all of the families we interviewed. Neverthe-less, among the families who discussed these issues with us (about half of our entire parent sample), a large majority felt that positive behavioral and/or psychological changes, post-implant, far out-weighed any negative changes. More specifically, about half of the parents we talked with about this issue (i.e., about a quarter of our sample) said their child seemed to have more self-confidence or assertiveness, appeared to be happier, or demonstrated more inde-pendence after getting used to the implant. In addition, a number of parents said they felt their child became less frustrated, less hyperactive (or more *manageable,* as one parent put it), and more outgoing after the implant was hooked up. Many also said that their child became more comfortable socially, although this was usually a very gradual process, particularly when the child associated with hearing friends. Others said their child's behavior, personality, and patterns of social interaction did not change much before and after the implant was activated (they had always been independent or self-confident or reluctant to use their voice, for example), and several mentioned that their child became somewhat more self-conscious after the surgery because of the visibility of the implant. As noted, some even stopped using the implant largely for this reason. Some of the comments from parents on these issues are presented below:

> The first year she didn't want to wear [the implant]. . . . And every chance she would have, she would take it off. She did not want to hear the sounds. . . . I think it scared her more than anything. . . . But then she started wearing [it]. Yes, it did take a while before she really, actually liked to hear the sound.
> *Mother of a teenage girl implanted in 1991*

The main reason he didn't want an implant for so long is that he felt very good about himself just the way he was. And he said, I've worked very hard to get here. I'm happy with myself. . . . But looking back, seeing that he's happy with the implant, I'm glad he decided to do [it].

Mother of a teenage boy implanted in 1997

Mother: He's so much more social. He's so much more comfortable going up to other people . . . and exploring a little more now.

Father: He became much less isolated [after getting the implant]. . . . It felt like he was connecting more with people around him and the world around him.

Parents of a 5-year-old implanted in 1996

A mother whose son stopped using his implant recently, but who is willing to try a behind-the-ear model when it becomes available, said:

Mother: Kids on the street [teased him] . . . [and at] the boys and girls club. I remember the day he would come home and threw [the implant] at me. And I said, What's wrong? And he said, Somebody made fun of me. And ever since that day he has not worn it at home; and it's been 4 years. . . . He would wear it at school, but not at home.

Interviewer: How do you feel about that [his wanting to stop using the implant]?

Mother: It bothers me a lot because his speech is so much better and he responds better when he's been wearing that. You can tell a big difference, but I don't want to force him to . . . wear [it] because then we are fighting each other. I don't want to do that. And I know how mean kids are and I know that's what caused this. I know it is. . . . People are cruel.

Mother of a teenage boy

Another mother, whose daughter had only been using the implant for about 10 months at the time of the interview, said:

First thing she does in the morning is take me to it and hand it to me to put on her. . . . From day one she has never tried to pull it off, not one time has she tried to pull it off or cried when we put it on as [she did] with the hearing aids. She was always pulling them off, throwing them around, trying to bite on them. But with this, even when it falls off, she's trying to get it on the right way.

Mother of a 2-year-old girl implanted in early 1999

When asked to elaborate on her daughter's feelings about the implant, one mother had this to say:

I think the main thing is that when she gets older she doesn't think she'll have it. Because she doesn't see many adults with [an implant]. . . . I think because she was implanted so young it's just a part of her. She's just as comfortable with it in as she is with it off. When we go to the park or go swimming we have the sign language to communicate. And then when she [has the implant] on we can communicate orally to her. She seems very well adjusted, and so does her [implanted brother]. . . . It feels like we're doing something right. . . . It seems like they're happy.

Mother of a 6-year-old girl implanted in 1996 and
a 5-year-old boy implanted at 27 months

You can be happy without it. I know that. But I just don't know anything else, and at this point in my life I'm really happy with [the implant]. I don't want to change it. . . . I view my deafness as a part of me, but a minor part of me. It's not the dominating part. . . . I don't let it run my life, basically.

College student implanted at age 12

A mother had this to say about her daughter's social interaction with hearing peers about 18 months after implantation:

I've noticed that it is hard for [my daughter] . . . when the other girls . . . down the street, who are hearing, come over. . . . They don't really know how to communicate with her. And they go chattering off, and [my daughter] doesn't really know what to do. . . . Sometimes I worry because she doesn't really have any hearing friends.

Mother of a 5-year-old girl implanted in 1998 and
a 3-year-old boy implanted in 1999

TABLE 6.1
Cochlear Implant (CI) Use Among Children in the GRI Study

	Response Categories			
Implant Use Question	Never	Once or Twice	Three to Five Times	Six Times or More
Since the initial "hook-up," how many times has your child not used the CI for more than a month?	84%	6%	3%	6%

	Response Categories			
Implant Use Question	Never	Once or Twice	Three to Nine Times	Ten Times or More
In the most recent year of CI use, how often did your child refuse CI use?	60%	18%	10%	10%

The GRI survey asked parents to respond to several questions regarding implant use. Two such questions were: (1) "Since your child's (initial) CI 'hook up,' how many times has your child not used the CI for more than a month?" (2) "In the child's most recent year of CI use, how often did your child refuse CI use?" Table 6.1 summarizes responses to these questions.

The GRI study also asked parents to estimate the extent to which their child interacts with hearing children during nonschool-related activities. Almost 90% of the parents said that their child socialized "fairly often" or "at almost all opportunities" with hearing children. Only 11% responded "almost never" or "very little."

As far as behavioral limitations with the implant are concerned, this is a fairly minor concern for almost all of the parents we talked with. Most parents do little more than try to restrict their child's activities in situations that are likely to cause the speech processor to malfunction (such as static electricity problems caused by plastic slides or other plastic playground equipment). In situations such as this, most parents simply remove, or ask their child to remove, the external equipment. Some parents do not even bother with that, and take the attitude that if the processor needs to be reprogrammed, then they will just have to deal with that (as some have had to do).

A few parents did not want their child involved in contact sports, such as wrestling, football, or soccer, but many parents had no problem with this as long as appropriate head protection was worn. Several children play basketball, volleyball, or softball even without disengaging the external equipment (and are looking forward to using behind-the-ear implants). Scuba diving is out, according to most parents, and one or two parents had concerns about going through security checks at airports (this is not a problem for the implant, per se, although it may set off the alarm). In short, beyond limitations related to the need to remove the external speech processor, microphone, and cords before swimming or using plastic playground equipment, and limitations on scuba diving, there are few hard and fast rules about what behavioral limitations are imposed by the implant. Presumably, over the years, as implant users experiment with different activities, and share their experiences in on-line discussion groups and in other forums, appropriate norms will emerge.

7

Educating a Child With
a Cochlear Implant

The issue of education is one that is of great concern to virtually all of the parents we talked with, and it occupied a prominent position in the Gallaudet Research Institute (GRI) questionnaire as well. Like most parents, parents of children with cochlear implants are concerned that the educational needs of their child will be satisfactorily met, whether in early intervention programs or at school. As will be seen, almost all of the children in our sample require some type of special services in their educational setting. Few are able to be completely mainstreamed in classrooms with hearing peers with no support services whatsoever.

One important consideration is how parents perceive the academic performance of their implanted child compared with both hearing children and other deaf children without implants. For some of the parents we interviewed, the relatively unimpressive reading and writing abilities of many deaf people was an important reason why they decided to implant their child in the first place. Although, as noted in the previous chapter, there is no evidence that early signing impairs later development of spoken language, many parents felt that initial instruction in a sign-based system, especially American Sign Language (ASL), would in fact make their child's later development of spoken English more difficult. Has the implant made it possible for the children of the parents we talked with to keep up with their hearing peers in terms of academic achievement (especially reading and writing skills)?

Early Intervention/Preschool Programs

The overwhelming majority of the families we interviewed enrolled their deaf child or children in some type of early intervention program. These programs varied considerably, however, with some children spending five days a week in such programs (or some combination of programs), whereas other children were only involved for an hour or so a week. Moreover, some programs included the parents while others did not. There is clearly no one "style" of early intervention that fits all, or even most, of the families with whom we spoke.

Early intervention programs (a nebulously defined concept, but usually taken to mean prekindergarten programs that are available until the child is about 5 years old) for children with disabilities have become increasingly popular in recent years in the United States. Public Law 94-142, the "Education for All Handicapped Children Act," which was signed into law in 1975, states that free and appropriate public educational services must be provided for all children with disabilities between the ages of 3 and 21. For political reasons, however, provisions of the law that applied to children aged 3 to 5 and 18 to 21 were seen as "permissive" rather than mandatory, and most states did not provide appropriate services for preschool-aged children (Heward, 1996; Moores, 1996). It was not until 1990, 15 years after PL 94-142 was signed into law, that legislation took effect and stipulated that states were required to fully serve all preschool (3 to 5 years of age) children with disabilities. This legislation, PL 99-457 (which was enacted in 1986, 4 years before it took effect), also encouraged, but did not require, states to provide special educational services to infants and toddlers from the time their disability was identified through 2 years of age. The 1990 reauthorization of PL 94-142 changed the name of the legislation to IDEA, the "Individuals with Disabilities Education Act."

What this legislation means is that parents of children as young as a few weeks old can now frequently take advantage of various publicly supported early intervention programs in which they might wish to participate. Whether these programs actually meet their needs, or whether, because of budgetary problems or other reasons, there are sufficient programs from which to choose, or whether the parents are even aware of all the options, are, of course, different questions. For some of the parents we talked with, their choice of program or programs often came down to what was available in their area, whom they happened to talk with about their child's deafness, what recommendations they received from family members, and so on. Other parents made choices based on a priori assumptions about what they wanted their deaf child to learn or be able to do. In this regard, some of these parents consciously sought out programs that emphasized Total Communication, whereas others were more interested in trying to locate a program where their child could, they hoped, develop some ability to use and understand spoken language. Other parents wanted programs that emphasized both of these approaches. Several parents even moved, temporarily or permanently, to get their child into the type of program they wanted. In addition, many parents opted to have their child in speech and/or auditory therapy in addition to group activities with other children their age. Many children, even very young children, and their parents were (and are) very busy.

The early intervention picture is further complicated by the fact that, in many of the families we interviewed, the children started in one type of program before receiving their cochlear implant. Then, after implantation at an early age, parents had to decide whether to leave their child in familiar surroundings or to move on to something new and different. Of course, for a number of children, their entire prekindergarten years were also part of their pre-implant years. Fifteen of the children in our parent sample received their implant after the age of 6. Nevertheless, it appears from our interviews that the early intervention experiences of these children were similar in many ways to those who were implanted at a younger age. They attended a variety of different types of programs, took advantage of home visits from itinerant teachers of deaf children, learned how to sign, and tried to learn how to use and understand spoken language, and so on. In one important way, however, the experiences of the later-implanted group were quite different: Parents did not have to worry about whether preschool teachers and other early intervention specialists knew how to deal with implant-related problems, such as broken cords or lost speech processors. As will be discussed in more detail, this issue is of some importance to many parents.

At least half of the families we talked with took advantage of more than one type of early intervention program for their child. Sometimes children were in different programs simultaneously (nursery school and a parent-infant program, for example). This was generally not very difficult to manage, because many early intervention programs were only an hour or two a week. In other cases, attendance at various programs with different goals and purposes was arranged sequentially, with parents opting to have their child involved in different programs at different times based on their changing needs and aspirations (of both the parents and the child). Some such programs are:

- Family education programs sponsored by state residential schools for deaf students, either at the school, a regional center, or at the child's home (typically called early-infant or parent-infant programs). These programs are usually once or twice a week, and a number of families used these services for several months or even several years. Most of these programs appear to be oriented toward Total Communication (signing and speaking), although speech and listening skills were by no means ignored. In parent-infant programs, the school representative typically works with both the child and the parents, helping them learn to communicate and otherwise adjust to having a deaf child in the family.
- Similar programs sponsored by county "intermediate units" or other public schools or publicly supported agencies not tied to a residential school for deaf students. These programs may provide parents with more options than are usually offered by residential schools. In Fairfax County, Virginia, for example, Cued Speech, Total Communication, and oral programs are all available for parents looking for an appropriate program for their child within the public school system. Home teaching is also an option supported by some public school systems.

A mother of a 7-year-old who was implanted in 1996 recalls that her daughter was able to attend a county intervention program sponsored by a neighboring county: *There were six Amish children in the class, a teacher and her aide, and these were 4-year-old kids just acting like 4-year-old kids. They were playing together. They were communicating. They were doing everything. They were singing . . . doing their alphabet. And each child used their voice to the best capability that they could. This classroom incorporated everything. It incorporated ASL, it incorporated Signed English. . . . They also got the kids to use as much speech as they could.*

- Publicly supported or private (sectarian or nonsectarian) preschool classes or groups—including child care and nursery school or playgroup arrangements—either with other deaf children only, other hearing children only, or some mixture of deaf and hearing children. Some of the parents we talked with wanted their preschool-aged child in a classroom or group environment with hearing children only so they could interact with, and, hopefully, "model" the speech of their peers. Some programs emphasize Total Communication, others use speech (auditory-oral) or listening (auditory-verbal) approaches, and some use ASL. A mother of a 10-year-old boy implanted in 1995 recalls her son's preschool experience before he received his implant: *He was barely 17, 18, months old at that time. And he went to school for four hours a day, and they had . . . a wide range of hearing loss [among children at the school]. It was really the only place available for hearing-impaired preschoolers in [city] at that time. . . . They did sign. And they used Signed English. And they spoke, and there was speech therapy that went on at the school. . . . And there was an emphasis on language.*

Some parents started in one program but, after determining that their child was not progressing as fast as they would like (in terms of spoken language development, for example), shifted to another program before implantation. Other families started with one program before their child was implanted and stayed with the same program after implantation. Most families gradually shifted to a more speech/listening-oriented early intervention program if their child was still young enough to participate in such programs after receiving the implant.

Not surprisingly, perhaps, given the dearth of information many parents initially had about the educational needs of their deaf child, sometimes parents were steered in what, in retrospect, is perceived as being an unfortunate direction by the preschool. The following example also makes it clear that sometimes the transition from the early intervention experience, where instruction is extremely individualized and child-centered, to a more structured classroom setting with a much less favorable teacher-student ratio, is not easy.

The mother of a teenage boy who is no longer using his implant said, when her son was nearing the end of his preschool years (several years before receiving his implant): *We were told that when he left [the auditory-only] speech school that they were totally opposed to any kind of special education. And we felt like they knew what they were talking about so we said No, we don't want any kind of special help for him [in first grade].* Later this mother added: *He was just overwhelmed. He was used to four or five children in the classroom at [the speech school] and one-on-one teaching. And he went from that to 30 children.* The father added: *The teacher put his desk . . . right up next to her desk. He sat away from all the other kids right beside her desk and his desk facing away from all the other kids . . . just totally separate from them. And, of course, that made for kids making fun of him because he wasn't around them, so he was kind of an outcast.*

- Speech and language or developmentally delayed preschool classrooms, as well as classrooms in which a speech therapist or other resource person works one-on-one with the child, are other types of preschool programs in which children participated. One mother recalls the experience of her 5-year-old son, who was implanted when he was 2 years old: *We ended up placing him in a speech and language delayed classroom. Because he was hearing tremendously well at this point with the implant, and he was starting to talk, although his sentences were just two or three words, phrases. . . . So he was seemingly more and more language and speech delayed than hearing-impaired.* The mother also added: *He had a very large vocabulary and conceptual vocabulary in sign language before the implant. . . . For him the transfer from sign language to spoken language was very beautiful to watch. It was very smooth. . . . When he has the implant off I sign to him.*

As far as the current educational placement is concerned, for about 20 of the 62 implanted children in our parent sample the early intervention or preschool setting is the current educational setting. Among these young children, all of whom continue to use their implant, about a third are in mainstreamed settings in which a teacher of the deaf or other specialized aide or assistant is also with them for at least part of the day. Some children in these main-streamed settings also rely on other support services, including assistive listening devices. Sign language is also a part of this instruc-tional environment for many of these mainstreamed children. Another third of the children whose preschool setting is their cur-rent educational placement are either in an oral program or main-streamed in a public or private preschool with no other deaf children. Signing is not typically found in such settings. Another third are in a variety of other programs, including playgroups, an ASL-only preschool setting, or a language-delayed preschool classroom.

In addition to their educational programs, many of these preschool-aged children also receive speech and/or auditory-ver-bal training at the school, from a private therapist, or from a cochlear implant center. Moreover, in many of these programs, the parents are quite involved in their child's early education. Some parents request lesson plans from their child's teacher, for exam-ple, so they can "preteach" some of the lessons to their son or daughter. Other parents spend a considerable amount of time "teaching the teachers" how to meet their child's unique needs.

Education After Preschool

A little more than half of the 40 or so children in our sample who are past preschool age are in mainstream public or private educa-tional settings all or almost all of the time. Some of them are now in college, but others are much younger. Only one person in this group of mainstreamed students is not currently using his implant. Moreover, within this group, only three or four of the children appear to be receiving no special services whatsoever. Either because their implant is working so well, or because they (or their parents) eschew any support services that might be perceived as curtailing their independence, this small group seems to be doing what many parents hope their child will eventually be able to do with the implant. As one parent of a 4-year-old who was implanted at 2 envisioned: *I would say, you know, 7 to 10 years old, you probably won't hardly notice a difference between him and any normal hearing or hearing child.*

Clearly, the vast majority of mainstreamed children with cochlear implants are receiving some type of special service, or services, in the classroom. There is no typical set of services, and assistance includes support such as the following: teacher aides or instructional assistants, itinerant teachers and other teachers of the deaf, amplification systems (whether personal assistive listening devices on the student's desk or "surround-sound" systems in the classroom), Cued Speech and sign language interpreters, "stenointerpreters" that type text onto laptop computers that also appear on the laptop computers of the students, resource or other support rooms, and note takers. In many cases, particularly for younger children, there is an extremely attractive teacher-student ratio, often one regular classroom teacher, a teacher of the deaf, or an aide for each child or two. In some programs, a teacher of the deaf and a regular classroom teacher may teach together. For some of the students, this support is not needed all day or in all classes, but in other cases it is. Some comments from parents on these issues are as follows:

> There's four deaf children in her classroom with 20 hearing kids and what a neat thing that we've seen. . . . She can communicate with her peers and they can talk to her. It's wonderful. And then when the teacher is up front lecturing, she has the interpreter so she knows exactly. You know, she can hear the teacher, but not good enough to catch everything.
> *Mother of an 8-year-old girl implanted in 1996*

> Real-time captioning cut her workload down. . . . [My daughter] has always prepared herself prior to classes, even in high school, that's how she got by . . . she'd always read things ahead of time. And finally, with real-time captioning, it [was] like, Wow, she heard every comment of every student. . . .
> *Mother of a college student implanted at age 16*

> DAUGHTER: I'll get captioners for the really important classes where I need them [for her third year of college]. . . . Might have a couple of note takers. . . . A lot of people always asked

me how I managed. . . . It's funny, all of my friends at [college] saw I did so well in history, English, painting, whatever, they couldn't understand how I managed. They didn't understand how hard I worked, hours and hours in the library. Five hours each night in the library. Some people drive me crazy! They do a paper in three hours! Me, it might take me 15 hours to do the same thing. . . . Friends at [college] didn't realize how I was constantly working.

The same college student implanted at age 16

I'm doing way above the average, but that's because I work so hard. It's unbelievable how hard I have to work in order to get the grades I do. And, CART [real-time captioning] and assistive devices help [me do] that. . . . With an assistive device I can be sure I'm going to get a good grade on something because I know the information.

Teenager implanted in the late 1980s

Although many parents hoped that their child would eventually be able to end up in a mainstreamed educational environment without support services, others realized that this might not be easily accomplished. Moreover, parents were generally aware of problems especially likely to surface in the later elementary school, middle school, or high school years—when hearing children might be less accepting of children with implants than they are in the early years of elementary school. One mother whose young daughter will probably be going to their local middle school in a few years discussed this issue.

INTERVIEWER: How do the other kids react to [her being the only person in the elementary school with an interpreter]?

MOTHER: So far, to my knowledge and to her knowledge, the other kids think it's cool. They actually have a sign language class two days a week during lunch period, and the interpreter and [my daughter] teach the class. And there's about 40 kids . . . [in] the class . . . My older daughter, who's in junior high, says, Well, when she gets to junior high she's not going to have the interpreter follow her around all day, is she? And I'm like, Well, yeah. So my oldest daughter thinks that's going to be a problem. [Later in the interview, the mother described

some of her daughter's previous educational experiences.]
Always with an interpreter. And first grade she was mainstreamed just for math. In second grade she was mainstreamed
for math and science. Third grade she was fully mainstreamed,
but at the school that housed the hearing-impaired program.
So she could still socialize with the kids that she had grown
up with in the hearing-impaired program. And then in fourth
grade she went to her home school.

Mother of a 10-year-old girl implanted in the early 1990s

This mother's reference to the "hearing-impaired program" refers
to programs that are commonly referred to as self-contained classes
for deaf students. In these classrooms, deaf and hard-of-hearing students are typically taught by a teacher of the deaf and other specialists, such as a teacher's aide or an instructional assistant.
Assistive listening devices may also be available in these classrooms.
Hearing children are not typically included in these classes,
although a few of the parents we talked with said that their child
participated in a "reverse mainstreaming" situation in which one or
two hearing children were in their child's self-contained class. In
some school districts, self-contained programs are found in elementary, middle, and high school "magnet schools," which draw
deaf and hard-of-hearing students from a wide geographical area.
Moreover, in some districts, parents and children can choose among
self-contained classes and programs that feature oral communication, sign language (usually Total Communication), or Cued Speech.
In other school districts, particularly in rural areas where the child
may be the only deaf child in the entire county, various options are
much less comprehensive.

In 11 of the families we talked with, their post-preschool-age
child or children are in a self-contained classroom for much, or all,
of the time. All of the 13 implanted children in these families continue to use the device regularly. The duration of implant use among
these children is 11 months to 7 years, a range that is typical for
the educational placements discussed in this chapter. (In other
words, there seems to be no simple relationship between duration
of implant use and likelihood of placement in all-mainstream programs.) Among the 13 children, about half are mainstreamed for
part of the day, and about half are in a self-contained class for all
or almost all of the time. Occasionally, some of the students in the

latter group may join their hearing peers for physical education or art; but, for the most part, all of their academic subjects are taught in self-contained classes. A mother whose daughter is in kindergarten and who has been using the implant for a little over a year said: *We chose for next year to keep [our daughter] in the deaf class and not mainstream her at all. So ... she's getting her speech therapy, she's getting her auditory therapy, she gets it from me and from her father and she goes to church school and she has an interpreter there. And she gets all kinds of input that we don't feel she has to be forced into mainstreaming yet.*

A half-dozen of the children in our parent sample attend a residential school for deaf students and one of them, who is having difficulty benefiting from the implant three years after the surgery, is still in a nonresidential (commuting) early intervention signing program at the school. Among the others in residential school settings, implant use varies—at least one child uses the implant regularly, some use the device occasionally, but others have stopped for one reason or another. Interestingly enough, one mother said her son uses his implant more at the residential school he attends than he did at his neighborhood public school. There is less teasing at the residential school, where implanted students regularly receive speech therapy, than there was at his "home" school. This mother added, *They are getting more out of him with it down there [at the state residential school] than they could up here. . . . He signed a contract that he will wear it in the classroom. All classrooms. He knows if he doesn't he will lose privileges.* A parent of a teenager who has stopped using his implant said, in response to a question about whether or not their state residential school is more accepting of kids with cochlear implants now than it used to be, *Yeah ... because ... the parents who have kids with implants [at the school] are very strong-willed, so they're going to participate in their education no matter where they go. And if they're there at [the school] they feel that's the best place for their kids. They've gone [to] other places and they've decided that's the best place.* Another parent, whose teenage son attends a state residential school and who still occasionally uses his implant, said, when asked if it was a mistake to keep him at a residential school after he got the implant, *Well, we discussed that, too. We had thought about maybe moving him to another oral school. There were other oral schools in St. Louis, you know, but we had this child who has been moved from oral to deaf and I felt like he had just been through enough moving. And we had, too. We had moved, we had picked up our family three different times for his betterment, we thought. And I, myself, just didn't feel like I could make another move.*

Educational Costs

A topic that has become a rather important issue in recent years is one that deals with the costs of educating deaf and hard-of-hearing students. A residential school education, for example, is not inexpensive, especially since a substantial physical plant needs to be maintained, administrator and teacher salaries need to be paid, and so on. Moreover, as the proportion of deaf and hard-of-hearing students attending such schools continues to decline, it is becoming more difficult for state legislatures to justify their continued support for these schools. Currently, only about 30% of deaf and hard-of-hearing students in the United States attend special schools or centers, which include both day and residential schools (Gallaudet Research Institute, 1999).

One of the arguments that is sometimes made by cochlear implant manufacturers, as well as implant centers and professionals, is that, in the long run, it is less expensive for the public to educate a child with a cochlear implant than it is to educate a nonimplanted child (Cheng, Haya, Rubin, Powe, Mellon, Francis, & Niparko, 2000; Francis, Koch, Wyatt, & Niparko, 1999; Niparko, Cheng, & Francis, 2000a). Although this may be true, especially if one compares a child who is mainstreamed, at least to some extent, with one who attends a residential school, it is also true that educating a child with an implant is almost invariably not cost-free by any stretch of the imagination. Clearly, almost all of the children in our parent sample, as well as most of the children in the GRI survey (see below), depend on some support services, even after implantation. Real-time captioning, which some parents and children already have and which more will undoubtedly request in the future, is expensive. Costs for this service include the equipment and the salary of the transcriber. Other services, ranging from instructional aides and self-contained classrooms to sophisticated amplification systems, although perhaps not as expensive as maintaining a residential school complex, are considerable. In one of our interviews, the following exchange took place:

> INTERVIEWER: One of the arguments is that if the kid gets an implant, then there's much more of a chance that he will be mainstreamed, which will save the state a lot of money for education. What do you think of that argument?
>
> PARENT: I think that's a very bad argument. I guess I'm at the point where, even though he got the implant, he still needs education. Whether he'll be mainstreamed further down the road, it's hard to say. But even a child with an implant, even if they are mainstreamed, they still have different issues than a regular hearing child.
>
> *Parent of a 4-year-old boy implanted in 1996*

It is also important to keep in mind that measures of cost savings for children with implants do not typically take into consideration the immense amount of time that many parents, particularly mothers, put into their child's educational and socialization experiences. Indeed, several mothers we talked with quit their jobs so they could help raise their implanted child or children. Although this may not be a direct cost of educating a deaf child with a cochlear implant, it is certainly an indirect and important one, particularly for the families involved, and is one that is easy to overlook in a simple cost-benefit analysis (and one that is, of course, not limited to deaf children with cochlear implants).

Parent Involvement

In general, whatever the educational setting, most of the parents we talked with are very involved in their child's education. Some parents are involved to the extent that they have a say in selecting their child's teacher and even their child's classroom. Other parents are not quite that involved, but most do maintain regular contact with the teachers and the school. This tapers off in high school and college, of course, but twice or thrice weekly visits to the school their child attends is by no means uncommon. Parents frequently indicated that their child's needs were their most important priority. As one father of an 8-year-old girl said: *[Our daughter] will show us what she's capable of. And if she has to go into a private school, then we'll go to private school. If she needs tutors to help her, we'll do that. Right now, yes, public school. But each year is a different year, and each year you have to re-evaluate what your child is doing.*

Among other things, most of the parents we talked with were actively involved in designing their child's IEP—"individualized education plan" (or IFSP, "individualized family service plan," which is the common designation when early intervention plans are being developed [Heward, 1996]). Individual education plans, ideally developed collaboratively between parents and school representatives, can cover just about any aspect of the child's public education. They typically include annual goals in subject areas, as well as social, cognitive, and emotional development, special support services that are needed to achieve these goals, and evaluation criteria. The IEP also requires annual reviews of the child's progress. In general, most of the parents seemed to be quite accommodating in their relationship with school representatives, and most said they were fairly satisfied with the instruction and support services that were available for their child. Other parents, however, had to work long and hard to get the services they thought were appropriate (school districts vary considerably in their enthusiasm about satisfying requests from parents). What follows is a sampling of some comments from parents concerning their IEP experiences.

PARENT: Although they are legally obligated to pay for the speech therapy that [our daughter] needs . . . they don't have the resources to do that more than three times a week. So what they say is she needs it three times a week. She does not need it five times a week like the Cochlear Corporation says, like her audiologist says, like her surgeon says.

INTERVIEWER: Have you thought about challenging the school system?

PARENT: Well, I've had friends that did that and you kind of wind up getting blackballed . . . you're a troublemaker. . . . And the school is doing such a wonderful job in so many other ways. It's kind of hard for me to go in here with this attitude like, You guys aren't doing enough for my child. We are the ones who chose for her to have the cochlear, so in a way it's our obligation to make sure she gets what she needs. But in a way

I really wish that the schools were given enough funds and enough resources to get [our daughter] what she needs.
Parent of a 6-year-old girl implanted in 1998

Interviewer: What kinds of things have you asked for?

Mother: Only what they give us. . . . When [my daughter] was in kindergarten she did have a sign language interpreter in the class. I don't know why it's different this year.

Interviewer: But could you ask for that in an IEP?

Mother: I don't know. I never thought . . . I thought they didn't let her have it because it wasn't there.
Mother of a 7-year-old girl implanted at age 4

I played the game real carefully, I didn't ask too much for them to say no. We bought our own FM system. . . . He used an FM system all the way through elementary school that he brought home and charged up every night. We didn't try to get them to pay for his [speech] therapy outside of school. . . . I had to choose what battles I was going to fight.
Mother of a teenager implanted at age 16

Mother: We're in the middle of a little battle now. . . . We want sign language. . . . Socially he's lagging a little bit. . . . Maybe he needs some social skills support group or some one-on-one play therapy. That's what I'm requesting now. . . . They want to take away our sign language services . . . they wanted to take away all our services.

Interviewer: They think he is doing just fine?

Mother: Right. . . . The recommendation [said] no more direct services. We'll call you in six months and see how he's doing. And I said, Nooooo way. No way.

Father: After all of the work we'd done, do we want to see him now slide back? . . . We have both spent time in the classroom with him, just watching. And it's clear that he's not . . . integrating into the classroom yet.
Parents of a 5-year-old boy implanted in 1996

FATHER: We select what teacher she gets next year. We look at the classroom ahead of time to see if there is any sound competition in the class . . . to make it as best we can.

MOTHER: Make sure there's no big glaring windows because that could affect how she lipreads. [A bit later in the interview, the following exchange took place.]

INTERVIEWER: Is there anything that you asked for that they said, We can't afford, or we're not going to give you?

MOTHER: Well, one time they did, about the itinerant teacher. They said, You can have it once a week. And we said . . . No, no, no, because her kindergarten year she had [it] three days a week. And first grade they tried to cut us down to one day a week, and we said no.

FATHER: Actually, we went out and spoke to a lawyer . . . who specializes in disability rights practice.

After the IEP hearing in which they paid to have an "expert witness" join them, the family eventually got what they wanted. They continue to support the public school their daughter attends and have paid for some of the things their daughter needs themselves.

FATHER: If your daughter needs something. . . .

MOTHER: . . . we expect it.

Parents of an 8-year-old implanted in 1993

A mother of a teenage boy who is no longer regularly using the implant said, concerning her effort to obtain services from her local school district about a decade ago:

MOTHER: [The county school system] said, You've got to find us at least seven children before we can get a program up. I got on the phone. I put notes in the newspaper, If you know of a hearing-impaired child, get in touch with me. I was looking for seven children. Didn't need it. . . . When I [understood] my parent rights, it said all I needed was one child for a program. I called [the] school board, I said, Let me tell you something, all I need is one child, and he's in my house. I'm bringing him to [the local school], I want a program. . . . They found a hearing-impaired teacher to hire. We met her, loved her. . . . [However,] I had not . . . talked with anyone about needing an interpreter. He went from first grade to fourth grade without one. . . . We . . . had another IEP, did an amendment. They would furnish him with an interpreter for the rest of his school years in this county.

INTERVIEWER: So, when you told them you wanted these things, what was their reaction?

MOTHER: They couldn't believe that I knew enough . . . that I had done some research. . . . I tell you, if it hadn't been for my family behind me pushing I would have given up. I mean, it drove me crazy. I was hitting a brick wall because I found out, dealing with school systems that are not for the deaf, they will do everything possible to keep you from knowing your rights. . . . I got what I wanted eventually, when I found out what I needed. It was a battle from day one.

We reconvened the case conference and I just said, Now you're going to give us this, you're going to give us the summer school, you're going to give us a third session of speech therapy every week. You're going to give [our son] an auditory trainer. And first it was, Okay we'll give you the summer school and that's it. We won't do the third session of speech because our speech therapist just isn't here three times a week. [I said], Then find a way. This is your problem, not mine. And lo and behold they found a way. And then they didn't want to get him an auditory trainer because, What will all the other kids' parents say? And I said, Ask me if I care what the other kids' parents say. And we threatened to do a due process hearing to which we were told, You don't want a due process hearing. And I said, Correction, YOU don't want a due process hearing. And the woman from the school system said, What makes you say that? Thanks to our advocate I had all of my numbers and I said, Okay, we'll go down the list. Win, lose, or draw. The due process hearing costs you $10,000 just to have the hearing take place. So right now you've spent $10,000. Now, I am assuming, I might not be correct, but I am assuming you are not stupid so you will have legal representation with

TABLE 7.1
Current Educational Placement

Educational Placement Characteristic	Percent
Type of school/program	
Public	72%
Private	28%
Current mode of communication	
Speech	51%
Sign	4%
Speech and sign	43%
Classmate characteristics	
Deaf	32%
Hearing	30%
Both	38%

you. That costs money. I know that I'm not stupid. I am also going to have legal representation and you will reimburse me for said legal representation when I win and you lose. So you can spend $20–$30,000 dollars and give me what I want or you can just give it to me NOW!

Father of an 11-year-old boy implanted in 1995

Educational Placements

A number of questions on the GRI survey dealt with the implanted child's educational placement. One question asked respondents to list their child's educational placement history. Table 7.1 summarizes the current educational placement of those responding to this question.[1]

1. It should be noted that the responses in table 7.1, as well as in other tables in this chapter, may include education-related information from a small number of parents (17 out of a total of 439 respondents [4%]) whose child is no longer using the implant, either temporarily, intermittently, or permanently. Since our parent interviews also include a few such children, and since we are interested in general trends in this book and are not performing sophisticated statistical tests, we have decided to include those responses in these tables.

It is clear from table 7.1 that only a small minority of children with implants in the GRI survey rely on signs only post-implant. However, it is also clear from the table, just as it is apparent from our parent survey, that sign language is far from forgotten or ignored after the implant. Based on our interviews and on the GRI data, it is reasonable to conclude that about half of the children with implants continue to rely on some form of sign communication in school after implantation. Moreover, most of the children with cochlear implants do not find themselves in educational settings in which they have little or no contact with other deaf children. Rather, more than two-thirds of the children in the GRI survey are in classroom settings with other deaf children or in settings with a mixture of deaf and hearing kids.

Parents also were asked to indicate if any of their child's school placements were made specifically in response to their child's cochlear implant use. Of the parents responding to this question, about one-quarter (24%) indicated that at least some of the child's educational placements (although not necessarily the current one) were selected for this reason.

The GRI survey also asked parents to describe their child's current educational environment. Table 7.2 summarizes these findings.

The "other" category in table 7.2 includes reverse mainstreaming (as noted, hearing children in a majority-deaf classroom), parent-infant groups or playgroups, deaf/hard-of-hearing private school, other self-contained classroom settings, and a number of other difficult to classify categories. In any event, it is clear that about one-third of the students are fully mainstreamed, and well over half spend a considerable amount of time with hearing peers during at least part of the school day. A fully mainstreamed educational setting may, of course, include some special services for the child, including assistive listening devices, interpreters, transliterators, and so on. Based on our parent interviews, it is apparent that there are very few implanted children who do not require any special educational services at all post-implant.

As far as special educational services are concerned, the GRI survey asked parents what "accommodations and/or special supports related to deafness or the CI does [their] child now receive in his educational setting?" Table 7.3 summarizes parent responses to this question.

TABLE 7.2
Current Educational Environment

Current Educational Environment	Percent
Fully mainstreamed with hearing children for all activities	34%
Partially mainstreamed with hearing children (only certain classes, activities, or times)	24%
Self-contained classes of deaf and hard-of-hearing children	13%
Commutes to residential school for deaf and hard-of-hearing children	10%
Live-in at a residential school for deaf and hard-of-hearing children	5%
Other	14%

The "other" category in table 7.3 includes such accommodations as preferred seating, a speech therapist, a laptop computer, and other accommodations, including "none," which makes it difficult to summarize this category succinctly. In addition, since some students in the GRI survey, like several students in our parent survey, undoubtedly take advantage of real-time captioning of classroom lectures and discussions that appear on their own laptop computer, it is likely that some of those responses are included in the "media captioning" category in table 7.3. It is also important to keep in mind that since the percent column adds up to considerably more than 200%, many students obviously take advantage of more than one type of accommodation in their current educational setting.

In the GRI survey, parents were asked to indicate whether they agreed or disagreed that the "professionals at my child's school understand my child's academic, communication, and social needs." The vast majority of parents either agreed (36%) or strongly agreed (50%) with this statement. This suggests that, although some parents are clearly unhappy with the outcome of the IEP process, a large num-

TABLE 7.3
Special Support Services Child Currently Receives in School

Special Support Service	Percent Receiving This Service
Sign language interpreting	40%
Teacher aide/assistant in the classroom	37%
Resource room help	28%
Media captioning (closed or real-time)	24%
Itinerant teacher support	22%
Remedial work/tutoring	17%
Classroom amplification system (e.g., a "loop" or infrared system)	16%
Personal assistive device (e.g., FM system or "pocket talker")	15%
Oral interpreting	13%
Note taker	11%
Cued speech transliteration	9%
Other	17%

ber appear to be satisfied with the IEP that they negotiated with their child's school system.

Parents were also asked to list two of the "greatest advantages," and two of the "most frustrating things," about their child's use of the cochlear implant in "the school or other instructional setting." Responses to this question are far too numerous to list and discuss here, but *awareness of sounds, hearing music, hearing language, better classroom participation, better communication,* and *hearing the teacher more easily* are among the greatest advantages cited by parents. Frustrating things include *lack of others' understanding that a cochlear implant does not make the child fully hearing, back-*

ground noise is a problem, hard to hear in a big group, recharge-able batteries do not last a full day, kids can be heartless at times, and *sometimes the head piece falls off.*

Parents responding to the GRI survey were also asked how often they met to discuss their child's progress with the staff at their child's school. About a quarter of the parents (24%) said they met with someone on the staff (not necessarily their child's teacher) at least every week. Another 17% said they met with someone on the staff each month. The remainder (59%) said that they meet up to six times a year with someone at their child's school.

In-School Activities

We asked parents about a variety of in-school activities, including their child's communication and interaction with peers and teachers within the school, the availability of speech therapy at the school, their perception of their child's academic performance, and the extent to which they feel teachers at their child's school are able to deal with implant-related problems. As far as communication and interaction are concerned, for the most part parents said that while some situations—such as recess, class discussions, and large classrooms with poor acoustics—were a problem, they were generally satisfied with their child's interaction with fellow classmates, whether deaf or hearing. General satisfaction, however, does *not* mean that communication with hearing peers and teachers is "barrier-free" and that their child does not miss anything in the classroom. In fact, only a handful of parents said that their child communicated easily and directly with hearing classmates and teachers. Rather, many parents seemed to feel that although there were still plenty of communication and interaction problems at school, they were pleased that progress was evident, and pleased that the implant frequently made it possible for their child to hear and understand conversations that were not possible with a hearing aid.

In addition to communication aids, such as sign language or Cued Speech interpreters, the children in our sample who were in mainstreamed environments sometimes relied on writing and gesturing when talking with hearing classmates, and, not infrequently, depended on speech- (lip-) reading to a great extent for satisfactory communication. Moreover, a few children communicated differently with deaf and hearing peers if both were present in the school. Despite these inconveniences, however, few parents felt that the communication and interaction in their child's school was such that a transfer to a different program was warranted. Some of the comments on this issue from the parents we talked with are presented below:

> There's so many deaf kids [in the school] . . . they have a pretty good group and all are different age levels. . . . But even the cochlear kids are just signing away at each other because I think it's easier for them, especially in the noisy running around kind of room they're in.
>
> *Mother of a 6-year-old girl in a magnet elementary school*

> INTERVIEWER: How does [your daughter] get along with [other students in the class, all of whom are hearing]?
>
> MOTHER: She does okay, considering. I've noticed that when they start playing "pretend" and it gets too much for her to understand, she kind of edges her way out and then she's not playing. . . . If they're not understanding everything she's saying, they'll accommodate for that and tell her to point or draw a picture.
>
> *Mother of a 7-year-old girl implanted in 1996*

> INTERVIEWER: How does [your son] communicate with the other kids; how does he get along with them?
>
> MOTHER: Well, one-on-one he does great. . . . But when you get into the little groups of children, he has difficulty. . . . I've seen that at school he'll try to get into one play situation, and he gets slightly rejected, and then he pulls back and plays by himself. He'll try again. And then, you know, then I see him just sort of wandering around the room, not quite in play with any of the children. And that's, well, that's very painful as a mother to watch that.
>
> *Mother of a 5-year-old boy implanted in 1996*

> This year has been a wonderfully improved year for her in terms of her socialization with some of her hearing classmates. . . . She's been invited for sleepovers, which she had

TABLE 7.4
Implanted Child's Interaction with Hearing Children at School

Frequency of Interaction	Percent
All opportunities	52%
Fairly often	23%
Very little	11%
Almost never	6%

> never had before. . . . This year she is beginning to have more closer friendships with some of her hearing peers.
>
> *Mother of an 11-year-old girl implanted at age 7*

Parents who responded to the GRI questionnaire were asked to indicate how often their child interacts with hearing children in his or her school setting. Table 7.4 summarizes the responses to this question.

This question on the GRI survey, of course, does not delve into the issue of the quality of the child's interaction with hearing children. From our data, it appears that the quality is quite variable, with some students communicating fairly well, and others, especially those in self-contained classes in mainstreamed environments, having, at best, limited and somewhat superficial contact with their hearing peers.

Speech Therapy

Many of the parents we talked with said that their child received speech therapy in school. We discussed this issue with about 30 of the parents, and in all but one or two cases parents said their child either had had some speech therapy at school in the past and stopped it, or continues to have it. For many parents, this speech therapy supplements private therapy, but for others in-school therapy is all their child receives. Some children, particularly those attending oral schools, constantly receive speech therapy throughout the day; others may see a speech therapist for a half-hour or an hour once or twice a week, or even less often than that. Some children have one-on-one sessions with a therapist, whereas others are involved in group therapy sessions. In addition, some students are pulled out of classrooms, whereas others prefer to arrange before or after school sessions so they do not miss activities in class.

Speech therapy is not limited to mainstreamed (or other non-residential) educational settings. In fact, such therapy is readily available for several children in a southern state who attend the state's residential school for deaf students. At another residential school in the west, however, a parent's request for speech therapy for her child was denied, apparently because of a lack of speech therapists at a school where ASL is the preferred mode of communication. For one family that lives in a rural part of the mid-Atlantic region, speech therapy at school is all that is available for the child; no other speech therapists are available in the county at all. Sometimes parents felt that the quality of speech therapy in school was not what they were looking for and specifically asked that it not be made available for their child. In these cases, other, private arrangements were made. In a few families, where the child was speaking quite clearly or because it was "time for a break," neither in-school nor private speech therapy was thought to be necessary, at least at the time of the interview.

In sum, a wide range of in-school speech therapy services are available for the children in the families with whom we discussed this issue; there is no obvious, discernible pattern linking implant user characteristics with frequency and type of in-school speech therapy. Some of the parents we talked with clearly felt that, at various times in their child's educational career, the public schools had not lived up to their commitment to provide their child with the speech training they had requested. Most of the parents, however, appeared to be more or less satisfied with (or resigned to) the speech therapy they were receiving from the school, particularly if it was combined with other public, private, or implant center resources.

Teachers and Cochlear Implants

There is a good amount of variability among the teachers and other professionals at the schools attended by the children in our parent sample in terms of their knowledge of cochlear implants, as well as their knowledge of the special needs of children with implants. Most of the parents said that they had to educate their child's teachers about implants, frequently by offering short in-service training workshops for the teachers, giving them brochures to read or videotapes to watch, or meeting with them individually before the school year began. Alternately, a teacher of the deaf, a representative from a cochlear implant center, or another resource person assumed this responsibility, which usually included providing information about how to make minor adjustments, such as changing or recharging the batteries, or replacing broken or lost cords. As a result of these efforts, a number of schools, particularly elementary schools, keep spare wires and batteries on site in case of an emergency. Older children, of course, are generally able to troubleshoot, make adjustments in their speech processing programs, or replace cords and batteries themselves during the school day. We discussed teacher-related issues with about 40 families, and most of the parents said they felt that, overall, teachers were generally accommodating and willing to do what was necessary to meet their child's needs. This frequently included preferential seating, using a microphone so that an amplification system would be available for the child, calling the parents if problems arose that could not be handled at the school, letting the child move around freely to find the best listening or speechreading situation, and so on. Interestingly enough, whereas some teachers were initially reluctant to wear a microphone, several parents said that their child's teacher had come to appreciate the benefits of amplification for all the children in the classroom, not just for the children with implants. This is particularly true for younger children.

One parent said she did not want her child's teacher to do anything special, because she was worried that her child would be singled out in a way that would not be desirable. In another case, the parents felt that their child's preschool teacher did not care if the implant was used or not and, in any case, was not willing to make any accommodations for the child. This child is attending a residential school, but the child's situation is such that the parents still feel this is the best placement for the child even though minimal benefit is derived from the implant (which is not used at school).

Several parents were able to select the teachers for their child or children.

I go the year before, and I will go two or three times throughout the year and sit in [the teacher's] classrooms and observe their styles. I observe their . . . facial expressions. I try to observe the quality of their voice. I try to observe all those things . . . their teaching styles. And then I go from there. And I usually try to pick the teacher. . . . I've never had any trouble [getting] the teacher I want.

> *Mother of a 6-year-old boy implanted in 1998 and*
> *an 8-year-old boy implanted in 1995*

Another parent of a teenager who was not implanted until he was in high school said that both before and after implantation:

We tried not to ask [teachers] to change much. We just asked that they would give him a chance to work with us and that they would try to get his attention before they started talking because he would also be speechreading. . . . I think it's hard for the teachers to have a deaf student in the class. They're not prepared for it. So I'm not a huge mainstreaming advocate for everybody. The classroom teachers cannot compare with the teachers in the special classes. I know that. But with the right family situation and the right kid . . . it really did work for us.

> *Parent of a teenager implanted in 1997*

Of those teachers who were not enthusiastic about meeting the special needs of the implanted child in the classroom, some did not want to wear a microphone and others made little effort to communicate clearly and directly. One 17-year-old girl who has used an implant for two years recalled some of the frustrations she has had in a mainstreamed high school environment: *One time I wasn't understanding anything. We were reading a book and I asked the teacher what she was talking about and she told me to look up the Cliff Notes.* Her mother added: *I took that note that [the teacher] wrote to her that said, Go read the Cliff Notes to my IEP meeting and [said] if they refused my real-time captioning [request] I was going to take that piece of paper to court. I thought, Something in writing!* Now a high school senior, her daughter enjoys real-time captioning in her classes.

Academic Performance

Parents are understandably concerned about their child's academic performance, and we discussed this issue in a very general way with about 40 of the 56 families. We did not have access to school records or results of standardized achievement tests, so what follows is primarily a discussion of parent perceptions of their child's language, reading, and other skills and abilities rather than an "objective" assessment of them.

Many parents readily admitted that their child's academic performance in many areas was not where they would like it to be. Roughly half of the children in the 40 families are experiencing delays to some degree, according to their parents. Some of these children are not reading at grade level, and some experience delays in other parent-identified areas such as expressive language, vocabulary, and mathematics. Some children are perceived by their parents to be at grade level in some areas but not in others. The other half of the children in the 40 families are, according to their parents, reading, using language, and otherwise performing at or above grade level.

It is difficult to make anything more than general observations from our interview data, but, as is the case with many of the other educational variables discussed in this chapter, there appears to be no simple, clear-cut relationship between implant user characteristics and academic success. Among the children who are not yet where their parents might like them to be academically, some were implanted at a young age (as early as 22 months) and some were implanted as old as 10 years; some have used some variant of sign language most of their life and others have used no signs at all; some have had access to auditory-verbal therapy, whereas others have not; some have used the implant for more than a decade, whereas others have been implanted for only a couple of years; some continue to use the implant, whereas others have stopped; and some may have central nervous system auditory processing problems that prevent optimal use of the implant.

Similarly, among those children whose parents perceive them to be performing at or above grade level, there is no clear-cut pattern. Some of these children were implanted at a very young age, whereas others were not implanted until they were teenagers (and some were doing very well academically long before implantation). Others have used sign language for years, whereas some do not sign at all. Some have even stopped using the implant. About all that one can conclude is that, collectively, variability seems to be one of the most predictable academic outcomes.

TABLE 7.5
Parental Evaluation of Child's Reading and Mathematics Skills
Compared with Child's Hearing Peer Group

Skill	Far Behind	Slightly Behind	About Equal	Slightly Above	Far Above
Reading or reading readiness	21%	38%	19%	13%	9%
Math or number handling	11%	26%	37%	19%	7%

Given the informal data we have on academic performance, it is not possible to say much more than this: Among children with cochlear implants, academic performance, including both spoken and written language proficiency, is clearly influenced by many different factors. These include such things as extent, quality, and type of early childhood communication, parental commitment and involvement, age of implantation and implant performance, quality of speech and auditory training; type and quality of a child's educational placement; the cognitive abilities of the child, and so on. It remains to be seen how these factors, as well as, no doubt, others, help explain variation in academic performance and language acquisition among implanted children (see chapter 9 for a comprehensive review of the literature on these issues).

The GRI survey included a few questions that focus on the child's academic performance. One question asked parents to comment on their child's reading (or reading readiness) and mathematics (or number handling) skills relative to those of their child's "hearing peer group." These results are presented in table 7.5.

If their child was judged to be "far behind" or "slightly behind" their peers, parents were asked to indicate if they felt the level of their child's progress in terms of reading or mathematics was "due mainly to your child's deafness." In both cases, most of the parents felt that, if their child was indeed behind, it was due primarily to his or her deafness. As far as reading or reading readiness is concerned, 83% of the parents felt this way. For mathematics, two-thirds

(67%) of the parents, felt that, if their child was behind, the delay was due to his or her deafness.

To be sure, many of the parents we interviewed were not overjoyed if their child was not reading, writing, or doing arithmetic (or math) at the level they might have hoped for when implantation was initially considered. But they were not depressed either, and most were optimistic that their child would continue to make progress and achieve many of the goals they had set for them. Given the current state of affairs, perhaps it is best to evaluate each child's academic success vis-à-vis individual goals rather than collective norms. Indeed, this seems to be what most of the parents we talked with do anyway. Some of the comments from parents concerning their child's academic performance are presented below:

> My daughter, [who is in a self-contained Total Communication kindergarten,] reads books that are like second grade level now; she can play the computer; she reads the closed captioning on the TV. . . . She comes home after school, she sits down at her little desk, she goes through her papers, she teaches her doll, she teaches her sisters . . . she just loves learning. . . . If she didn't have the cochlear she'd probably be in the same place she is now. . . . She wouldn't be speaking . . . but I still think she'd be at the same academic level because she is so bright.
>
> *Mother of a 6-year-old girl implanted in 1998*

> I wish there were other deaf kids that were at his level . . . with language. . . . He has been a high-functioning deaf kid. He's always done really well. . . . He's a normal kid, but his language levels were always a lot higher than his peers. . . . I [also] wish there would be other . . . kids that were at the same level as him so he would have more interaction with other deaf kids. . . . Now he's kind of separated from a lot of the deaf students . . . because he's mainstreamed [in high school] all the time and . . . because a lot of these kids are just . . . [Father finishes the thought] . . . not interested in the same things, you know.
>
> *Mother of a teenager boy implanted in 1993*
> *who no longer uses it*

Stepfather: So, overall, she's almost to sixth grade. . . . [Her previous oral school] did not encourage any use of sign language and they did not encourage academics either.

Mother: [After they moved with her daughter to a new state when she was 13, the new school] tested her . . . and she was at the first grade level in everything. And within six, seven months the principal called us for a meeting . . . and he looked at us and he says, [Your daughter] is very, very intelligent, she's practically caught up with the rest of the children [in a self-contained Total Communication sixth grade class].

Parents of a 14-year-old girl implanted in 1991

I'd say she's probably about one to two years behind still, her language skills, especially written. Her written skills are still behind. But she speaks well, I mean you understand her, [but] sometimes she leaves out articles when she speaks. [Later in the interview, this mother said:] I thought by this age that she would be caught up with her peers.

Mother of a 14-year-old girl implanted in 1988

At [an infant hearing center] they use a developmental scale which summarizes what normally hearing children would be doing at certain age ranges. It is broken down into categories like communication, receptive and expressive, developmental abilities, cognitive abilities, etc. Once a quarter we sit down and compare what [our son] is doing to those norms. When [he] was 23 months old he was performing between 25 and 30 months old in all areas. And in a lot of ways he's just been kind of astounding to us because he already knows all of his letters, he knows numbers almost through 20. He knew all of his colors.

Mother of a 2-year-old boy implanted at 19 months

Satisfaction

The last issue related to education that we discussed with parents dealt with their satisfaction with their child's educational placement. We discussed this issue with about half of the families and, overwhelmingly, parents were quite happy with their child's educational situation. Not only that, most of the parents said that the current educational placement, whether in the mainstream, at a residential school, in a self-contained class, or at an oral school was the best situation for their child. What this probably shows is that whenever parents found that the educational setting was not what they wanted, they made a change to something they deemed more appropriate. In fact, a number of parents expressed great dissatisfaction with some of their child's previous schools, classrooms, or teachers. But, given the fact that most of the parents we talked with were quite involved in their child's education, they were generally quick to remedy what was perceived to be an unsatisfactory situation. As noted previously, some families moved to a different school district, or even a different state, to find a better educational environment for their child. When dissatisfaction with their child's current educational setting was expressed, it was generally about issues such as class size, a desire for more listening therapy, or other issues that could perhaps be satisfactorily resolved at their next IEP conference. What follows are some of the comments from the parents we interviewed on this issue.

> One thing we really liked about this school is it's very individualized and the teachers are able to address special needs for each child. That's pretty special when they help you with that.
> *Mother of a teenager partially mainstreamed in a magnet public high school*

> [The school] is wonderful compared to what I've had in the past.... Our [local] school system had never had a deaf child so they didn't know how to do it. They didn't know how to educate the deaf. Down there at [the state] school for the deaf they know what he needs.... It's speech ... it's physical ed., the life management classes.... He washed his own clothes ... he knows how to clean ... he's had cooking classes down there, he has learned how to ... manage money, what a checkbook is.... They are teaching life-skills down there that he would never have up here.... They teach him how to sew and they teach him how to cook.
> *Mother of a teenager attending a residential school*

> [My daughter is] in a very good place.... I would like her to be further along, but the only reason that she's not further

along is because the professionals misled us. They led us to believe that signing was bad for [my daughter]. The only thing that I would . . . ever change for [her] would be, I would have started signing with her from the very beginning. And I would have checked into a cochlear implant sooner instead of later.

Mother of a 7-year-old girl implanted at age 4

Conclusions

The parents of children with implants that we talked with, as well as those who responded to the GRI survey, were very concerned about their child's education. Of course, this does not mean that all parents of children with cochlear implants are equally involved in their child's education. But we suspect that given the commitment most parents are asked to make upon deciding that implantation is the course of action they wish to take, extensive involvement in their child's education is likely to follow. To be sure, parents are frequently frustrated with the educational roadblocks through which they have to navigate. By and large, however, they are persistent, and most appear to be satisfied with their child's current educational situation. If one of the assumptions parents bring to the entire cochlear implant decision-making process is that their child will have more options in the future with an implant than without, then one of the courses of action that follows from this assumption is that parents will tend to be very involved in their child's educational program.

It is clear, however, that there is no magic formula for educating children with cochlear implants. Rather, as many parents reminded us, each child is different, and what might be an appropriate situation for one child may be completely inappropriate for another. For one child, a post-implant signing environment might delay progress toward the goal of spoken language development. For another, a classroom setting with some signing or other type of visual communication might be indispensable for progress toward the same goal. Constant vigilance (and sensitivity) on the part of both parents and teachers is certainly essential.

8

Looking Back: Overall Progress and Satisfaction

Almost all of the parents we talked with put a considerable amount of time and energy into the cochlear implant decision, as well as their child's post-implant habilitation, and we wanted to know whether, in retrospect, they felt it was "worth it." Are they pleased with the decisions that they made, sometimes in collaboration with their child? Would they do anything differently if they were going to do it all over again?

Most of the parents we talked with are clearly pleased they made the decision to implant their child. This conclusion is perhaps not too surprising, given the nature of our sample. As noted previously, the families we talked with are undoubtedly skewed toward the "success" end of the pediatric implant success-failure continuum. Even though success stories are overrepresented, parental retrospection is nevertheless useful since a number of interesting issues emerged in our discussions with parents on this point that might have otherwise remained obscure.

Parent Perceptions

Although most parents are generally pleased with their child's over-all progress with the implant, more than half of the parents we talked with also said they wish their child could have gotten a cochlear implant earlier. This is especially true for parents of some of the children who were not implanted until they were 5 years of age or older. However, even a few of the parents of children who were implanted as young as 2 said that, if they could do it over again, they would try to have their child implanted at a younger age. Early implantation, in their mind, would presumably make it easier for their child to develop spoken language.

Even so, many said that, occasionally, they still have second thoughts about the procedure, even if, on balance, they are glad they did it. Other parents said they wish they had been more aggressive in seeking out the services, such as speech and/or auditory training, they now realize were initially insufficient. Some said they wish they had started signing earlier, even before their child received an implant, so that language development could have started much sooner than it did. A few parents said that their child's earlier educational situation could have been better. And, not surprisingly perhaps, several parents said that they would try to find a more knowledgeable or understanding pediatrician if they could rewind the tape and start over.

A small number of parents said that, since their child was not benefiting very much if at all from the implant, they wish they had not gotten the implant in the first place. In addition, the one parent we talked with who decided against implantation remains pleased that the family made that decision.[1]

Some of the comments from parents on these issues that we present below do indicate that looking back does not always bring complete peace of mind, even for parents who are pleased with their decision. We often saw expressions of regret for "what might have been" among parents whose children experience very different degrees of success with the implant.

---

1. On this point, readers may be interested in an account of another family's decision against cochlear implantation (Peters, 2000). We did not interview this family.

MOTHER: I don't know if I would still make the same decision. Now [my husband] will say something different, but I don't know if I would still make the same decision that . . . we've got to get you this implant so that you have the opportunity to hear. Which I still think is good, but after meeting so many deaf people and learning more about the [residential] school and opportunities . . . I don't know if I would make the same decision now. But I'm happy we did it. I still think we needed to give him every opportunity that we can, that we could. I think we're happy with it.

FATHER: The most important thing was that he needed to be able to speak, to communicate. . . . In order for him to be successful in the world, not just in the deaf community, but in the world, I really felt that he needed spoken language. And that might be a little narrow-minded, but I'm his father and I can be narrow-minded if I want to. . . . And I still feel that way. . . . [However,] there's a very good chance that he's going to be an active part of the deaf community and if that's the case he's going to have to sign. . . . If we had known, if we knew then what we know now, we would have stuck with sign language from the very beginning and really concentrated on that.

Parents of a 4-year-old boy implanted at age 2

I wish every day that she could have gotten [the implant] earlier. I wish I had known she was deaf from the second I [adopted her], because I do think that would have helped her in her development in language. . . . In terms of having the implant I never, never regret it for a second, honestly.

Mother of a 7-year-old girl implanted in 1994

If she had been implanted two years ago she probably would be speaking and hearing a lot better now, and things would be easier for her. On the other hand, I'm glad she has the Nucleus-24 [cochlear implant] with the behind-the-ear unit. . . . People with the [Nucleus-] 22 don't get the behind-the-ear for another six months or a year. So in some ways I'm happy that we waited and in some ways I wish she'd had it sooner.

Mother of a 6-year-old girl implanted in 1998

MOTHER: [The implant] has helped him. I mean it really has helped him with his speech overall a lot. So I mean ... it hasn't met ... all of our expectations, but I think it has met some.

INTERVIEWER: You don't regret making the decision?

MOTHER: No.

FATHER: Oh no, no.
> *Parents of a teenager implanted in the early 1990s*
> *who no longer uses his implant regularly*

I had days where I was convinced we'd done the right thing and I had days where I was convinced we did the wrong thing. And I don't have ... days anymore where I think we did the wrong thing.... We developed a certain relationship [with our son], and that relationship died.... The relationship that ... I had with him up to 2 years old, that relationship kind of died.... For as miraculous and wonderful [as the implant is], there's this whole other side that nobody really prepared me for or talked to me about.
> *Father of a 5-year-old boy implanted in 1996*

A mother was asked if she would have gotten an implant for her daughter at the age of 2 if one had been available:

We would have done that, absolutely.... It would have [made a difference] because [my daughter's] life is so much easier [with the implant].... She had to work twice as hard as everybody. Now, at [a university], she's on the dean's list. She doesn't have to work so hard and so, yes, she has done great, but with a great price.
> *Mother of a 20-year-old young woman implanted in 1996*

The daughter, who participated in the interview, added:

I would have, like hands down, loved to have had the implant [years ago] if that would have been the case.... There's nothing wrong with having hearing aids, but if I had it to do over again I would definitely choose the implant.

A mother who left her home on the East Coast with her son and lived in another city for several years so her son could attend school there said:

It was hard living apart from my husband for four and a half years, and he came to see us every two to three weeks. But I would do it again tomorrow if I had to.

Mother of a teenage boy implanted in the late 1980s

With the implant, it's opened up his world, I feel like. . . . It's just been a phenomenal experience . . . and we would do it again.

Mother of a 2-year-old implanted in early 1999

MOTHER: He was about 13 years old at the time [of the surgery]. . . . I feel like now, looking back, that he was old enough to tell us then, whether he would like it or not, and he told us that he didn't want it. But we felt like we knew what was best for him so we went ahead with it. And it's been a struggle, it's been a fight between us and him . . . because we disagree on a lot of things about it. I believe if he had been 3 years old at the time he was implanted it would have been good.

INTERVIEWER: So, if he's not really using it now, why don't you just stop?

FATHER: 'Cause daddy won't let him. Daddy's still, I'm still at the point where I feel like it could do something good for him if he would use it regularly and try it rather than just saying, No, I don't want it, and turn it off. So, I guess that's me. [Later the father added:] When you're 18 and you're out on your own and you're making your own living, doing what you want to do, then you can turn it off if you want to. But as long as you're home I feel like . . . he needs what hearing it gives him, whether or not it improves his speech.

Parents of a teenage boy implanted in 1995

MOTHER: I was not led to believe that one day we would sit down and not have to use sign language, and I would understand everything and he would understand everything. No, I think I wanted that to happen, and I still want that to happen. I want him to be able to sit down with a group of people, hearing and nonhearing, and understand everybody.

Interviewer: Do you think that is going to happen?

Mother: He might understand from reading lips. He won't understand from hearing it.

Later in the interview the following exchange took place:

Interviewer: Do you wish things could have been different?

Mother: There's times when, yeah, I wish things had turned out different. There's times when, you know, things I can look at and I say, Okay, you know, we got it pretty good. He's done great, he's done good because I see some [children] that haven't done as well. . . . He's got some speech. You know, it's just, it's so tough. It's tough making these decisions and not knowing how he is going to feel. . . . They [asked] me at [the implant center], What are you going to do when he looks at you one day and says, Mom, why did you do this to me? And, you know, I thought, okay, I'm just going to tell him this, I thought it was the best thing for you. I wanted to do the best that I could for you and I thought this was it. [Later she added:] Maybe if I had that option [earlier implantation] I would have done it, [but] no earlier than age 4 because I don't think a child needs it earlier than that. It's a traumatic surgery.

> *Mother of a teenage boy implanted in the late 1980s*
> *who occasionally uses his implant*

I can only put myself in [my daughter's] shoes and look back and say, in retrospect, If that was me, what would I want my mother to do? And I would want my mother to have done that for me. No doubt about it. . . . I would rather have her give me the implant than not. And to do the method to try to get me to speak instead of signing.

> *Mother of a 2-year-old implanted at 19 months*

When asked if she would do anything differently, a mother of a young boy said:

Mother: I think the only thing I would do differently . . . is to teach others to slow down and don't sweat the small stuff. Like just work it day to day . . . and lose the guilt. I was right along there with [my husband] when we first found out, you know. Why was I screaming at this child to do something if he really couldn't hear me? I tortured myself.

FATHER: I was in no rush to have [the surgery] done . . . because I wanted to find out more and I was convinced, and I still am, that if he didn't have it he would be okay, he'd be fine, and he would adapt to his situation. People would still love him and he'd be successful at whatever he decided to do when he gets older and he would make his way in life. So the time issue I don't think was as critical. I don't think if we had known three months earlier that we would have scheduled the surgery or whatever, because I was a little apprehensive about it and wanted to give myself time to think everything over and also find out as much about it as I could. So I think the timing, I'm pretty pleased with [it], and sometimes pretty proud of the way that we handled it. Because given our situation I don't think, for me, there is anything that I would do any different, except for maybe be a little easier on myself and my son.

Parents of a 4-year-old boy implanted in 1997

Several questions on the Gallaudet Research Institute (GRI) survey deal with parent perceptions of their child's success with the cochlear implant. One question was, "How satisfied are you with your child's progress to this date [date of the survey] in the development of spoken language skills (including correct use of grammar)?" More than 80% said they were either satisfied (39%) or very satisfied (43%) with their child's progress. Moreover, slightly fewer than half of the respondents said that both parents and the implanted child now use "all speech" as the predominant form of expressive communication in the home. Interestingly enough, a slightly higher percentage of parents said that the child used only speech at home (46%) more often than did they, the parents (44%). The second most frequently used form of communication at home, for both parents and children, is a roughly equal balance between signs and speech.

Parents were also asked to respond to the statement: "I understand my child's spoken communication all of the time, most of the time, about half of the time, some of the time, or hardly at all. About three-quarters of the respondents (78%) said they understood their

TABLE 8.1
Parental Satisfaction with Child's Cochlear Implant Progress

Parental Satisfaction with Child's Overall Progress	Percent Satisfied	Percent Very Satisfied
After the first year with the cochlear implant	33%	54%
At the present time	21%	67%

child all or most of the time. The same response categories were also available for the following statement: "When using his/her CI, my child seems to understand my typical spoken communication . . ." Again, about three-quarters (73%) of the respondents said that their child understood the parent's communication.

Several questions on the GRI survey asked parents to take a retrospective look at their family's experience with the implant. One question was: "In retrospect, how realistic were your pre-implant expectations of your child's performance with the CI?" Parents overwhelmingly said that they felt their expectations were either somewhat realistic (36%) or very realistic (55%). The vast majority of parents also said that, at the time of the implant, they were fully aware (56%), or almost fully aware (26%), of the "personal and material resources that [our] family would need to commit toward promoting [our] child's ultimate success with respect to communication, academic, psychological, and social development."

Parents were also asked to indicate their satisfaction with their child's overall progress after the first year with the cochlear implant, as well as their satisfaction at the present time. Table 8.1 summarizes these responses, which include communication, social, medical, and psychological satisfaction.

It is clear that almost 90% of the parents are satisfied or very satisfied with their child's overall progress in both situations. It also is apparent from table 8.1, however, that the percentage of those who are "very satisfied" is appreciably greater after the child has used the implant for a few years.

Additionally, three-quarters of the parents (75%) reported a "vast improvement" in their child's quality of life as a result of cochlear implant use; another 15% noted a "slight improvement" in this area. Similarly, over 80% of the parents responding to the GRI survey said that their child either relied "an enormous amount" (66%) or "quite a bit" (16%) on the implant. Furthermore, 88% said that, in their opinion, their child was either "very satisfied" (67%) or "satisfied" (21%) with the implant.

One concern that we discussed with some of the parents we talked with dealt with the issue of appearance, and whether or not embarrassment, self-consciousness, and similar feelings were evident when their child used the implant. For the most part, our findings were somewhat mixed: Some children, particularly teenagers, often expressed an interest in a behind-the-ear implant model so that their use of the cochlear implant would not be immediately obvious. Others, including some teenagers, did not appear to be overly concerned about the aesthetics of their implant. In the GRI survey, over 90% of the respondents said that, in their opinion, appearance was either of negligible or no concern to their child (66%), or of concern only occasionally (26%). To get a more accurate assessment of a young implantee's feelings on this point, it would probably be a good idea to focus primarily on the children and adolescents themselves rather than rely on parental perceptions.

Parents in the GRI survey were also asked to respond to a list of statements regarding the timing of their implant decision. Table 8.2 summarizes the responses to this question, which asked parents to select one statement that they felt was MOST true.

Parent Expectations

One question we asked virtually all of the parents we talked with was: "Would you say that the cochlear implant has exceeded your expectations, met your expectations, or failed to meet your expectations?" Well over half of the parents said that, overall, the implant has exceeded their expectations. In some cases, the parents were clearly ecstatic; as one parent said, their child's use of the implant has *exceeded our wildest expectations.* For other parents, exceeding expectations simply meant that, because initially they did not expect their child to do much more than hear environmental sounds with the implant anyway, they were pleased that the child was able to do more than that. A number of parents said that they

TABLE 8.2
Looking Back: Parental Decisions About Implantation

In Retrospect, "I wish ..."	Percent Agreeing with This Statement
...I would have, or could have, gotten my child implanted sooner.	62%
...I had waited to get my child implanted a little later, to take advantage of recent technological advances.	2%
...I had waited to get my child implanted a little later, when my child was older.	2%
...my child had never received the CI.	1%
I am happy that my child received the CI at the time (s)he did.	32%

had fairly low expectations, but higher hopes, primarily because the implant center cautioned them against expecting too much from the implant. In addition to the majority of parents who said the implant exceeded their expectations, about a half-dozen parents with whom we talked said the implant did not meet their expectations, and about a dozen said that it simply met their expectations. What follows is a sampling of parent comments on this issue:

> It's just definitely been a miracle for us in all the ways that it could be. ... It's not perfect, life is not perfect, it doesn't work that way. ... Did I expect he would be finishing first grade and doing what he's doing? I mean he just finished first grade, he just turned 7 ... no, I didn't expect any of these things.
> *Mother of a 7-year-old boy implanted in 1996*

> She's exceeded. I remember thinking if I could just get [my daughter] to read, if she could just learn how to read. And when she was first [diagnosed as] deaf I was scared that I

would never be able to teach her to read. . . . She's exceeded
my expectations.

Mother of an 8-year-old girl implanted in 1996

It exceeds them. . . . I did not for the life of me ever thought
that she was going to speak, or that she was going to hear
me . . . I never thought it would happen, and it did. . . . I mean
to me, in all honesty, I really believe it's a miracle. I really do.

Mother of a teenage girl implanted at age 6

MOTHER: . . . failed to meet my expectations.

FATHER: Mine, too.

INTERVIEWER: What exactly did you expect?

MOTHER: I expected him to grow to love it like he liked his
hearing aids, and being better than the hearing aids. I felt
like everything would be better because of it.

FATHER: I expected he would have speech, improved speech,
more speech.

INTERVIEWER: Is there any way that it met your expectations?

FATHER: Just that it brought his hearing up to a mild to moderate loss from a profound [loss].

MOTHER: But, just because he can hear the sounds does not
mean that he understands.

Parents of a teenager implanted in 1995

Still a Deaf Child?

We also asked parents if they saw their child as deaf after receiving
the implant and what their reaction would be if their child stopped
using the implant at a later date. Perhaps somewhat surprisingly, the
vast majority of the parents said that, in their eyes, their child was
still deaf after implantation and, if their child decided to stop using
the implant later, that was basically their decision. Of course, given
the enormous amount of time, effort, and expense they put into the
obtaining and making sure that their child benefited from the implant,

most of the parents we talked with would certainly be disappointed if their child stopped using it. But, at the same time, parents realized that this was not something they could force the child to use, especially as the child became older. Here are some observations from parents on these issues:

> I don't think we used the word *deaf* much before. And now it doesn't bother me, because he . . . was certainly deaf enough to qualify for an implant. . . . The surgery does take away your residual hearing. So when he took his hearing aid out, there was still a sense of something. He could put on a really loud headphone and hear something. But now he takes [his] implant off and he knows there's nothing. So I think he went through a phase of really facing deafness with the implant.
>
> *Mother of a young man implanted as a teenager in 1997*

> Just the other day [my daughter] said to me if her friend . . . slept over in her room on a sleepover, which she's never had yet, we would have to take the [nocturnal] hamster out of the room because it would wake [her friend] up. [My daughter] was laughing, I'm so lucky, she said to me, Right, mommy? It can't wake me up, I can't hear. I take my processor off and I can't hear. I'm so lucky, right mommy?
>
> *Mother of a 7-year-old girl implanted in 1994*

> I know my child is deaf, but her being deaf does not say that's who she is. She's a child first. . . . Deafness is a part of her, it's not her. . . . [The implant] doesn't fix the problem. The child is still a deaf child [be]cause you take the implant off every day. . . . Since [our daughter] has started signing, kids want to learn. Kids love learning sign language. A local elementary school started a program in the morning, and the kids love it. . . . They want to communicate. And why not teach them? And the more kids that know, then maybe later on down the road it won't be such a big separation . . . it'll be more of a mix, where people can communicate together. And it's done very well for her that way, definitely.
>
> *Mother of a 7-year-old girl implanted in 1996*

> [My daughter] might have better speech if pressured to wear it more and not allowed to sign. But I opted for a well-adjusted

happy signing and verbal child who I could relate to.
Mother of a teenager implanted at age 6

In response to the question about whether they see their implanted child as deaf, this couple replied:

MOTHER: No.

FATHER: Oh, no.

MOTHER: I mean we see him as a child who has hearing loss, a child who has a problem with his ears, no different than a child who has a problem with their eyesight.
Parents of a 2-year-old child implanted in 1998

When asked if he sees his recently implanted son as deaf a father said: *Yes, I mean, although [the implant] gives him the opportunity to process speech, my son is deaf. We know that. He will ... never be a hearing child, and we know that. This isn't a fix.* When asked how she would feel if her son stopped using his implant later, one mother observed: *That would probably bother me a lot, but it's just like if he got a tattoo or something. It's a child who you try and give them their foundation, but they're still gonna make choices that you're not going to like throughout their whole life, whether they're hearing-impaired or not.*

Another parent, when asked how she would feel if her son stopped using the implant someday, said:

MOTHER: That would be his choice.

INTERVIEWER: What if he decided to go to Gallaudet University ... and decided to stop using it?

MOTHER: I would be disappointed. I think that having the implant helps him to learn, and I wouldn't want him to give that up.
Mother of a 10-year-old boy implanted in 1995

If she decides when she's old enough that she doesn't want to use it, and she wants to be completely sign, live in the deaf community or not, Hey, fine with me. ... Our goal is to offer her every opportunity that was available.
Mother of a 10-year-old girl implanted in 1996

A father laid down the law: *When she becomes 18 she might throw it away. I think I can live with that. Until she's 18, I'm god.*

Another father said:

We were even told by the child psychologist that the day may come when he tells us he hates us for having done this to him . . . and, well, I hope that doesn't happen, but if it does, then, Gee, I'm sorry, we did what we thought was best. You don't want it, don't use it.

Father of an 11-year-old boy implanted in 1995

If he stopped now I wouldn't be happy. But I don't want him to stop. I know I can't be with him all the time. I can make him put it on in the morning before he goes to school, and he can have it turned off before he gets out of the car. And that may be the way it happens. I don't know. But I would like for him to continue using [it] . . . but I can't make him.

Father of a teenager and intermittent implant user

FATHER: When my child gets older and he wants to be part of the deaf community and he doesn't like wearing his implant, if he doesn't get enough benefit off of it, he can take it off. That decision is back to him. And it's true that it's a surgical procedure, but at that age [2 years old] they're not able to make a decision about what they're going to have for lunch so, of course, you can't expect them to make a decision about something like that.

INTERVIEWER: I don't think the argument is that you should ask them when they are that young, but you should wait until they're old enough to make the decision.

FATHER: Right, but the brain is developing at this young age when there is a window of opportunity for speech to develop; . . . if you . . . learn how to talk later, it becomes much more difficult.

Father of a 4-year-old boy implanted in 1997

Parent Advice

We asked parents to speculate about what factors they felt were important for determining the success of any child trying to benefit from a cochlear implant. Parents stressed the importance of such things as early implantation, parental commitment and family support, having realistic expectations, developing a good language base by talking and reading to the child as much as possible (*bathing them in language,* as one parent said), speech and listening therapy, a good school and good teachers, being an advocate for the child, taking the time to investigate different types of programs to see which one might be best for the child, and making sure that the implant itself (including the mapping) is working properly.

We also asked parents if any other parents had asked them for advice about whether or not their deaf child should get an implant. Many parents said that they have, in fact, discussed implantation with others seeking advice from them. Some parents we talked with have made a conscious effort to become available (by establishing or participating in a parent-support group, or participating in on-line discussion forums, for example), whereas others have taken a more low-key approach and have only responded when asked. A few parents have never been asked by others for advice or for a recommendation. For the most part, it appears that parents are not proselytizers and most refrained from taking an "If we can do it, you can do it" attitude. They generally realized that children have myriad experiences with the implant and hesitate to try to impose their views on anyone else. Rather, parents said that, when asked, they usually told other families about their experiences, how and why they made the decision they did, and why it is important to thoroughly investigate all options before making a decision. Some parents told others seeking advice about the surgical risks involved, as well as the fact that, in rural areas, it might be difficult to consistently get the necessary post-implant audiological and habilitation support. Some parents suggested that inquiring families meet their child, or other children with cochlear implants, and see how they are using the implant. A selection of comments related to these issues from the parents we talked with are presented below:

> Make sure they [other children] learn how to listen with it. . . . It's not putting it on them and expecting them to recognize and understand the sounds that . . . we hearing people have learned to listen for since birth. . . . Making them aware of what a cricket sounds like, or what water sounds like running. All those sounds that they've never had. It's just teaching them how to listen for those sounds.
>
> *Mother of a 6-year-old boy implanted at age 5 and*
> *an 8-year-old boy implanted at age 4*

> We could survive without the therapy, and I think she would do fine. It's nice to have the therapist guide you because you run into stumbling blocks and that sort of thing, but it's the parents. I mean it's your responsibility to make sure that they are getting the input and getting stimulated.
>
> *Mother of a 3-year-old girl implanted at age 2*

> Everyone says we don't know why [implants] work for one person and why they don't work for another. Well, I know why! I mean, are we all idiots? You know what I mean, look at the parents who know what they are getting involved in, and who have researched it, and committed to it, and look at their kids. [Implants] are just amazing . . . but they are only for people who know how to use them. They are just a tool. . . . It's not going to teach your kids to talk, it's not going to teach your kid to hear, it's not even going to make your child hear . . . You have to teach them how to hear with it. It's not natural hearing, you know.
>
> *Mother of a 4-year-old girl implanted at 19 months*

> Developing a confidence level to speak to other people. . . . She needs opportunities. Do set-ups like I do with the neighbors so that she can gain the confidence. And that's something that I think parents need to be very, very aware of. They can learn to talk, and they can talk to you. But they might be afraid to talk to anybody else. That would be an important thing.
>
> *Mother of a 10-year-old girl implanted at age 7*

What [an auditory-verbal program] has taught us is [that] you expect him to be a hearing child, and you put those expectations out there and treat them like they are. And they . . . use that implant to fulfill those expectations. . . . You expect them to hear and you talk to them like they can hear.

Father of a 4-year-old implanted shortly before age 2

He wanted it to work . . . he wanted to hear. He realized he couldn't . . . so he wanted to use the cochlear implant. And I think he has worked very hard himself at learning how to use it. [Later the father added] I remember this girl's mother talking to me one time, telling [me] that . . . they weren't happy with how things were going and that the child had said, I'm tired of this, all it does is hurt me. I don't hear anything with [the implant] and I'm deaf and I want to live like a deaf person. And her mother said, What should I do? And I said, Well, unfortunately you've gotten nowhere having her live as a hearing person, so maybe it's time to grant her her wish. And she's a bright kid; she seems to be doing fine since they stopped using it.

Father of an 11-year-old boy implanted in 1995

Let your children help you decide what is right. Don't force the issue too strongly because you're liable to have rebellion. . . . But also, that they know that you love them, and you think this is good for them. . . . And talking things through, pointing things out. . . . Try to take opportunities to teach the language as you're doing things. These children won't always learn it incidentally like your other hearing children. Abstract concepts aren't always so easy, so things have to be talked through.

Mother of a 5-year-old boy implanted in 1996

As parents, you all play with your children, so it is just taking the situation and highlighting certain words or repeating certain words more frequently than you would if you were just engaged in a completely natural conversation. Like, when I was playing with [my son] this afternoon, with his trains. He is working on colors, so we were talking, Where's the green train, where's the blue train ... the red train? Highlighting the color words; that's an example.

Mother of a 2-year-old boy implanted in 1998
and a 6-year-old girl implanted in 1996

It's not just putting in the device. It's the follow-up care. It's the audiology. So if you don't have a center with all of those things, and you get some kid in there, and they diagnose deafness, and then the ENT [ear, nose, and throat doctor] recommends an implant and off the family goes, that's a terrible disservice to that child. So there's reason for caution, and if the deaf community has to be that voice, that's important.

Mother of a young man implanted as a teenager in 1997

If we've learned nothing else through this whole process we've learned there is a need for compassion and understanding. ... I think you have to take individual situations for each family, for each child, and ultimately give the parents the choice. ... Even though we may have strong feelings about this and the success of it, I'm not going to tell someone that this is the answer, because for them it might not be.

Mother of a 2-year-old implanted in 1998

One mother we interviewed wrote a paper several years ago explaining why she and her family decided not to get an implant for their child. We asked her what advice she would give parents who decided to get an implant for their child if she were writing the paper today. She replied: *I would somehow try to reach out to them and say, [that] it doesn't have to be an either-or. You know, you're not going to get no benefit from the device just because you allow your child to sign also. There are many times the implant isn't going to help. You know, when the child is swimming [and] in a crowded room.*

Conclusions

It is clear that the parents we talked with and the parents in the GRI survey are basically pleased with the way things have turned out. It seems reasonable to conclude that 80%–90% of the parents in these two samples are quite happy with their decision. Some, of course, would like to change a few things if they could do it all over again. In this regard, implantation at an earlier age is something that many parents would find attractive.

Our interviewees (and the respondents in the GRI survey) are not necessarily representative of all parents of children with cochlear implants. In fact, they are probably not representative. Consequently, there is no way of knowing if the large percentage of satisfied implant customers that we found is true across the board. Future research studies might want to ascertain the extent to which a random sample of parents of children who have received a cochlear implant are satisfied with the progress that has been made.

9

Language Development of Children With Cochlear Implants

Patricia Elizabeth Spencer

"Oh, she's still deaf, but now she can talk."

The comment above was made by a hearing father of a deaf child about two years after she received a cochlear implant (P. Spencer, 2000a). This child, just like her parents, was a fluent signer before getting the implant. And, according to her father, the family continued to use sign language after she was implanted. This child's results from the cochlear implant are excellent: Before the implant (at age 4), she neither understood nor produced spoken language; using the implant, she has learned to recognize spoken language and to produce it intelligibly. However, sign language remains an easier and more reliable way for her to communicate. With it, she can receive the full "signal," or complete information; relying on the cochlear implant, she cannot always receive complete information and often has to ask for repetitions and clarifications to "fill in the gaps."

I greatly appreciate comments and suggestions from Barbara Cone-Wesson, Debra Nussbaum, Ron Outen, and Amy Lederberg, who read and reacted to earlier versions of this chapter. In addition, I thank John Christiansen and Irene Leigh for their insightful editorial suggestions.

There is much individual variation in how well children learn to understand the information they receive through their cochlear implants, and not all children benefit as much from using a cochlear implant as the child above. This child is special in yet another way: Her parents are working hard to maintain her signed language skills and the family's contact with deaf people. As will be discussed later in this chapter, there is considerable argument about whether sign language promotes or, instead, interferes with children's learning to understand the information their cochlear implants provide. Using a cochlear implant, this particular child has increased her ability to communicate with nonsigning members of the general public, while maintaining her ability to communicate using signed language and keeping an identity as "deaf."

Most parents who obtain cochlear implants for their children do so with the goal of having the children learn to recognize and produce spoken language (Kluwin & Stewart, 2000) so that they can interact freely with hearing people. However, as Pisoni (2000) pointed out, the signal received from a cochlear implant typically provides "highly degraded and impoverished sensory input" (p. 76) compared with the auditory information received by a hearing child. Only parts of the auditory signal available to the hearing child are accessible by a deaf child using a cochlear implant. Asking a child to make sense of, and be able to reproduce, spoken language received only through a cochlear implant is somewhat like asking the child to recognize and draw a picture of an exotic animal never seen before that is standing behind a tall picket fence. Only parts of the strange animal are visible through the spaces between the wooden slats of the fence. The child must complete the image in his or her mind, imagining the shape of parts of the animal that are not directly visible. How successful are children at recognizing spoken language through the "picket fence" of partial information provided by a cochlear implant? How successfully do children use this partial signal to build a spoken language system? What characteristics of children and their environment predict the level of success they will have? These questions are addressed in this chapter, using information from published research, plus some new information based on a study of children in Australia who received cochlear implants by the age of 3 years (P. Spencer, 2000b, 2000c).[1]

Before proceeding, it is important to note some difficulties in interpretation of studies of effects of cochlear implants on children's language development. One complication arises from the fact that much early research, especially that represented in many papers published in the 1980s and early 1990s, was clinical in nature and included relatively small numbers of children with varied characteristics. Because the children in this study often differed in cause of hearing loss, age at which the loss occurred, and presence of conditions (such as learning disabilities) that might interfere with language learning, it is difficult to generalize the results. That is, results for one group of children may not be representative of results for other children. In some reports, researchers failed to provide information about potentially important characteristics of child, family, and habilitation or education programs that would be important for interpreting results.

Interpreting studies of children's performance with cochlear implants is also complicated by the fact that the technology continues to advance at a rapid rate. Important changes have occurred since the 1980s in both the hardware used in the implants and the software used to process sounds in the speech processors (see chapters 1 and 2). An initial difference occurred when multichannel cochlear implant systems became preferred over single-channel systems. Because the former are used most often and appear to provide significant advantages for children, this review focuses on reports of use of the multichannel implants. Ongoing upgrades in the software used in the speech processing systems of the implants add a further complication. In many studies, newer processing strategies are used by some but not all children. In fact, some researchers report that individual children changed from one to another processing strategy during the course of the study. Information about differences in this component of the cochlear

1. Financial support for the study of Australian children with cochlear implants was provided by the Australian-American Education Foundation and the J. William Fulbright Foundation. I wish to thank Elizabeth Barker, Shani Dettman, and Rod Hollow of the Cochlear Implant Clinic, Royal Victorian Eye and Ear Hospital, for significant assistance in the conduct of this research. In addition, I am most grateful to Peter Blamey, Barbara Cone-Wesson, and Graeme Clark of the Bionic Ear Institute, University of Melbourne, for their support and assistance.

implants used by children in a study is sometimes, but not always, included in the background information provided by researchers.

The research literature, surveyed over time, also reflects the fact that children are getting cochlear implants at increasingly younger ages, and many researchers suggest that age of implantation affects the results obtained. Because many existing reports of progress with cochlear implants are based on children who received cochlear implants at relatively older ages, those reports may not reflect the experiences of more recently implanted children. Thus, the degree to which information is current and reflects current practices is especially important when interpreting results of research related to cochlear implantation.

Finally, interpreting the research related to children's results with cochlear implants requires attention to the specific kind of skills studied. Researchers have tended to address one or more of the following aspects of spoken communication: speech perception, speech production, and language. *Speech perception* includes awareness of sounds, knowing that one speech sound is different from another, and recognizing speech sounds in the context of various syllables and words. It can be tested in either a *closed-* or *open-set* situation. (*Closed-set* testing often includes tasks in which a child must listen to a spoken word and then point to a picture of it among an array of other pictures. In *open-set* testing, the examiner may ask the child to respond to questions or to imitate a word, phrase, or sentence.) *Speech production* is the ability to produce individual speech sounds, syllables, and words accurately. Assessment of *language* typically includes recognition and production of vocabulary, as well as reception and expression of syntax, sometimes called grammar. (Syntax includes use of word order in sentences, use of tenses and plurals, and use of other rules for combining segments of words and words in utterances.)

In fact, the skills of speech perception, speech production, and language are tightly intertwined, with each influencing the other in complex ways (O'Donoghue, Nikolopoulos, Archbold, & Tait, 1999; L. Spencer, Tye-Murray, & Tomblin, 1998). Although these associations have always been theorized, research with children with cochlear implants has helped to establish them more clearly. Advances in one area tend to be associated with advances in the other areas. Because of these associations, no attempt is made in this chapter to separate studies that focus on one instead of another of these areas of development.

Despite all of the complications, much is known about the effects of cochlear implantation on deaf children's speech and language development. Research conducted in centers around the world and with various groups of children has provided opportunities to compare results in different settings and under different conditions. Although the following sections of this chapter will highlight areas of continuing disagreement, it is now possible to reach a number of conclusions about the effects of cochlear implants for children. Cochlear implants provide many, but not all, deaf children with access to information that can help them develop understanding and production of spoken language. However, the range of benefits experienced is large and the factors that influence the benefits received by an individual child are still being investigated.

How Does Development of Language-Related Skills of Deaf Children Using Cochlear Implants Compare to That of Deaf Children Without Implants?

A question asked frequently in research about cochlear implants is whether they provide more support for the development of speech perception, production, and language skills than other kinds of aids and technologies. For example, some researchers have compared the relative effectiveness of cochlear implants and tactile aids, which produce vibrations on the skin that are modulated to indicate loudness and frequency (or "pitch") of speech sounds. The results of these studies have not been conclusive. For example, Ertmer, Kirk, Sehgal, Riley, and Osberger (1997) reported data supporting the conclusion that cochlear implants are more effective than tactile aids, especially related to children's production of vowel sounds. In contrast, Eilers and her colleagues (Eilers, Cobo-Lewis, Vergara, Oller, & Dolan-Ash, 1995; Eilers, Cobo-Lewis, Vergara, & Oller, 1997) failed to find differences in speech perception benefits from cochlear implants compared with benefits from the use of tactile aids.

There is much more agreement on the benefits of cochlear implants compared with use of conventional hearing aids. Numerous researchers have concluded that cochlear implants provide more assistance to developing speech perception and language. Geers and her colleagues (Geers & Moog, 1994; Geers & Tobey, 1992) conducted a series of analyses comparing speech production and both receptive and expressive spoken language of children who used cochlear implants with children using either conventional or tactile hearing aids. They concluded that profoundly deaf children with hearing loss greater than 100 dB performed better with tactile aids than with conventional hearing aids. However, the speech and language performance of children with cochlear implants was even better than that of the children using tactile aids. The researchers concluded that use of a cochlear implant allowed children with very profound hearing loss (greater than 100 dB) to process auditory information much like children with lesser hearing losses (in the 90 to 100 dB range) who use conventional hearing aids effectively. Meyer, Svirsky, Kirk, and Miyamoto (1998), although finding a somewhat lesser advantage than that reported by Geers and her colleagues, concluded: "On average, children with hearing loss in the 101–110 Db HL range . . . would receive greater speech perception benefits from a cochlear implant than they do from their hearing aids . . . " (p. 855). Svirsky and Meyer (1999) provided further support for this advantage in a report that compared 75 children using hearing aids with 222 children using Clarion multichannel cochlear implants.

More recently, Blamey et al. (2001) reported that profoundly deaf children using cochlear implants performed on speech perception as well as receptive and expressive language tasks at a level similar to that of children with severe hearing loss using hearing aids. In fact, these researchers concluded that "an average cochlear implant user with a hearing loss of 106 dB HL performs like an average hearing aid user with a hearing loss of about 78 dB HL (p. 278)." Blamey and his colleagues suggested that these results were somewhat better than those reported earlier because of recent advances in implant technology and because the children in their study had, on average, used the cochlear implants longer than those in earlier studies.

Children's development of English grammar skills using either cochlear implants or conventional hearing aids was the focus of a recent report by Tomblin, L. Spencer, Flock, Tyler, and Gantz (1999) on 29 children in a public school Total Communication (simultaneous speech and signed language) program. The children ranged in age from 3 to 13 years when they received their implants. The children's understanding of sentence structure was assessed by their performance on the Rhode Island Test of Language Structure, a test of sentence comprehension normed for deaf children. (Sentences were presented in speech plus Signed English.) Results showed that all but one of the children with cochlear implants scored very high on the test, well above the average expected for deaf children and near the ceiling (highest score possible) for the test. In addition to this receptive language measure, the children's ability to use expressive grammar (syntax) correctly was assessed using a story retell task. A second group of deaf children, matched with the cochlear implant group in degree of hearing loss and other background characteristics but without cochlear implant experience, also participated in the retelling task. An examiner presented stories, using sign and speech, to individual children. Each child retold the story using his or her preferred communication mode(s). The retellings were videotaped, transcribed, and analyzed using a scoring system to assign points for production of noun and verb phrases, questions, negation, and complexity of sentence structure. The children with cochlear implants performed significantly better than those not using implants. In addition, the children with implants tended to use speech (without signs) for a larger percentage of their words than did the children without implants, although both groups continued to use both modalities simultaneously for the majority of their productions.

Grammatical morphemes (sound segments connected to base words to indicate plural, possessive, verb tense, and so on) have long been known to be especially difficult for deaf children to recognize and produce. This is true whether the children use oral language or English-based sign systems (Bornstein & Saulnier, 1981; Bornstein, Saulnier, & Hamilton, 1980; Quigley & Paul, 1990; Schick & Moeller, 1992). However, L. Spencer et al. (1998) studied children in Total Communication programs and found that 25 children with cochlear implants used grammatical morphemes more often than a group of 13 children who used hearing aids only. In addition, the implanted children tended to use speech without sign for expressing these morphemes, even though they continued to produce the majority of their whole words using both speech and sign simultaneously. (There were individual differences, of course, and one child with an implant used no grammatical morphemes.) This indicates that, in general, the children using implants could perceive the sounds in these morphemes when spoken by others. That perception led to the children's incorporating the grammatical morphemes into their expressive language. The researchers also noted that the order in which the morphemes were integrated into the language system and used expressively was the same as that reported previously for hearing children. Thus, despite their language delays, the deaf children with implants were acquiring the grammatical morphemes in the typical order.

These along with many other studies have indicated that cochlear implants provide better support than conventional hearing aids for most profoundly deaf children's development of speech perception and spoken language skills. This is not surprising. In contrast with a cochlear implant, hearing aids can only amplify sounds that the child already has the ability to hear at some level of loudness. For many children with profound hearing loss, these will be only the lowest frequency sounds—sounds that do not provide much information about speech.[2] In contrast, a cochlear implant can supply information about sounds in the higher frequency range that help children recognize more of the sounds that occur in spoken language. But does this improvement in access to sounds in the speech frequency range assure that a deaf child will develop speech and language skills at a rate and level typical for hearing children? This question will be addressed in the next section of the chapter.

Does a Cochlear Implant Allow a Deaf Child to Learn Language Like a Hearing Child?

Most researchers report that, despite the benefits of cochlear implants, deaf children using them continue to have more difficul-

---

2. Much of the auditory information needed for understanding speech is found between the frequencies of 1000 and 4000–8000 Hz. Most profoundly deaf people cannot hear sounds in those frequencies, and conventional hearing aids typically do not provide information at these frequencies that is loud enough to be perceived. This range of frequencies, and the loudness levels at which they are typically perceived, is often shown in an audiogram within a bent oval shape that is sometimes called the "speech banana." Cochlear implants can provide profoundly deaf persons with information about sounds in the speech banana range.

ties with speech and spoken language development than do hearing children. In addition, most researchers emphasize the great variability, or individual differences, they find among children with cochlear implants. For example, Osberger, Robbins, Todd, and Riley (1994) assessed speech intelligibility scores of children who had used cochlear implants for at least two years and found an average intelligibility rate of 48%, a level considerably below that which would be expected for hearing children at the same ages. However, the speech intelligibility ratings for individual children ranged from a low of 14% intelligible to a high of 93% intelligible. Considering only the group average rate would obscure the experience of both the least and most successful children, some of whom performed almost like hearing children.

Blamey and his colleagues (1998) also reported generally delayed language skills, but wide individual differences, for 57 children between 4 and 12 years old with cochlear implants. The researchers measured language skills by administering the Peabody Picture Vocabulary Test (PPVT) to assess receptive vocabulary and the Clinical Evaluation of Language Fundamentals (CELF-3 and CELF-Preschool) to assess understanding and production of English grammar. Both of these tests have norms for hearing children but not for deaf children. The PPVT does not require children to actually speak. Instead, they listen and point to a picture of the word spoken by the examiner. In contrast, portions of the CELF require children to produce spoken language in response to the items. On average, the children with cochlear implants performed at 45% of the expected level for hearing children on the CELF and at 62% of the typical hearing child's expected level on the PPVT. However, some children had extremely low scores on the tests, whereas some others scored in the average range compared with hearing children.

Svirsky, Robbins, Kirk, Pisoni, and Miyamoto (2000) administered the expressive language sections of the Reynell Developmental Language Scales to test vocabulary, as well as structural complexity of the language of children with cochlear implants. They confirmed that development occurred, on average, faster than predicted for deaf children without cochlear implants. However, 18-month follow-up data available for 23 children showed that some continued to have severely delayed expressive language compared with hearing children, whereas other children with implants performed close to average compared with hearing children. For the more successful children, Svirsky et al. concluded that use of cochlear implants prevented their pre-implant language delay from increasing after receiving implants. Furthermore, after implantation, some of these children actually made progress at a rate typical for hearing children. Bollard, Popp, Chute, and Parisier (1999) reported a similar phenomenon occurring in 10 young children with implants. Their scores on vocabulary, language comprehension, and language use increased at a rate equal to or faster than that of hearing children at their language level. (Of course, those hearing children would be chronologically younger than the deaf children using implants.) Even after 18 months of faster-than-average language growth, however, the deaf children remained delayed compared with same-age hearing children. This was attributed to the fact that the language of deaf children was significantly delayed prior to implantation.

Overall, despite the advantages provided by cochlear implants compared with other types of amplification, even recent research indicates that the performance of children with implants rarely reaches the average range expected for hearing children of the same age. Furthermore, the range of benefits children receive from cochlear implants is striking. Some children make significantly greater progress with implants than they would without them. Others, however, seem to get little benefit from the implants.

What Factors Predict Individual Differences in Benefit from a Cochlear Implant?

Researchers have proposed a long list of factors thought to influence children's outcomes from cochlear implantation. These factors include the length of time the implant has been used, the length of time the child was deaf before getting the implant, the age of the child at the time of the implant, language (and listening) skills before getting the implant, cognitive and attention abilities, the intensity of the therapy (or habilitation) after getting the implant, and the kind of language programming (oral, auditory-verbal, sign, and so on) provided after implantation. In addition, factors related to the intactness of the child's neurological system and the resources and involvement of the child's family have been suggested to affect progress. Because these factors are often interrelated, and because children differ so much on each factor, it is difficult to determine the effects of each of them. However, there have been significant numbers of investigations of the following factors.

Duration of Deafness and Age at Implantation

In general, the longer a person is deaf before obtaining an implant, the less effective the cochlear implant is likely to be (Blamey, 1995). Thus, late-deafened adults tend to receive more benefits from cochlear implants than do adults who have been deaf from birth or their early years. This may be due in part to physiological changes that occur in the auditory neurological system when it no longer receives input (Ponton, Moore, & Eggermont, 1999).

It has been reported that duration of deafness is an important factor affecting the progress children, as well as adults, make with cochlear implants (e.g., Dowell, Blamey, & Clark, 1997, Tomblin et al., 1999). However, others (e.g., Barker et al., 2000) have found that duration of deafness does not significantly predict progress of *prelingually* deaf children with a cochlear implant after age at implantation is taken into account. In fact, for children who are born profoundly deaf, duration of deafness before receiving a cochlear implant will be the same as the age at which the child is implanted. This is one reason that many clinicians and researchers believe that earlier implantation allows better results for these children.

Another reason that age at implantation is thought to influence speech and language growth is related to the concept of a "sensitive" or "critical" period for language development during the first few years of life. It is widely accepted by professionals in language development that language is learned more rapidly and easily during the first 3 to 5 years of life than afterward. This has been supported by studies of bilingual hearing children, in that a second language can be learned more completely if it is acquired early in life (e.g., Johnson & Newport, 1989; Patkowski, 1980). It has also been supported by studies of the acquisition of American Sign Language (ASL), in which it has been noted that early experience with sign language is critical for natural and complete learning (Morford & Mayberry, 2000). In a brief review of the literature on age effects for learning ASL, Morford and Mayberry conclude: "When language exposure is delayed, even by as little as a few years, language processing deficits become apparent" (p. 113).

These deficits are found in the phonology and in the grammar of the language. (In contrast, vocabulary development does not seem to be strongly affected by age of acquisition, thus possibly explaining the fact that deaf children tend to perform better on tests of vocabulary than on grammar.) In addition, Morford and Mayberry report that early learning of a first language supports later learning of a second.

Studies of children with cochlear implants can shed light on the concept of a "critical" period early in life for access to and development of spoken language. Although it was initially thought that implantation before 2 years of age was not possible due to continuing growth of the skull and cochlea (Brown & Yaremko, 1991), it has now been shown that there is no greater risk for surgically related complications at this early age (e.g., Waltzman & Cohen, 1998). This has resulted in a wide age range at which children receive cochlear implants and has allowed researchers to make systematic comparisons among the progresses of children implanted at different ages.

Evidence across studies indicates that children implanted earlier in life have a greater chance of learning to use and benefit from the device. For example, Dowell et al. (1997) studied children who ranged from 1.9 to 19.9 years old at the time of implantation. They found that when deafness was congenital, early implantation ages predicted better speech perception progress. Similarly, Tye-Murray, L. Spencer, and Woodworth (1995) reported data on speech production skills of three groups of children implanted at different ages: between 2 and 4 years of age; between 5 and 8 years of age; and between 9 and 15 years of age. Initially, the older children had better speech production skills than the younger children. However, after two years with a cochlear implant, the younger children matched the older children's skills. This indicates that the children implanted at a younger age made faster progress than those who were older when implanted. This result is consistent with a report by Nikolopoulos, O'Donoghue, and Archbold (1999), who found that, in a group of 126 children, the older children initially tested better than the younger children on both speech perception and production. However, after three or four years of implant use, the children who were younger at implantation outperformed the older children.

Barker et al. (2000) compared speech production of 10 children implanted even earlier—before 2 years of age—with that of seven children implanted between the ages of 4 and 6 years. After at least four years of cochlear implant use, the two groups of children produced isolated speech sounds with about the same level of correctness. However, the group implanted before 2 years was better at producing speech sounds as part of intelligible language instead of just as isolated sounds. The researchers concluded that implantation before the age of 4 leads to better speech production outcomes. Similar results have been reported by Waltzman and Cohen (1998) for children implanted before the age of 2 years. Cheng, Grant, and Niparko (1999) conducted a "meta-analysis" in which they compared results across many published papers that focused on children's development of speech perception skills using cochlear implants. They concluded that the results of those studies supported the idea that earlier age at implantation leads to more rapid increases in speech perception skills for congenitally deaf children.

These and most other reports indicate an advantage for groups of congenitally deaf children who receive cochlear implants early in life, compared with those who receive implants later. However, it is important to emphasize that age at implantation does not always predict the outcome for an individual child. This is shown by the wide range of functioning within the younger as well as older groups reported in the studies summarized previously, with frequent indications of overlap among the groups. In addition, some researchers have presented data showing that many older children can also benefit from cochlear implantation. For example, Osberger, Fisher, Zimmerman-Phillips, Geier, and Barker (1998) assessed speech perception of 30 children who received an implant after 5 years of age. They found that cochlear implants provided more access to spoken language than conventional hearing aids even for this older group of children. Gary and Hughes (2000) also presented data indicating benefits in a group of children who obtained implants between 8 and 14 years of age. Some of these children showed increased rates of improvement in receptive and expressive language skills, including speech intelligibility and ease of communicating orally.

Thus, overall, research results fail to demonstrate any specific age during childhood beyond which a cochlear implant cannot provide increased support for development of speech perception and production. As Dowell et al. (1997) concluded regarding speech perception: " . . . a child who has a congenital profound hearing loss or is deafened early in life will have a much better chance of learning to understand speech if . . . implanted as young as possible. [However] the results do not suggest that there is a crucial age, beyond which implantation is not useful, but that the chances of developing good open-set speech perception decrease with age . . . . " (p. 301).

The studies summarized here focused on age at implantation and addressed speech perception and production, not language skills. However, associations previously found among these areas suggest that findings about age of implantation will also be reflected in achievements in vocabulary and grammar. Overall, the data related to development of children with cochlear implants support a hypothesis that language is learned easier and more completely when it is learned early (e.g., Tait, Lutman, & Robinson, 2000). At least prior to adolescence, the ease of language learning seems to decrease in a gradual way, with no absolute "cut-off" age beyond which increased input will not support language growth. Furthermore, age at implantation alone does not reliably predict an individual child's outcome with a cochlear implant. Other factors must also play important roles.

Language Modality

The kind of language program (signed or oral/auditory-verbal) in which children participate has also been proposed to influence speech perception, speech production, and spoken language skills after cochlear implantation. However, reports comparing the development of children who are in different types of language programs typically consider the program to be a *cause* of the rate of progress with a cochlear implant. It is often forgotten that program placement may be a *result* of children's sensitivity to auditory information—both before and after cochlear implantation (A. R. Lederberg, personal communication, November 2000). In fact, some researchers have indicated that a number of children move from one kind of program to another during a study (e.g., P. Spencer, 2000b, 2000c; Tomblin et al., 1999). And the movement occurs in both directions—from oral/auditory-verbal to signing programs and vice versa. Both the selective placement of children in different language program types and the frequent movement from one to another program need to be kept in mind when studies of "effects" of language modality are interpreted.

Concerns about the type of language modality used in programming stem from the observation that children require large amounts of exposure to auditory language after implantation to learn to use information received through the implant. This has led to concern that, especially given the incomplete "picket fence" nature of auditory information provided by implants, children will focus predominately or exclusively on visual language input if it is available. The results of a number of studies appear to support this concern, reporting that children in Total or Simultaneous Communication programs make less (or perhaps slower) progress in speech and spoken language skills after implantation than do children in oral or auditory-verbal programs: On average, children from oral or auditory-verbal programs have been reported to show faster gains than those in Total Communication programs on speech intelligibility (Geers et al., 2000b; Osberger et al., 1994), on speech perception or recognition (Geers et al., 2000b; Hodges, Ash, Balkany, Schloffman, & Butts, 1999), and on language (Gary & Hughes, 2000; Geers et al., 2000b; Osberger et al., 1998). However, this apparent advantage for oral/auditory-verbal children is only relative: Children using implants who are in signing programs also show advantages when compared with deaf children not using implants. As a group, children with cochlear implants (regardless of program type) have been reported to increase speech perception, production, and spoken language skills at a faster rate than is typical without implants (Osberger et al., 1998; Svirsky et al., 2000; Tomblin et al., 1999).

In fact, some researchers have *not* found language advantages for children in oral/auditory-verbal programs. For example, Svirsky et al. (2000) compared language skills of children with implants in oral programs and programs using signs, and found no difference between the groups when signed as well as spoken language was considered. However, the orally trained children had more intelligible speech and therefore expressed their language skills more effectively in that mode than did the children who used signs.

Connor, Hieber, Arts, and Zwolan (2000) presented results of a well-controlled study in which a primary goal was to determine the influence of type of language programming on the children's language growth, speech production, receptive vocabulary (oral), and expressive vocabulary (oral and/or signed). This study included 147 children with cochlear implants: 66 were in programs using signs (primarily Simultaneous Communication programs) and 81 were in oral programs (including auditory-verbal). The children received their implants between the ages of 1 and 10 years and had used them for lengths of time between six months and 10 years. The children had been in one or the other type of language program (oral or signing) for at least three years; children who switched programs were excluded from the study. (This means, unfortunately, that children who had been deemed to need to switch programs were not included in the study; however, it ensures that children included in the study had time to benefit from the program in which they were participating.) The researchers collected data from the children at several points over time and calculated "growth curves" for the three skills assessed. In determining effects of language modality on growth, they controlled for effects of hearing experience before implantation, age of implantation, the type of implant device and processing strategy used, and whether electrodes had been fully or partially inserted in the cochlea. Age at time of testing, as well as length of time using the implant, was also controlled.

The outcome of this study provides additional support for effects of age of implantation on subsequent speech and language development. Children implanted before 5 years of age performed, on average, better than those implanted later. In addition, effects were found for the type (modality) of language programming. However, those effects were not simple: Outcomes with the implants depended on the type of language programming *in combination* with other variables. For example, the type of language programming did *not* seem to affect gains in speech production (production of consonant sounds) for children who received implants during the preschool years. However, if the implants were received during elementary school years, children in oral programs made more gains than those in signing programs. Age also combined with type of language programming to influence receptive vocabulary scores. Even though receptive vocabulary was assessed using oral language (without signs), children in signing programs performed significantly *better* than those in oral programs if implants were obtained during the preschool years. Neither group showed an advantage, however, if the implants were received at later ages. Finally, children in signing programs performed better than those in oral programs on expressive vocabulary (using their choice of modes for responses) if implants were received during either preschool or early elementary years. Connor et al. (2000) conclude that cochlear implants increase speech and language skills, regardless of the modality of language programming provided. They point out, however, that the programs using signs in their study also provided significant amounts of speech and oral language training. They also found that, as expected, outcomes were positively affected by having the complete electrode array inserted, by having some hearing sensitivity prior to implantation, and by using newer technologies for speech processing.

As the previous discussion illustrates, conclusions are mixed about the influence of language modality used with and by a child after cochlear implantation. Although a number of studies indicate an advantage for children in oral/auditory-verbal programs, recent well-designed studies have failed to find such an advantage. Other factors, such as age at implantation and the technology used in the implant, may interact with the language system used to influence speech and language development in complex ways.

All of the studies cited here compared effects of oral versus signing programs by focusing on children in Total or Simultaneous (signing plus speaking) Communication programs. It is not yet known how participation in a bilingual/bicultural ("bi-bi") program affects the amount of benefit from a cochlear implant. Most programs that use a bilingual approach to language development for young deaf children focus on written instead of oral representation for the language that is spoken by the hearing community. Such an approach might not provide sufficient exposure to spoken language to allow children to learn to use the implants. In fact, results presented for a small number of children participating in such a program using Swedish Sign Language and Swedish (primarily print) were discouraging (Preisler, Ahlstrom, & Tvingstedt, 1997). However, special speech training was provided for most of the Swedish children for only half an hour twice a week; so, it appears that overall exposure to spoken language was quite limited.

Evolving approaches to bilingual programming adapted for children with cochlear implants would provide more frequent, natural access to spoken language on a regular basis. Continuing trends for more and younger children to obtain cochlear implants (see chapter 1) will allow for further systematic observation of children's language development when signed and spoken language are presented separately. One issue to be addressed is the frequency and character of oral language input required to allow children to use information from cochlear implants effectively. Another important topic for research is whether attaining one language early (signed or spoken) has facilitative effects on learning a second language.

Other Factors

Even when considered in combination, the factors described here fail to explain sufficiently the individual differences in speech and language outcomes of children using cochlear implants. For example, Dowell et al. (1997), in a study of 52 children and adolescents implanted between the ages of 2 and 19, found that the duration of profound hearing loss, age of implantation, etiology and age of onset of hearing loss (i.e., whether hearing loss was congenital, caused by meningitis, or was progressive), experience with implant, and the type of language used in postoperative educational programming accounted for only about half of the variance (individual difference) in open-set speech perception. More recently, Blamey et al. (2001) accounted for 60% of the variance in speech perception scores of a group of 106 children by using a combination of factors, including hearing experience before implantation, vocabulary knowledge, and age of onset of profound hearing loss. Summarizing a similar analysis, Hodges et al. (1999) concluded " . . . the variation in speech perception . . . among implanted children cannot be explained by one or even several factors. Other more difficult to quantify factors such as family motivation, the child's own communication characteristics, different teacher and therapist effects, and learning styles probably contribute significantly as well" (p. 34). This is undoubtedly the case for speech production and spoken language as well as speech perception skills.

Factors currently being investigated include children's auditory experiences and skills before getting an implant, children's general cognitive and attention skills, and family characteristics related to providing an environment supportive of language development in general. In addition, integrity of the cochlear implant itself, the kind of speech processing strategy used, surgical factors such as the placement of electrodes in the cochlea, and factors related to function of the auditory system beyond the cochlea (e.g., the auditory nerve, as well as processes in the brain itself) probably impact individual progress made post-implant (Pyman, Blamey, Lacy, Clark, & Dowell, 2000). Given all of the factors that are suspected to influence the outcome of cochlear implants in children, it may never be possible to predict with mathematical certainty what the result will be for an individual child.

Individual Patterns of Outcomes With a Cochlear Implant

Information presented in this section of the chapter was obtained in Melbourne, Australia, where I had the opportunity to interview parents and assess the language skills of children who had received a cochlear implant by the age of 3 years. I was interested in patterns of language development after cochlear implantation and in child and family characteristics associated with those patterns. Although data were collected for 20 children and families, only 13 children were old enough to participate in the formal language testing described here. Despite this small number, and despite the fact that these families volunteered and therefore were not randomly selected, the group represented many of the characteristics of the population of children with hearing loss in Melbourne. They differed on many characteristics that have been posited to influence development of deaf children, including those with cochlear implants.

The children showed a wide range of nonverbal cognitive problem-solving skills. Eight of the children attained Leiter "Brief IQ" scores greater than 90 (in the average or above average range), and the other five obtained scores between 70 and 90. About half of the children were in oral or auditory-verbal programs; the others were in Total Communication or bilingual Australian Sign Language (Auslan) and English programs. At the time they were assessed for this study, the children ranged in age from 3 to almost 8 years of age. They had received multichannel cochlear implants between the ages of 13 and 38 months. All but one child (who had meningitis and was implanted at 32 months) had used the implants for at least two years. Seven of the children were girls and six were boys. Four of the children had delays in motor skills, slightly below average nonverbal cognitive skills, or suspected learning disabilities. Eleven of the children had profound hearing loss from birth; the child who had meningitis had a profound loss subsequent to the illness. The child implanted at 38 months of age had a less than profound hearing loss and had begun to use some spoken language before getting the implant.

Most of the children's parents had the equivalent of a high school or high school plus vocational training educational level; but, in several families, the parents had attended or graduated from a university. There were several single parent (female-headed) families. Diverse ethnic and cultural groups were represented, including Asian, Middle Eastern, and Southern and Northern European. Several parents had immigrated to Australia during childhood or young adult years.

Data on children's receptive vocabulary were obtained using the PPVT-IIIb. Grammar skills were assessed with the CELF preschool edition.[3] The language method used in the child's class-room was used for administering the tests. A speech teacher at one school and an aide at another helped to administer the tests in Australian Signed English or Auslan signs using English word order for children in signing programs. The PPVT was administered a second time, using voice only, to children who were in signing programs so that their performance with and without sign support could be compared. In addition, parents were interviewed about their children's language development.

To accommodate age differences, scale scores were used for PPVT performance, and a "percent of age" score was calculated on the CELF. PPVT scale scores ranged from 40 (extremely low) to 96 (average), with a mean of 71. CELF scores ranged from 35% to 75% of that expected for age, with a mean of 50% (excluding one child who was unable to respond to this test). The PPVT scores of all but one of the children in programs using signed language dropped precipitously when the test was administered using voice only.

Vocabulary performance of this group of 13 young children is consistent with results reported earlier by Blamey et al. (1998) for somewhat older children. The finding that vocabulary performance exceeded performance on the expressive and receptive language instrument (CELF) that included grammar skills was also consistent with earlier reports. The following profiles for individual children illustrate in more detail some of the

3. As noted earlier in this chapter, PPVT is the Peabody Picture Vocabulary Test and CELF is the Clinical Evaluation of Language Fundamentals test.

characteristics that are thought to impact on performance with a cochlear implant. (Children's names have been changed to protect their identity.)

Jimmy and Barbara

These two children scored consistently higher than the other children on both vocabulary and grammar assessments. They had several characteristics in common: Both had parents who had university degrees; both children had cognitive skills in the average range or above; both were in oral programming. Most importantly, these two children had developed some spoken language skills before getting a cochlear implant. Despite these similarities, their stories are quite different.

Jimmy was born hearing and was already talking in short sentences when he developed meningitis at the age of 2. As he was recovering from his illness, his family noticed that he no longer responded to sounds. He had continued to talk; however, his utterances became shorter as time went on. A diagnosis of profound hearing loss was soon obtained, after which an itinerant teacher of the deaf visited the family. According to Jimmy's parents, the teacher presented them with few options, and apparently made a strong case for the use of sign language before the parents had a chance to adjust to the diagnosis of hearing loss and all that it implied.

After an unsuccessful trial with hearing aids (which Jimmy resisted), and a visit to another family whose child had already gotten a cochlear implant, the family decided to get an implant for Jimmy. It was important that the implant not be delayed for long because meningitis can cause ossification (growth of spongy or bony tissue) in the canals of the cochlea that can interfere with implanting the electrodes. Within months, Jimmy had his cochlear implant. The surgery was without complication. However, Jimmy showed no sign of hearing any sounds until 3 weeks after the implant had been turned on and tuned. At that time, he turned around when his mother said his name and then he imitated her. After that, his spoken language skills began to return. Jimmy, at the age of about 4, scored on the PPVT within the range expected for typical hearing children. His scores on the CELF, which primarily assesses grammatical skills, were approximately 1 year below his age. He understood and produced basic English sentence structures and was very accurate with word order in sentences. He knew many words for important concepts and used grammatical morphemes to express plurals and some verb tenses correctly. However, more complex grammar was difficult for him.

Jimmy's pattern of development is a bit different from that of many children who get meningitis. First, his spoken language was advanced for his age before he became ill. Second, unlike many children who become deaf from meningitis, Jimmy never stopped talking after he lost his hearing. Both of these characteristics suggest that Jimmy is "language oriented" and has innate strength in that area. It can be predicted that Jimmy's language skills will continue to develop well, although it is not clear whether he will be able to function in a regular classroom without some kind of special assistance. Even in a small group setting, he must occasionally ask for repetition, and he does better when he can see (and speechread) the speaker in addition to listening.

Barbara was a bit over 5 years old when she was assessed. Like Jimmy, Barbara's score on the vocabulary measure was within the normal range for a typical hearing child of her age. Again, her score on the test that required knowledge of grammar was somewhat lower. Barbara was born with a hearing loss in the severe-to-profound range. Because she has an older sibling who has a cochlear implant, her parents were knowledgeable about the devices and believed that an implant would provide more assistance to Barbara than just a hearing aid. Despite the fact that Barbara benefited from her hearing aid and was beginning to talk, she was given an implant at the age of 38 months.

Barbara was shy, and it took some time and sensitive support from her mother and teacher before she was comfortable with the testing. However, she clearly enjoyed using spoken language and eventually enjoyed the assessment tasks. Despite her below-age score on the test involving grammar, she displayed very strong skills in that area for a child with a hearing loss. Like Jimmy, she was strong in the kinds of skills (word order, sentence structure, plurals, simple verb tenses) that develop earliest in hearing children. She showed relative weakness in more complicated grammatical usage, such as complex verb tenses (third person singular, future tense) and sentence structures (passive) that typically develop later.

Barbara was participating in a program in a school designed for deaf children that integrates deaf and hearing children in the classrooms. It is clear that her parents hope that she will be able to attend school in a regular classroom as she grows older. It is not clear to what degree using the cochlear implant has accelerated Barbara's language skills. However, given the delays in language typical even for children with mild to moderate hearing loss (Davis, Elfenbein, Schum, & Bentler, 1986), Barbara's skills are impressive.

Most of the time, I could understand these children's spoken language. Most of the time, they could understand me when I used an appropriate level of language. Given their personal and family strengths, it is probable that these two children would be successful in any kind of program for deaf children, regardless of the language or the language modality used.

Ginny

Like Jimmy and Barbara, Ginny and her family have many strengths to use to assist her language learning. Although Ginny's parents are separated, extended family members live with her and her mother and provide significant support. Also in common with the other two children, Ginny has cognitive skills in at least the average range.

Ginny differs from the other two children in that her hearing loss is both congenital and profound. Her language history is complicated in part because her family is originally from Asia, and English is not her mother's first language. In addition, Ginny has moved from one kind of language program to another. I originally thought that Ginny had always been in oral programming, but discovered when I interviewed her mother that she had, in fact, been in a signing classroom until the most recent school year. Although Ginny and her mother communicated clearly in spoken language while I observed, her mother also occasionally used signs. She explained that before and after the cochlear implant, she felt that signs had been necessary for clear communication with her daughter. Only after Ginny showed evidence that she was hearing and understanding spoken language with the implant did her mother agree to move her to an oral-only classroom. Her mother and teacher judged that Ginny was successful in the oral classroom, and she was using speech more since moving to that classroom. Recently, Ginny had demonstrated that she was beginning to understand her mother and grandmother's first language in addition to English.

Almost 5 years old when she was assessed for the study, Ginny had gotten a cochlear implant before she was 2 years old. Because I was unaware of her history using sign language, Ginny was assessed using oral language only. Her score on the PPVT showed vocabulary skills at the borderline between average and moderately low when compared with hearing children her own age. Her score on the CELF showed more delayed skills, indicating functioning at about 2 years below her actual age.   Although she knew many words for important concepts and had good knowledge of sentence structure and word order for English, Ginny was only beginning to understand and use words and morphemes to indicate pronouns, verb tenses, and other grammatical markers.

During the assessment, Ginny spontaneously used spoken English. Some of her utterances included: *I pour full. What's that in that? Two little shoes. My brother tall. I, uh, computer with my brother.* Despite her delay in spoken language compared with hearing children, she had made excellent progress compared with most children who are deaf.

Peter

Peter was a bit more than 7 years old when he was assessed. He has a congenital profound hearing loss, and although his family is supportive and he attends a highly regarded school, his progress has been slower than that of the first three children discussed. Peter received his cochlear implant at a bit over 2 years of age. Although he had started his schooling in an oral-only program, lack of progress in oral language led to his moving to a Total Communication program. I was able to understand some of Peter's spoken utterances, and he obviously understood some of mine. However, signing significantly increased ease of communication.

Peter seemed to have problems both attending to and making sense of the auditory input that his cochlear implant provided. In fact, his attention skills were less consistent than expected for his age even during nonverbal tasks. Although he performed at age-appropriate levels on nonverbal cognitive tasks involving matching and figure-ground discrimination, he had problems with tasks that involved sequencing and predicting patterns, even for visual material. On the vocabulary assessment, Peter scored significantly below age level when it was administered using Simultaneous Communication. His performance decreased even more when the test was given using oral language only. His performance on the CELF was more delayed than that on the vocabulary test, and he scored at less than half his age compared with hearing children. Although he had good understanding of word order, he had much difficulty using the grammatical words and morphemes of English. This was the case even when they were represented visually.

Peter shows a profile of skills that would predict language delays even for a hearing child. Although the cochlear implant allows him to detect sound and to understand some oral language, he continues to face significant language learning problems.

Liz

Liz was born with a profound hearing loss and some mild motor disabilities. Her mother reported difficulties obtaining a diagnosis of Liz's hearing loss, and feels that she had to be quite assertive to ensure that Liz would be in a signing program before and after getting her cochlear implant at the age of 2. At the time she was assessed, Liz was in a bilingual classroom that included both a deaf and a hearing teacher. During her assessment, at about 5 years of age, Liz depended primarily on signed language. However, both her teacher and her mother report that she can speak intelligibly, albeit with immature speech sound patterns and sentence structures. When tested using signed language plus speech, Liz scored just slightly below the average range for age on the vocabulary test. This matched her performance on nonverbal cognitive tasks. When tested using oral language only, her vocabulary score dropped significantly; however, she still recognized many words. Her performance on the CELF was significantly lower than on the vocabulary measure. In addition, the difference between the two tests was greater for her than for most of the other children. She was not able to understand or to use many English grammatical words and morphemes, whether using signs or speech.

Amber and Philip

Both Amber and Philip have congenital profound hearing losses. Both also have evidence of significant developmental difficulties. One child has a neurological anomaly that is expected to slow learning in general; the other had very delayed development of motor and other skills related to overall functioning levels. These children's parents and the professionals who have worked with them felt that it was important to give them cochlear implants in hopes that they would learn to process auditory language and therefore have more ways to compensate for their other difficulties. Amber was 5 years old when assessed and had received a cochlear implant at age 2. Philip was almost 6 years old when assessed and had received an implant before he was 2 years old.

Both of these children performed in the below average range on the cognitive tasks. However, Amber performed much better on the language tasks than Philip did. Amber's scores were significantly below that expected for a hearing child her age, with the expected pattern of vocabulary scores higher than grammar. Philip was unable to provide enough answers to permit scoring of either test.

Neither child expressed or seemed to understand spoken language. However, Amber was in a program using signed language, whereas Philip continued in an oral program. Of course, it would not be right to claim that Amber's better performance was solely because of her exposure to signed language. However, Philip had not had the opportunity to develop language using signs up until the time of this assessment. Recently, at home and at school, some signing was being introduced. It was too early to determine how effective that might be.

Summary

The cases presented here reflect individual patterns of progress that may be obscured in studies focused on group trends or averages. Cochlear implants allowed some of the children to acquire spoken language skills at near average levels expected for same-age hearing children. More success was experienced by children who had the ability to process some auditory information prior to getting a cochlear implant, and higher levels of nonverbal cognitive skills were associated with higher language skills. When the children who had some hearing experience before getting the implant were removed from the group, younger age at implantation was related to better language performance. This was true even though the range of age at implantation in this study was quite restricted, with all the congenitally profoundly deaf children receiving implants before the age of 3. Participation in an oral language program seemed to be associated with better spoken language. However, a closer look disclosed that children with higher cognitive skills and from more educated families were overrepresented in the oral programs. In addition, one "oral" child was found to use signed language at home and had moved to an oral program only in the most recent school year. One "signing" child had only recently moved to that program after years in an oral program. It was not possible, therefore, to determine any association between type of language program and spoken language progress in this group. It is possible that these kinds of complications confuse the results of many efforts to evaluate the effects of language program on spoken language outcomes with a cochlear implant.

Conclusions

Easterbrooks and Mordica (2000), reporting on teachers' perceptions of the performance of children with cochlear implants, summed up their view of the effects of cochlear implants this way: "If the greatest hope of conventional wisdom is that the implant will be a bionic ear, curing deafness, and if the worst fear is that implants will eliminate Deaf culture altogether, then implants are a resounding failure, as neither scenario has resulted" (p. 55).

This quote exemplifies one inference to be drawn from the studies summarized in this chapter: Despite the benefits provided to many children, cochlear implants do not provide a "quick fix" for the language development challenges faced by deaf children and their parents. Although cochlear implants seem to help very profoundly deaf children, on average, function more like hard-of-hearing children, the results are highly variable. Some children show no discernible benefits, whereas others come to function almost like hearing children. Two conclusions can be drawn from data now available: (1) Many children have acquired language through use of cochlear implants. That is, cochlear implants allow a significant portion of very profoundly deaf children, who would not otherwise have been expected to be able to hear or produce spoken language, to do so. (2) Cochlear implants do not, on average, provide enough benefit to allow a child born profoundly deaf to learn spoken language as easily or as quickly as is typical for a hearing child.

In general, the prognosis for oral language skills is best for a child with the following characteristics: (1) a short time between the onset of deafness (or birth, if the deafness is congenital) and implantation; (2) ability to benefit to some degree from a conventional hearing aid in the time between onset of deafness and implantation; (3) at least average cognitive skills for age and (probably) good attention skills; and (4) home and school environments that provide extensive exposure to spoken language. Of course, there are exceptions, with some children who would be expected to do well failing to receive benefits from the implants and others who have a less positive prognosis actually receiving useful input from the implants. As the technology of the implants continues to improve, and as data become available from very young children who have received implants, the incidence of positive results is expected to increase.

However, it is important that guidelines be developed to identify children who are not benefiting from cochlear implants while they are still young enough to acquire language through other means. Even if there is no specific early "critical period" during which language must develop or be forever lost, the overall cognitive and psychosocial development of children will be negatively affected if they do not have access to a shared language system with which to communicate with family members, other children, and other adults during their early years.

Tait et al. (2000) recently reported that some of the individual difference in outcomes with a cochlear implant can be predicted from young children's preverbal communication skills prior to or soon after receiving an implant. Children who were most likely to make original contributions to a communicative interaction at the preverbal level were also the most likely to have good speech perception and production skills three years after implantation. In addition, these researchers reported that children who receive significant input from cochlear implants show this by changing from mostly gestural preverbal communications to mostly oral preverbal communication signals within a year of getting the implant. Thus, they suggested that early pre-language behaviors can predict children's outcomes. More information of this kind can help parents and service providers identify early the children who need more or different kinds of support for language development and to feel more confident about those who appear to be making good use of input from a cochlear implant.

PART

III

Current Issues

The Deaf Community: Perceptions of Parents, Young People, and Professionals

"In an ironic twist, a medical device is being rejected by many members of the community it was ostensibly designed to serve."

(Clay, 1997, p. 1)

Despite the barrage of publicity outlining the intense negative reaction of many in the deaf community to cochlear implants, pediatric implantation has continued to increase exponentially. As noted in chapter 1, well over 35,000 people the world over have received the implant, and about half of those are children under the age of 18. This is clear evidence that many parents are *not* listening to opponents of pediatric implantation who caution the public regarding the alleged lack of information on long-term social, psychological, technological, or medical implications. To better understand this phenomenon, we asked the parents we interviewed for their reactions to statements and opinions expressed by the deaf community and whether or not they had any contact with deaf people during the decision-making process.

Additionally, we report on interviews with deaf adolescents and young adults who have had both positive and negative experiences with cochlear implants. In those interviews, we inquired about their relationships with the deaf community. We also met with several administrators of schools for deaf students, several psychologists, and with prominent deaf community members to solicit their observations of the cochlear implant debate. Finally, we include results from a survey of opinions on the cochlear implant that was distributed to a small sample of Gallaudet University faculty, staff, students, and alumni. Although Gallaudet University is often viewed as an institution that speaks on behalf of the deaf community, its official position is that it does not speak on behalf of everyone who is deaf (Byrd, 1999). Gallaudet University's viewpoint is that it is a university whose mission is to welcome diversity and encourage critical scrutiny of the varied perspectives brought to bear on any issue, including that of cochlear implants. This is a mission not fully understood by many who perceive Gallaudet to be a bastion of the hardcore anti-implant community.

To put our findings in perspective, we first need to describe the deaf community, how it has evolved, and the reasons many of its members oppose pediatric implantation.

The Deaf Community

The process of adapting to life as a deaf person has often encouraged connections with the community of deaf people, based in large part on shared experiences, feelings of differences with the majority hearing society, and proximity to other deaf people. Current estimates are that of the approximately 28 million people in the United States who are deaf or hard-of-hearing, mostly due to age-related progressive hearing loss (National Institute on Deafness and Other Communication Disorders, 1996), over two million are deaf, and approximately 400,000 (Schein, 1989) or more may be connected to the deaf community. Those who identify as deaf usually have a severe or profound hearing loss (as opposed to a mild or moderate loss).

For many people within the deaf community, "deaf" is less about audiology than it is about life and culture (Brueggemann, 1999; Lane et al., 1996; Wrigley, 1996). Individuals who identify as culturally deaf (in contrast to audiologically deaf) perceive themselves as a linguistic minority group because of their use of American Sign Language (ASL), a visual language with its own grammar and syntax. Their visual orientation, which differs from the reliance on sound by those who hear or those who depend completely on aural amplification, has facilitated shared ways of behaving that reinforce the bond with the deaf community (Padden & Humphries, 1988). Consequently, many downgrade the importance of speech and hearing aids. They see themselves as possessing none of the negatively toned characteristics that accompany the term "disability" as it pertains to deafness, such as linguistic deprivation, powerlessness, incompetence, and deviation from a norm that focuses on "hearing" as an essential characteristic (Davis, 1995; Olkin, 1999). Instead, these individuals identify themselves as a normal part of the spectrum of human diversity that exists throughout the world. The rationale for their objection to the use of the phrase *hearing-impaired* is that it emphasizes disabled functioning in the guise of broken ears that need fixing rather than an achieved way of functioning in daily life.

What is often overlooked is the fact that the deaf community in the United States and elsewhere is not a homogeneous entity. Rather, it reflects social, political, cultural, linguistic, religious, regional, racial, ethnic, and especially communicative variations (Corker, 1994; Humphries, 1993; Lane et al., 1996; Leigh & Lewis, 1999; Padden, 1980; Rosen, 1986; B. Tucker, 1998a). As Nancy Bloch, Executive Director of the National Association of the Deaf (NAD), unequivocally states, many in the deaf community "wear hearing aids, converse in sign language, enjoy listening to music, talk on the telephone, order food in restaurants, and interact daily with hearing persons" (Bloch, 1999, p. 5). An exploration of major deaf community publications reveals a wide range of opinions expressed by deaf community members on any one issue. Even the issue of whether a deaf culture exists is not sacrosanct. In 1992, Larry Stewart (a deaf professional well known for his outspoken advocacy for deaf children, their parents, and the deaf community) wrote that the phrase "deaf culture" was developed for political purposes and to deny deafness as a disability was nonsensical (Stewart, 1992). Many members of the deaf community do acknowledge that they have a disability, i.e., deafness (Solomon, 1994; B. Tucker, 1998a). They frequently miss out on, for example, airport announcements and other forms of spoken dialogue.

The existence of differences within the deaf community flies in the face of the typical assumption made by many writers that the deaf community has only one "collective" voice (e.g., Nevins & Chute, 1996). Although this assumption clearly is wrong, many people, both hearing and deaf, nevertheless view the deaf community as having one voice. The question then becomes, why has this one voice become so prominent?

Humphries (1993) describes this phenomenon as emerging out of the frustrations many deaf persons have experienced of being dominated by the greater hearing society. It goes without saying that to be deaf is often to be viewed as less intelligent, or less capable than might otherwise be the case because of limitations in communication, whether oral or signed (Biderman, 1998; B. Tucker, 1998a). The 1988 Deaf President Now movement (which culminated in the appointment of the first deaf president at Gallaudet University) reflects a visceral collective reaction to this negative perception and a concerted effort to demonstrate its fallacy (Christiansen & Barnartt, 1995; Gannon, 1989). This "voice of the deaf community" has come to symbolize the struggle by deaf people to control the direction of their lives, to control how they are portrayed by the media and within educational settings, and to have a stronger say in how deaf children should be raised. The fundamental rationale is that deaf people themselves are the experts, having experienced growing up deaf. This collective voice is now being tested by the emergence of cochlear implants, a technological development that many in the deaf community have up until now seen as the antithesis to their lives as healthy, well-adjusted deaf persons. This development has engendered a struggle intense enough that at times families with hearing and deaf members can be emotionally torn apart by the cochlear implant issue.

Initial Reactions to the Cochlear Implant

When cochlear implants emerged on the scene, a vocal part of the deaf community took a hard-line stand against pediatric implants. The targets of the protest were the medical establishment, the media, and parents who were considering cochlear implants for their deaf children. Ancillary to this protest, adult deaf persons who chose the implant were seen as beyond the pale and therefore ostracized because of their so-called desire to be "hearing." Implantation was interpreted to be a rejection of deaf cultural values that incorporate pride in being deaf (Markon, 1998), even if the implanted individuals continued to sign.

Beginning in the 1980s, national organizations of the deaf in different parts of the world, as well as the World Federation of the Deaf, went on record as staunch opponents of pediatric cochlear implants because of the inadequacy of information on social and psychological implications, as well as long-term medical consequences, for young deaf children (Andersson, 1994; Bloch, 1999; Lane et al., 1996). In the United States, the NAD position paper ("Cochlear Implants in Children," 1991), written by Harlan Lane, a hearing spokesperson, deplored the decision of the Food and Drug Administration (FDA) to approve pediatric cochlear implantation as "invasive surgery upon defenseless children, when the long-term physical, emotional and social impacts on children from this irreversible procedure—which will alter the lives of these children—have not been scientifically established" (p. 1). There was concern that parents were poorly informed about alternate options, as well as risks related to pediatric implantation. Additionally, concern was expressed that parent commitment to aural/oral training meant a delay of the family's acceptance of the child's deafness and use of sign communication.

In the early 1990s, protests against pediatric implants took place in Australia, Canada, and Europe (Gibson, 1991; Lane et al., 1996; Montgomery, 1991; "Demonstrations Against Childhood Implants," 1994). Leading advocates for the deaf claimed it was "brutal to open a child's skull and wind wires through the inner ear, or cochlea, just to rob that child of a birthright of silence" (Barringer, 1993, p. 1). Deaf community publications published cartoons lambasting hearing "oppressors" who forced their methods on powerless deaf children (Barringer, 1993). There were cries of cultural genocide and comparisons to Nazi-like medical experiments (Niparko, 2000b; Solomon, 1994). One deaf community member even found her tires slashed after she refused to speak out against the cochlear implant (Yaffe, 1999). Examples such as these served to reinforce the general public perception that the deaf community was extremist in nature, relying as it did on inflammatory, even inaccurate portrayals, to get their points across.

As recently as 1997, Nancy Bloch of the NAD testified before the FDA that: "Oftentimes implants on children may be performed for the wrong reasons. Often parents want their child to be hearing and see this implant as the 'magic' answer. . . . Cochlear implantation for use on children two to seventeen years remains a questionable procedure, without sufficient scientific basis. Furthermore, procedural, longitudinal, and bioethical issues remain unexplored" ("Testimony Before the FDA," 1997, p. 6). The FDA subsequently proceeded to approve a new cochlear implant device for use in children. However, an article in the *NAD Broadcaster* reported that, in contrast to previous FDA panels, the panel members appeared more amenable to considering the different perspectives, and the need for more rigorous data, that were suggested in the testimony provided by the NAD and other deaf community representatives ("Testimony Before the FDA," 1997). This reflects a concerted effort by the organized deaf community to be heard, and to be perceived as rational and reasonable, rather than as an angry, irrational, and unreasonable group of people who were rejecting pediatric implants out of hand.

Barbara Brauer (personal communication, May 9, 2000) and Allen Sussman (personal communication, May 9, 2000), Maryland psychologists who are deaf and faculty members at Gallaudet University, believe that the anger demonstrated by many in the deaf community comes not necessarily from the expressed fear that the culture of deaf people will disappear, but rather from the tendency of many medical personnel (including FDA panel members, as well as professionals at cochlear implant centers), the media, and hearing parents of deaf children to focus on the cochlear implant as a way to enhance the quality of life, as if deaf people's lives were inherently lacking and unfulfilled without the implant. According to Brauer and Sussman, the result has been a mindset, at least until now, in which the dissenting viewpoints of deaf people who are concerned about potentially adverse long-term medical and psychosocial implications have been deemed inconsequential in the process of evaluating the effectiveness of the cochlear implant. The NAD's 1991 position paper opposing pediatric implants can be seen as a protest against this mind-set. It states that the "FDA's failure to consult deaf spokespersons represents, if an oversight, gross ignorance concerning growing up deaf in America, or, if willful, an offense against fundamental American values of individual liberties, cultural diversity and consumer rights" (p. 1). Moreover, during the 1995 National Institutes of Health Consensus Development Conference on cochlear implants in adults and children (see chapter 1), there were no deaf organization representatives in the formal program. After the program went to press, a concerted effort resulted in the public comment session subsequently being extended to accommodate the requests of those who wished to offer opposing, as well as supporting, perspectives, including representatives of national organizations of deaf people.

Cochlear implant centers throughout the country, such as The Listening Center at Johns Hopkins University (Baltimore) and The Cochlear Implant Center at Lenox Hill Hospital (New York City), as well as at least one cochlear implant manufacturer, have in the past several years begun to disseminate information about the deaf community in response to requests that all alternatives regarding language, amplification, and communication be presented to parents. The parents we interviewed confirm this. However, Bienenstock's (1998/1999) series of interviews with professionals and parents of children with pediatric implants in Texas indicated that the deaf community was "not even considered a significant factor by the implant team" (p. 15).

There are ongoing complaints that the media tend to misrepresent, ignore, or minimize viewpoints of representatives from the deaf community (Bloch, 1999; Brauer, 1993; "Debate Continues," 1997; J. Tucker, 1996, 1999). Basically, the media tends to glorify one side, specifically the cochlear implant as a "miracle cure" for the "tragedy" of deafness, which reinforces the perception that the lack of sound destroys the lives of deaf people. This continues despite the current lack of research data on long-term linguistic and psychological effectiveness, and ignores the numerous accomplishments of many deaf nonimplant users.

Solomon (1994) acknowledges that the media have portrayed the NAD as propagandizing the danger of cochlear implants in an alarmist and inaccurate fashion. Many deaf people report that vital points regarding opposition to pediatric implants—including the unhappiness of many older implanted children and deaf adults, the existence of deaf culture and of a vibrant language (ASL), and the value of deafness as contributing to a diversity to be cherished rather than fixed and erased—have been deleted from their interviews with print and broadcast journalists (Rosen, 1992; B. Stewart, personal communication, April 3, 2000). Additionally, Dale Atkins (personal communication, March 30, 2000), a New York City psychologist who works with oral cochlear-implanted children and their families, expresses serious concern about misleading perspectives generated by several promotional films covering hearing and speech for deaf children, which tend to show cases reinforcing the idea that the implant will restore full hearing, a fallacy naive parents may latch on to. Clearly, exceptions notwithstanding, many people in the deaf community feel maligned by media distortions emphasizing limitations in the lives of deaf people and focusing on the cochlear implant debate in simplistic oppositional perspectives without sufficiently portraying the diversity of opinions expressed by various deaf people.

Concerning parents, Alec Naiman (personal communication, April 2, 2000), a Nassau Community College (New York) professor who is at home in the deaf community, comments that:

> Parents assume that we don't want to walk on the bridge to
> them. Many of us do want the access to the hearing world. It
> is not that we don't want the access, as mistakenly perceived.
> Parents assume that deaf culture is substandard to their culture
> and we are resisting something better. Maybe our deaf culture
> is just as good, but they don't get it. What worries me is that
> we don't know the long-term implications. Parents are too
> eager. The cochlear implant is really a parent issue, as parents
> are trying to deal with the fact their child is deaf. There is a
> difference and they are trying to eradicate that difference.
> They want to undo what they perceive to be the nightmare.

This observation reflects the tendency of many in the deaf community to comment that parents too quickly frame the cochlear implant as a means of dealing with the deafness, without approaching different deaf people themselves and evaluating how their lives are lived. Even if parents do so, their mindset, assumptions, and cultural backgrounds will generally predispose them to search out ways their deaf children can participate in the majority culture.

In sum, a number of people in the deaf community feel their views have been poorly or inaccurately represented. Many still see the procedure as highly experimental for children despite medical assurances to the contrary. They note the limitations of current studies on speech and language development in children with implants, which generally do not include those who have discontinued use of the implant and therefore potentially minimize the variability of results (see chapter 9). They question whether children with implants learn English (or any other spoken language) any better than they would with a hearing aid or no aid (Lane & Bahan, 1998a). They also feel that an implant will delay a deaf child's eventual acquisition of sign language and assimilation into the deaf community. They wonder why there is such an obsession with the sense of hearing in the development of the deaf child and why there is a perceived need to "fix" the deaf child's ears (Carver, 1990; Yaffe, 1999). They worry about long-term educational and mental health implications for some of the implantees, such as language delay, identity confusion, possible psychological trauma, and social difficulties (B. Stewart, personal communication, April 3, 2000; J. Tucker, 1996).

Winds of Change

However, winds of change are in the air. Advancing technology is changing the nature of the implant itself. Universal infant hearing screening, which is rapidly spreading across the United States, will lead to earlier diagnosis of deafness. In addition, the age for pediatric implantation is becoming increasingly younger to maximize auditory input and development of spoken language (Bykowski, 2000), even though results continue to reflect outcome variability. The number of pediatric implantees is rapidly increasing. Most likely, previous studies on performance with cochlear implants will be rendered obsolete as time goes on.

Although individuals like Phil Bravin, a nationally renowned leader in the deaf community and moderator for the video *Covering the Basics: Cochlear Implants* (2000), states that cochlear implants are not ready for "prime time" (personal communication, May 7, 2000), the deaf community is nonetheless beginning to face the reality that the cochlear implant (or some variant thereof) is here to stay, their protests and concerns notwithstanding. Sharon Applegate (personal communication, April 2, 2000), assistant executive director at the New York Society for the Deaf, notes that the deaf community is changing as more deaf people express curiosity about the implant. She now has close friends who have undergone the procedure, though she herself would not consider the procedure unless it more closely replicates normal hearing. A letter to the editor of a monthly deaf community newspaper, *Silent News* (Hill, 1999), titled "Confessions of a Burned-out Deafie," describes the author's denial of, and ultimate confrontation with, her frustrations as a deaf person who was tired of missing out on noncaptioned TV channels and first-run movies, tired of having to be aggressive just to make herself understood by store clerks instead of merely assertive, and tired of the inability to communicate freely within hearing family encounters. This encouraged her to explore the cochlear implant. As she wrote "Even though I am acquiring a CI, I will still consider myself to be deaf and a member of the deaf world. If my deaf friends should choose to abandon or exile me from their 'society,' then I am sorry that they should have to be so insecure that they feel threatened" (p. 4).

There are people like Myrna and Phil Aiello of Maryland who are comfortably ensconced within the deaf community and who cherish sign language. They were not tarred and feathered when they got their cochlear implants, although they did initially encounter some criticism. They are living evidence that deaf persons can be curious about what it is like to hear, get implanted, take pride as deaf community members, and take advantage of new technology (Byrd, 1999). As an example of the latter, one of the authors recently attended a party where signing implanted deaf adults compared notes about how to use cell phones with their cochlear implants![1]

At the 1998 NAD convention, a cochlear implant panel consisting of one deaf researcher and two signing individuals with cochlear implants drew a standing room only audience, and the majority of questions were technical in nature rather than confrontative (Leigh, Sullivan, Graham-Kelly, & Aiello, 1998). Branton Stewart (personal communication, April 3, 2000), a deaf activist who was a delegate to that convention, came to the recognition that the NAD was no longer interested in political-type moves against the cochlear implant when his anti-implant resolutions

---

1. One author, John Christiansen, recently got a cochlear implant himself and has received no criticism at all from students, colleagues, or deaf friends. In fact, almost everyone, deaf and hearing, has been very supportive. It should be noted that all of the research and writing for this book, except for final editing and proofreading, was completed before his implant was activated in April 2001.

were not supported. In the fall of 1998, the leaders of the NAD withdrew the 1991 position paper against pediatric cochlear implants because of adverse media portrayal, and what they described as the ethical and educational complexities of the issue (Bloch, 1999). An ad hoc cochlear implant committee—consisting of hearing and deaf parents of deaf children, deaf and hearing professionals from a variety of fields, including medicine, and consumers—was formed to develop a new position paper. During a cochlear implant workshop run by Phil and Myrna Aiello at the 2000 NAD Convention, implant issues were discussed by an interested audience (Aiello & Aiello, 2000). At this convention, Advanced Bionics Corporation, a cochlear implant company, had an exhibit of its products.

All of these activities were forerunners of the new NAD position statement on cochlear implants that was released in October 2000 (National Association of the Deaf, 2000b). Its primary focus is that of "preserving and promoting the psychosocial integrity of deaf and hard-of-hearing children and adults." This means, in part, that deafness is not to be denigrated or defined as a burden, nor that it needs to be "fixed" with cochlear implants. The current statement views cochlear implants as one of a multitude of options to be considered for the deaf child. Pediatric implantation is described as an option that must be thoroughly explored before a final decision is made by parents, and the right of parents to decide based on unbiased information from a variety of sources is emphasized.

The World Federation of the Deaf is also working on a new position paper (National Association of the Deaf, 2000a). Gallaudet University is now encouraging open discussion of cochlear implants and their place in education and the deaf community. Cochlear implant forums held at Gallaudet during 1999 and 2000 have focused on increased awareness and collaboration (Christiansen, 1999; Mahshie & Nussbaum, 2000). This reflects a change from 1993 when a cochlear implant forum was canceled due to potential student unrest on campus (Niparko, 1999).

Additionally, Gallaudet University has recently established a cochlear implant center at the Laurent Clerc National Deaf Education Center (which consists of preschool through high school programs). Jane Fernandes (2000a, 2000b), Gallaudet University provost, envisions this as an opportunity to develop strategies for educating children who rely on visual learning along with children who depend on auditory input. This is a critical issue for schools with sign language programs that are increasingly welcoming students with cochlear implants. Some, including the Maryland School for the Deaf (J. Tucker, personal communication, May 31, 2000), Lexington School for the Deaf in Queens, NY (O. Cohen, personal communication, April 3, 2000), and P.S. 47 in New York City (M. Florsheim, personal communication, April 4, 2000) have developed collaborative endeavors with centers that offer specialized services for students with implants.

All these changes, and more, have led Carol Padden, author of major writings on the deaf community and deaf culture, to comment on the need to write a new description of the deaf community in the face of technological innovation, as well as population diversity and migration (Padden & Rayman, 2000).

Parent Perceptions of the Deaf Community

Since the beginning of the cochlear implant controversy, parents of children with implants and the deaf community have had an uneasy coexistence. Although many in the deaf community have attempted to reach out to parents, such efforts have often backfired in the face of statements such as the following: "Deaf adults love Deaf kids; they know that most hearing parents make a botch of having a Deaf child—frequently they had hearing parents themselves" (Lane, 1993, p. 23). Comments such as these did not endear Harlan Lane, a Northeastern University professor who is widely perceived as a hearing spokesperson for the deaf community, to many parents of deaf children, even though he qualified his comments by adding that he wanted to spare parents from imposing needless suffering upon their child. His purported unwillingness to speak with implanted children or their parents (Arana-Ward, 1997) serves to reinforce the general parent impression of the deaf community as close-minded and not open to dialogue and mutual learning.

In a written debate on pediatric cochlear implants in *Hearing Health* magazine, Larry Fleischer, a prominent deaf community activist and professor of deaf studies at California State University at Northridge, concluded: "Somehow, the idea must be conveyed that human rights for deaf children, based on the wealth of the deaf experience, must supersede the notion of birthrights for deaf children born to hearing parents," whom he considered to be "ill-informed, ill-prepared, ill-advised, ill-founded, and ill-fated" (Fleischer, 1993, p. 23). In return, Rick Apicella, a hearing parent of a deaf child, countered that: "The hearing parent is bypassed, dismissed as an insignificant factor in his own child's growth and development. . . . To blindly proclaim that cochlear implants are universally wrong for all children and that parents are either incapable or unable to make that decision for their own children demonstrates a total lack of understanding of the parent/child relationship" (Apicella, 1993, p. 19).

More recently, in reaching out to parents, Lane et al. (1996) affirm in their book, *A Journey into the Deaf-World*, that parents are natural advocates for their language and culture, but make the point that their deaf child as an adult will likely be part of deaf culture. Hence, parents should be especially cautious in weighting their views of childhood implantation more heavily than the views of deaf community members. Nancy Bloch (1999), NAD executive director, acknowledges that the original NAD position on childhood cochlear implants has driven parents away from the American deaf community (as substantiated by the parent interviews reported here). The NAD now aims to ensure that parents receive "balanced, unbiased, and resourceful" information to make informed decisions for their children (Bloch, 1999). In addition, the American Society for Deaf Children, a parent organization, encourages hearing parents to interact with the signing deaf community. This is similar to what the Alexander Graham Bell Association for the Deaf does in bringing parents together with oral deaf adults.

Parent Interview Findings

We discussed the views of the deaf community with the parents we interviewed, and a question on the Gallaudet Research Institute (GRI) survey also dealt with this issue. In view of the fact that a large number of the parents in our sample have signed or continue to use some form of sign communication with their children, it might be logical to assume that many hearing parents felt comfortable about approaching deaf people for advice. This was not necessarily the case. In the GRI survey (see table 3.2), 54% of the parents reported that they did not meet with any deaf adults prior to implantation. As for the other parents, 29% got direct information from deaf adults opposing pediatric implants, 24% met deaf adults who supported the procedure, 16% met with deaf adults who were neutral, and 6% met with adults or parents of children who had discontinued cochlear implant usage. Our interview data basically supports these results as well. Most of the parents did not meet deaf adults for advice, whether oral or signing, prior to the decision to implant their child. Many did not know any deaf adults to begin with. A few were concerned about how they would communicate with signing deaf persons because of their limitations in sign communication. For some, the literature they read made them hesitant to contact deaf people. Others felt they knew the deaf community perspective, so did not follow-up on contacting deaf individuals. In addition, the deaf community perspective as portrayed on television seemed to have a powerful impact on some of the parents we talked with. As the father of a young boy, who signs and speaks, states:

> One of the things we noticed with that *60 Minutes* program, with Caitlin's story, was that when Roz [Roslyn Rosen] was talking, she wasn't able to communicate unless she had an interpreter, whereas little Caitlin was doing everything on her own, and it seemed so black and white, like, What's the matter with this woman? . . . . Why would you want to try and put a roadblock up for somebody that wanted to go out there and do this? And it just boggled our minds.
>
> *Father of a 7-year-old boy implanted at age 5*

It is particularly noteworthy that the questions related to parent observations of, and contact with, the deaf community drew some of the most emotional responses in our interviews. This was primarily because these parents felt they were being attacked by individuals who assumed the parents had not done their homework and were cavalier about their decision, when in fact the parents felt they had investigated the cochlear implant issues thoroughly and had agonized about their decision to have their children undergo surgery. In reading through these responses, it is apparent the parents frequently described the signing deaf people they encountered or read about as judgmental, misinformed, and unwilling to enter into mutually respectful dialogue. This heightened their feelings of being threatened. Some examples of these feelings are presented below:

They actually scared us away, basically. It's like these guys are just too intense.

Mother of an 8-year-old girl implanted at age 2

When we spoke to the deaf community about the cochlear implant . . . certain members of the deaf community . . . their feelings were so angry and so hurtful. I mean, we were called child abusers . . . and butchers.

Parents of an 8-year-old girl implanted at age 2

I just had a lot of pros and cons and I think it was a week before surgery and I got something from . . . the deaf community. They sent me fliers of people that were against it and they kind of had pictures in there of kids that were all wrapped up and said that if I did that I would be a failure as a mother and that was a wrong decision to make and that the doctor was nothing but just a neo-Nazi that was going to cut into the brain and make her Frankenstein. It was pretty ugly letters.

Mother of a 7-year-old girl implanted at age 4

Some of these people are really closed-minded to these different avenues of improving your hearing. So that really kind of turned me off, too, when they would tell me I'm not admitting my child's deaf, when I feel that I'm just giving him more opportunities.

Father of a 16-year-old boy implanted at age 10

Parent fears about the deaf community even extended to the researchers themselves and to the Gallaudet setting:

I even wrote to my friend . . . that went to Gallaudet, before I responded [to our request for an interview] and gave you directions to the house, because I . . . just wanted to be sure this is okay, that, you know, this person's not going to come to the house and be very upset because we did this to our child.

Mother of a 3-year-old girl implanted at 22 months

My son is deaf. He should feel comfortable enough to go over to Gallaudet to look around. . . . I'm afraid for him to go over there.

Mother of a 14-year old son implanted at age 3

I've heard so many [stories] that I wouldn't want to send her there [Gallaudet]. Right now my feelings are because she is not a generational deaf child that I hear in order to be really accepted at Gallaudet, you need to be that generational deaf child. And I think that's wrong; it's absolutely wrong. You're having a brand new generation of children who are getting cochlear implants and I don't know if they're going to choose Gallaudet because of what's going on now.

Mother of a 9-year-old girl implanted at age 4

A good number of the parents who took the time to read about deaf community perspectives or communicate with deaf people reacted with concerns about the validity or logic of some of the points that were made.

The idea that [my daughter] belonged to strangers [the deaf community] more than she belonged to her blood family is a very disturbing logic.

Mother of a 15-year-old girl implanted at age 2

How can they say I should give over my deaf child to a deaf person to raise because she is deaf? . . . . I did read about the controversy, and I thought, I guess perhaps you don't know what you don't have.

Mother of a 10-year-old girl implanted at age 7

I didn't quite understand [the suggestion that deaf parents should also have the right to make their hearing children deaf] because they can sign to their child, and their child can sign to them, and be raised in the deaf culture, but their child also has an ability that they don't have, which is to hear. And why would they want to deny that? So I tried to understand both worlds, but I feel it is hard.

Mother of a 4-year-old son implanted at age 2

Some were even influenced to get an implant *because* of the information they received from the deaf community.

They really tried to turn us away from it. . . . If we did this, that it was denying the child his right to deafness . . . . I couldn't agree with that and I still don't agree with it. And it may have even leaned me a little more towards the implant.

Father of a 4-year-old boy implanted at 22 months

Whenever the 1991 NAD position paper was brought up, whether by the parents or the interviewer, it invariably elicited negative responses such as the following:

> Yeah, NAD came out with that paper saying how it was child abuse. Well, we thought that was really out of line.
>
> *Mother of a 13-year-old boy implanted at age 7,*
> *now a nonuser*

> I was kind of upset [by] the paper, the position paper, because it was so old, number one, it was almost 10 years old, so a lot of the things that I thought they were saying could easily be refuted by current statistics because it's been so long. And I was really angry at some of the statements that were made in it like, Nazi-like experimentation on children; that really made me angry. But this is America and people are entitled to their opinion.
>
> *Father of a 2-year-old boy implanted at 18 months*

The 1991 NAD position paper does not include comments about Nazi-like experimentation and the phrase "child abuse" is not mentioned. The parents clearly have associated the position paper with popular, as well as deaf-related, publications that have covered different perspectives on the cochlear implant issue. Several parents were able to recognize that the militant perspectives garnering the most publicity were not necessarily reflective of the deaf community as a whole.

> At first I thought that's what deaf culture was, was just totally anti-speech, anti-listening. And I have found since that time that it's not. It's just a real militant minority, but they're the one that gets press.
>
> *Mother of an 8-year-old girl implanted at age 2*

Others noted the need to understand the rationale for these perspectives and some even spoke of the constructive nature of the deaf community's historical opposition to pediatric implants:

> Their opinion is more of a political stand than a realistic determination for our child . . . . I think that if we've learned nothing else through this whole process, we've learned there is a need for compassion and understanding.
>
> *Mother of a 2-year-old boy implanted at 19 months*

It was the summer after my daughter lost her hearing that the Gallaudet movement [Deaf President Now protest in 1988] happened, and we were overjoyed. You know, anything that was about deaf pride we were thrilled, and then we kind of woke up to a lot of the internal politics of that.

Mother of a 15-year-old girl implanted at age 2

It's important for the voice of the deaf community to keep people cautioned or aware of wait a minute, slow down this speeding train.

Mother of an 18-year-old son implanted at age 16

We have in the past had deaf adults come [to our parent group] so parents can build that kind of relationship and understand some of the challenges that our children will face as they grow older. Because we hear, we don't fully appreciate those challenges . . . . You understand, there isn't anything wrong with the deaf community and people that only sign or whatever, for a lot of people that was their choice . . . . But the technology we have available makes it possible for our children to have exciting choices, real choices.

Parent of a 6-year-old girl implanted at age 2 and a 2-year-old boy implanted at 18 months

Most of the parents we interviewed were not aware that the NAD had retracted the 1991 position paper. Those who were informed felt this augured positively for the deaf community's eventual acceptance of their children as deaf children with cochlear implants.

I honestly try to keep openhearted about a bridge between the two cultures. And I really hope that maybe their softening on the implants will make them appear more accepting, too. I've never had bad experiences with deaf people, and I've been a little worried sometimes that they don't accept me or my son, and so if we can work from both sides, you know.

Mother of an 18-year-old young man implanted at age 16

And so I've talked to them [deaf people] about what it is, and they question me, Why did you get her an implant? Why did you do this? Why did you do that? And sometimes it's just education. They don't understand. That's why they're not accepting. And once they've gotten some of the information, it doesn't mean that they're fully on my side, but at least they understand why I made my choices.

Mother of a 7-year-old girl implanted at age 4

The NAD admits it has a huge task to convince parents and mainstream programs in the direction of positive awareness about what the deaf community is and what it can offer. In turn, some parents acknowledge that difficulties in communicating with deaf people who sign do hamper the effort to create bridges to understanding.

I honestly believe that the only reason that there's a big separation between the deaf and hearing world is because so many people don't know how to use sign language.

Mother of a 7-year-old girl implanted at age 4

Here deaf adults sign exclusively, and so we didn't really have a way to communicate with them. There was a barrier that we didn't know how to overcome, you know, because we didn't know how to sign.

Mother of a 6-year-old girl implanted at age 2 and
a 2-year-old boy implanted at 18 months

I talked with the [local] Association for the Deaf a little bit. It's intimidating . . . because of their sign—I don't know.

Mother of a 10-year-old girl implanted at age 3

The comments here indicate that these parents tend to blame their own inability to sign rather than the deaf person's inability to talk. There are hearing parents who have become fluent in sign language and are immersed in deaf culture (Barringer, 1993). However, if parents such as those cited here are not made to feel welcome, their own communication limitations notwithstanding, their desire to help their children forge bonds with the community of deaf people can potentially be dampened. This is a concern that has been articulated by Oscar Cohen (personal communication, May 30, 2000), former superintendent of the Lexington School for the Deaf in New York City. He reports that, among the hearing parents attending the 1999 National Symposium on Childhood Deafness in Sioux Falls, South Dakota (sponsored by the NAD), many had children with cochlear implants and, being from fairly isolated areas, were seeking support from the deaf community regarding the parents' desire to both embrace cultural aspects of deafness as well as their choice to have their children obtain cochlear implants. Many of these parents expressed disappointment over their perceived lack of support and acceptance from many of the deaf participants.

In our interviews, one parent said:

> We really had a bad experience with the signing community, too, when we sent our son to summer camp one time in [a western state]. It was really a bad experience. They looked at us like we had really done something terrible. We thought, well, summer camp would be kind of a fun place, kind of a safe environment for him to learn more sign, be with more deaf [peers] that are not oral kids, get comfortable with that before he starts in a classroom. I said he's just learning sign language, he's been in an oral program; they said great, you made a good choice, send him, we'll be patient with him . . . . We drive in. And they ignored us and . . . we're trying to talk to these people and they knew that we didn't know sign language. We had said that. We were hoping this program would help him become familiar with it and [my husband] says, What! Are we invisible here? What's happening? And then one lady at the table said, Why don't you come over here (under her voice), you know, come over here and I'll help you out. Yeah. So we came this close to saying, forget it . . . . But my son jumped right in and started playing with the kids; he was fine.
>
> *Mother of a 16-year-old son implanted at age 10*

There are parents who would like more interactions with deaf adults. Some find them within church settings and other deaf community activities. Others meet deaf adults in school settings. Those reporting that their implanted children had deaf teachers, whether within mainstream settings or at a school for the deaf, appeared satisfied with this arrangement.

In our interview sample, at least nine parents came right out and commented on the lack of information exhibited by the deaf people they talked with. Specifically, the deaf individuals did not appear to understand what the cochlear implant was, nor did they have accurate information on the technology and the process of implantation. For this reason, their arguments regarding the negative role of cochlear implants in a child's life were not convincing.

> The only thing that bothered me, and it's better now, is that there was so much lack of information by other deaf people. I found hearing people were very open to learning all about the different things.
> *Mother of a 20-year-old young woman implanted at age 17*

> A lot of it was misinformation that they [deaf people] were not informed of exactly what went on. You know, they thought that it was a big surgery and that we were implanting a device [to make] her hearing and things like that. They were misinformed and everything that I was able to tell them, they couldn't rebut back to me, because they had not had the information. I even brought brochures in and things from, you know, this is what it is and they had not read, they did not know. So that was disappointing to me.
> *Mother of an 8-year-old girl implanted at age 4*

> Before we got the implant, and . . . we were deciding what direction we wanted to go in, we received a lot of urging from the deaf community . . . not to go in that direction . . . .You know, they . . . didn't ever really give a reason other than, you know, She's beautiful the way she is. Why do you feel you need to change her? She's part of a lovely group of wonderful, warm, supportive people. Why do you want to destroy that? That sort of thing. And I think maybe people were not accurately categorizing the nature of the surgery, you know, making it out to be perhaps more risky than it was, more dangerous than it really was, and so forth. And an inaccurate portrayal of staff at implant centers . . . also, we were warned that a lot of children who have the implant really don't do very well with the implant. And I think a lot of that was based on very old studies.
> *Parents of a 4-year-old girl implanted at 18 months*

Martin Florsheim (personal communication, April 4, 2000), who is deaf and serves as principal of P.S. 47 in New York City, concurs with these parents that the deaf community is not fully informed about cochlear implant developments. He often finds himself in the position of having to explain things to them.

Much rhetoric from the deaf community is related to basic concerns about how the psychological and social lives of deaf children may be negatively affected post-implant. In a study of peer relationships of children with implants, Bat-Chava and Deignan (2001) report on interviews with 25 families attending an intensive communication therapy program focusing on mainstream education and oral communication. They note three themes: (1) most parents reported significant improvement in their children's relationships with hearing peers after receiving the implant, based on improved oral skills and a change in the child's personality in that the child became more outgoing and confident; (2) problems in social relationships with hearing peers did not disappear due to residual lags in oral communication skills, difficulties in group interactions, the attitudes of hearing peers, and their low level of familiarity with deaf implantees; and (3) ongoing relationships with deaf peers were supported by one-fourth of the sample who realized the importance of these relationships in socialization experiences. In a telephone interview study with 35 parents of children with implants, Kluwin and Stewart (2000) found that the socialization of children who had a large circle of friends or at least one single close friend pre-implant did not change. Those children whose primary playmates were siblings or who had other types of friendship groups prior to implantation generally branched out to new friends afterward.

In our sample, the parents who addressed personality aspects (roughly 20) mostly noted stability or improvement in social relations post-implant (see chapter 6). They saw their children as manifesting a better sense of self or improvement in relating with others, whether family or outsiders. One father came right out and talked about his child as a child first and foremost:

> The implant is not what she is. The implant is just a thing, okay. And she's a kid. And some days she's great, and some days she's trouble. But she would be that whether she was deaf, whether she had an implant, whether she had sign. That's just her.
>
> *Father of an 8-year-old girl implanted at age 2*

Very few parents remarked on psychological difficulties after implantation. These difficulties were generally related to children getting the implant when closer to adolescence and not being happy with it.[2] Unquestionably, adolescents need to undergo a thorough evaluation to ensure that they have a realistic need for the implant, and that they possess the auditory skills and commitment required to potentially benefit from it (see chapter 11 for further discussion). How they may feel about the implant afterward is variable. For example, one mother reported on how her adolescent endeavored to hide his implant. Another mother of an adolescent implanted at age 13, a difficult age for most teenagers, admits she went ahead with the decision to implant despite his resistance, and he has not adjusted well to the implant. In contrast, one father wryly recounted how his son purposefully got a buzz cut, since showing his scar was "cool."

In addressing whether parents truly accept their child's deafness, parents we met overwhelmingly stated that they still identify their child as deaf (albeit audiologically deaf rather than culturally deaf) after the implant and accept their child's deafness. However, a couple of parents said:

> As soon as he's out of the pool, we get him showered off and put his clothes on, put his implant on, and he's a normal hearing kid again.
> *Father of a 4-year-old boy implanted at 22 months*

> She's almost hearing, like I hear.
> *Mother of a 20-year-old college student implanted at age 17*

Acceptance is reflected in part by parents' awareness that their deaf children will benefit from contact with deaf peers. As noted in the following examples, most of the parents we interviewed are comfortable to varying degrees with their deaf child having deaf as well as hearing friends.

> I wanted to make it really clear . . . we were not pulling her out of the school. We were not taking her away from her deaf peers because that is a part of who they are. We realize that. . . .
> We were not taking away the sign language. . . . So our goal was not to like rip her away from [deaf peers]. . . . We didn't look at the cochlear implant as the miracle cure. . . . It's not. It's medical

---

2. The reader is reminded that this sample is weighted toward parents of children who continue to use the cochlear implant. Parents of children who minimally benefit from the implant may have been less likely to participate in the study.

technology . . . . There's so many more children who are implanted now at the school.

> *Mother of a 10-year-old girl implanted at age 4 and*
> *an 8-year-old boy implanted at age 4*

That's important to know that there's other people in the world and other kids your age that are deaf, that they're the same, that understand you. . . . If he'd have been implanted earlier, he still would have been in a Total Communication school because I feel that he is deaf, and he's going to rely on sign language for a lot of things.

> *Mother of a 17-year-old young man implanted at age 8,*
> *now a nonuser*

We have to get him involved with other nonhearing children . . . to let him be with his own kind, so to say, because . . . if he has problems, he can say this is bothering me.

> *Father of a 5-year-old boy implanted at age 2*

I know that she will be involved with the deaf world to some extent.

> *Mother of a 7-year-old girl implanted at age 2*

Those deaf peers, they love to sign, and I can't take that away from her.

> *Mother of an 8-year-old girl implanted at age 5*

Socially what saved her when she was in a rough time was a very close bond with other hearing-impaired children on weekends.

> *Mother of a 20-year-old young woman implanted at age 16*

The goal for many parents is to have their child part of the hearing community as well as the deaf community, and some do think hard about this:

When that implant is not on, he's deaf; it's as easy as that. So he's really part of the deaf community. When he's wearing the implant, if it works out, he will be part of the hearing community. So it's kind of like he is really part of both.

> *Mother of a 4-year-old boy implanted at 21 months*

We didn't want to make this decision for him and all of a sudden at 18 be left out. To be left out of the hearing world, left out of the deaf world. I think the hardest thing for us was feeling that we were alienating him. Were we truly helping him? Or were we alienating him from the majority of what he truly is? He is deaf. He will always be deaf. An implant does not make him not deaf. I worry less about him being alienated when he gets older because the number of children and adults accepting this is growing. By the time he gets older, the community of cochlear implant folks will be huge.

Parents of a 4-year-old boy implanted at age 2

Others confront more directly the issue of being caught in the middle or struggling with communication.

He came home last year, first time, and said, Mom, some of those [deaf] kids pick on me. . . . Well, they tell me to shut up and not to talk. . . . At one point he felt very much in the middle because he really isn't a hearing person and he really isn't immersed into the deaf community. . . . And I told him you are kind of in the middle, . . . and I told him why we made that decision—so that he could learn to talk and listen. . . . And he says I like that.

Mother of a 16-year-old boy implanted at age 10

One last point we need to make is that some deaf parents are now proceeding to have their deaf children implanted. One set of parents in our interview sample is deaf. Other parents have been identified through personal contacts. In one segment of the documentary film *Sound and Fury* (Aronson, 1999), Peter and Nita Artinian, the deaf parents who decided against the implant, interview deaf parents with an implanted child. During one of our interviews, a hearing mother whose parents are deaf said:

My deaf brother said, They don't work, they don't work, and now that he has seen that they work, he said, If I have a deaf child, I want my child to have an implant.

Mother of a 2-year-old boy implanted at 18 months

These individuals have not been overtly attacked by deaf peers. This may be yet another significant reflection of the winds of change blowing through the deaf community.

Adolescent and Young Adult Perspectives

Parent perceptions are important. So are the perceptions of the newly emerging generation of young people who have grown up deaf and experienced the cochlear implant. Our interview sample of 27 adolescents and young adults consisted of the following: (1) 14 continuing users, of whom seven were interviewed without parents present and the rest were interviewed together with their parents; and (2) 13 who have stopped using the implant or use it only intermittently, of whom seven were interviewed without parents present. These seven included six Gallaudet University students and one recent Gallaudet graduate. The eighth student in the Gallaudet sample was still using the cochlear implant. All but one stopped because they felt they derived no benefit from the implant. The Gallaudet students came from a mixture of mainstream programs and schools for the deaf. One of them had received a single-channel implant at age 4; two were implanted at age 7, with one being reimplanted at age 11; and the remaining five were implanted between the ages of 13 and 20. The non-Gallaudet students who had stopped regular use of the implant had been implanted at ages from 5 through 13. They were primarily attending schools for the deaf. The age at which continuing users were implanted ranged from age 2 to late adolescence. Not surprisingly, the great majority of these were in mainstream programs.

It is clear from our full sample of interviewees that a large majority see themselves as deaf. This includes both implant and nonimplant users. The Gallaudet student, who is still using her implant and is 1-year post-implant, labels herself hard-of-hearing, having functioned that way all her life. Interestingly, she does not feel stigmatized at Gallaudet, even when people discovered she was still using her implant. Moreover, results of the Gallaudet University survey (reported in the next section) indicate that students with implants are no longer rejected outright. One other 14-year-old implant user, who uses sign, was uncertain, having replied, "I don't know," when asked if she saw herself as a deaf person.

Self-perceptions as deaf do not necessarily translate into desire for connections with other deaf people. However, most of the 14 implant users indicated they had deaf friends and desired contact with both deaf and hearing peers. A good number see themselves as affiliated with the deaf community. A sampling of their comments is presented here:

The cochlear implant is not about being hearing. . . . It's making life easier and I can still be part of the deaf community anyway. [She also mentioned that some of her friends accept it; others don't, but respect her choice.]

17-year-old young woman implanted at age 16

Actually, I have a friend. . . . He complains to me, Why are you, why do you have that cochlear implant? You are not a real true deaf person. . . . And I am like, Well, having a cochlear has nothing to do with being involved with the deaf world. . . . The cochlear implant just means that I want to hear things and not be stupid as he is.

14-year-old girl implanted at age 2 and again at age 9

I want to be able to hear, and plus I don't want people, my friends, to think that I am like some machine, . . . or some kind of a person that would, like, want to go away from the deaf community. I want to be with both worlds as well. I've been raised by a hearing family and I'm learning how to be with the deaf community because I am going to be with the deaf because I am deaf too when I take off my aids, so there's no big difference.

15-year-old girl implanted at age 13

I feel like I've kept one foot in the hearing world and the other foot in the deaf community, so I feel I can interact with both, okay?

18-year-old young woman implanted at age 15

I'm glad I'm deaf. I like the hearing world a lot. And I'd like to stick with it [interacting with both deaf and hearing peers within the school setting].

13-year-old boy implanted at age 3

I'm a pretty social person. . . . I have lots of hearing friends and I keep in touch with my deaf friends through e-mail and that's really great. . . . Two of my deaf friends live pretty close to me, and that's really nice. I know a few odds and ends of sign, and whenever I'm in a situation where I'm with deaf signing people, I always manage a way to communicate with them, basically through lipreading.

15-year-old girl implanted at age 2

I was really lucky. I started going to the A. G. Bell conventions and I became friends with a couple of hearing-impaired girls who helped me think I wasn't different .... I had this close clique of (hearing) girlfriends and we were the popular girls.

20-year-old young woman implanted at age 16

Everyone has got to have a form of support, from people like themselves, just like I have a form of support from the other oral deaf community.

18-year-old young man implanted at age 12

One 20-year-old female respondent who received her implant at age 17 reported she was in touch with other people who had implants. She knew nobody who signed and was not in a signing environment while growing up, even though she attended a school that had a self-contained hearing-impaired program.

Those who use the implant intermittently or not at all socialize mostly with deaf peers, either by choice or because they are in a deaf school setting. For example, a 15-year-old girl who is now considering intermittent use of the implant after having stopped for a while very much prefers her experiences with other deaf students rather than being in a complicated social setting with only hearing peers.

The seven Gallaudet nonimplant users made it clear they are interested in being part of the deaf world. One mentioned seeing students with cochlear implants accepted at Gallaudet University, and knows at least four students still using their implant on campus. Another said her best friend still wears it. She also emphasized that it was possible for a person with a cochlear implant to be part of the deaf community. Another interviewee said:

Getting the cochlear implant doesn't mean you turn hearing. No. You're still deaf and part of our community.

18-year-old young woman implanted at age 7,
but stopped when she became a high school sophomore

In response to the common observation ascribed to the deaf community that deaf children are pressured to be "hearing," one implant user had this to say:

My parents never forced me to be hearing ... but I have been confronted in several situations where people, either parents of children whom they raised as deaf and signing, or deaf people who sign themselves, who have said, Oh, I feel so sorry for you, and basically my response is, Don't be sorry for me. I'm very happy.

15-year-old girl implanted at age 2

A couple of Gallaudet nonusers said:

My dad was the only one who wanted me to have a cochlear implant because he wanted me to become hearing, so . . . he expected me to be able to hear him. That's what he says. . . . My dad did not accept me being deaf.

18-year-old young woman implanted at age 13,
stopped at age 15

I wanted to think like a hearing person, and I looked at deaf people as inferior. I was trained to think that way since I was little.

22-year-old young woman implanted at age 14,
stopped at age 16

Two of the Gallaudet nonusers express concern about misinformation among those in the deaf community:

It really bothers me when they don't get their facts straight. They have exaggerated many times. You lose people's respect when you don't use research facts.

28-year-old young woman implanted at age 20,
stopped at age 21

Deaf people are still following primitive beliefs about the implant. These are things that are not happening any more.

22-year-old young man implanted at age 4,
stopped at age 17

Survey of Gallaudet University Faculty, Staff, Students and Alumni

Even though Gallaudet University takes no official position regarding whether cochlear implants should be used, information about the opinions of individuals connected with Gallaudet will indicate how this group perceives cochlear implants. Hampton (1997) developed a survey on cochlear implants specifically for Gallaudet University faculty, staff, and students, as well as a separate survey for professionals working for institutions with strong cochlear implant research and education programs. Results for the 38 Gallaudet respondents indicated that those who identified themselves as culturally deaf showed minimal or no support for pediatric implantation, whereas those respondents who leaned toward supporting the implant for children tended to be hearing or hard-of-hearing. Additionally, the Gallaudet respondents showed comparatively more support for implanting teenagers, deaf adults, and late-deafened adults. The group consisting of 46 professional (medical community) respondents indicated very strong support for pediatric implantation and relatively less but still strong support for implanting teenagers, deaf adults, and late-deafened adults.

To obtain current perspectives of individuals connected with Gallaudet University, a survey incorporating nine statements about cochlear implants for which respondents could indicate agreement, disagreement, or no opinion was sent out to a random sample of 110 faculty and staff, 120 students, and 125 alumni, as well as a non-random sample of 20 Gallaudet summer school students in the spring and summer of 2000. There were a total of 138 respondents (37% response rate); the general composition of the respondents is summarized in table 10.1.

In addressing the first statement: "When using his/her cochlear implant, an implanted person can usually hear as well as a hearing person," 74% of the respondents disagreed, whereas 5% agreed, and 21% did not know. This general rate of disagreement held true across the deaf, hearing, and hard-of-hearing subgroups. Concerning the next statement, 51% overall agreed it was "possible to have a cochlear implant and still retain one's identity as a Deaf [culturally deaf] person," whereas 30% disagreed, and 20% had no opinion. Within the subsample who identify as deaf, opinions are roughly equally divided between agreement (37%) and disagreement (39%). The hard-of-hearing (71%) and hearing (81%) groups strongly support the notion that it is possible to have a cochlear implant and still have an identity as a culturally deaf person. Relevant to pediatric implantation, 56% of the full sample disagreed with the statement that "hearing parents should be permitted to get a cochlear implant for their child under the age of 5 if they study the issue

TABLE 10.1

Composition of the Gallaudet University Sample

Hearing Status		Gallaudet University Affiliation	
Deaf	63%	Faculty/staff	38%
Hard-of-hearing	12%	Students	33%
Hearing	23%	Alumni	29%
Gender		Race/Ethnicity	
Male	35%	White	80%
Female	64%	African American	9%
Not reported	1%	Asian/Pacific Islander	1%
		Native American	1%
		Multiethnic	1%
		Unknown	1%
Deaf Community Affiliation		Age	
Yes	75%	15–20	4%
No	16%	21–25	12%
Not sure	8%	26–35	29%
		36–50	31%
		51+	20%

carefully and believe this to be the best decision for the child and the family," whereas 35% agreed, and 10% had no opinion. It is noteworthy that although a large majority of the deaf respondents (72%) did *not* agree with this statement, 78% of the hearing and 53% of the hard-of-hearing respondents did. It was on this question that the clearest evidence of disagreement among deaf and hearing respondents was apparent.

A statement about whether "Gallaudet University should do more to encourage students with cochlear implants to attend" drew 59% agreement and 23% disagreement, with 17% expressing no opinion. Most of the deaf (54%), hearing (71%), and hard-of-hearing (65%) respondents agree. Concerning the statement about whether "Gallaudet should establish a cochlear implant center to help meet the needs of students with cochlear implants," 53% agree, whereas 26% disagree, and 21% express no opinion. The hearing (78%) and hard-of-hearing (71%) subgroups show much stronger agreement than the deaf subgroup (41%). Asked whether such a center "should provide information for people interested in learning more about cochlear implants," 52% agree, whereas 38% disagree, and 10% express no opinion. Although 59% of the hard-of-hearing and 74% of the hearing subgroups agree, only 44% of the deaf subgroup agree with this statement.

In considering the statement that "faculty and staff should be encouraged to sign with voice whenever possible in order to make the University more 'user-friendly' for students who use voice communication more than sign, as many cochlear implant users do," 51% of the full sample disagree, whereas 34% agree, and 15% don't know. Not surprisingly, in comparison with hearing (31%) and hard-of-hearing (24%) respondents who disagree, a much higher proportion of deaf respondents disagree (63%).

The eighth statement asks respondents to rate whether "the deaf community in America will eventually disappear because so many children are getting cochlear implants." In response, 58% disagree, whereas 25% agree, and 17% don't know. Half of the deaf sample disagrees, whereas the rest (34%) agree or don't know (15%). In contrast, over 70% of both hearing and hard-of-hearing samples disagree, less than 10% agree, whereas the rest don't know. The last item, which asks whether "the cochlear implant may be appropriate for a late deafened adult who does not want to be a part of the deaf community," elicited a 69% agreement, whereas 12% disagreed, and 19% expressed no opinion. Over 90% of the hearing respondents supported this, in comparison with 41% of the hard-of-hearing respondents and 66% of the deaf respondents.

Additionally, deaf and hard-of-hearing respondents were asked whether they had ever considered getting a cochlear implant. Of the 105 respondents who answered this question, an overwhelming majority, 87%, reported no; and 13% said they had considered getting one. A sampling of comments on this item follows:

It will affect my nerve. Nor do I want metal in my head. I am not interested in shaving part of my head off and having a life-long scar on it.

I considered it once when I was a child. I was not proud of being deaf and wanted to hear. I went for an evaluation and was determined eligible, but my parents declined because they felt it was not right.

I come from a deaf family. I have been deaf all my life. If I get the cochlear implant, I would lose my identity as a deaf person.

I am happy with the way I am. I believe that as technology increases, so will hearing aids. I am perfectly pleased with my hearing aid right now. The cochlear implant is not an option for me. I accept to be a deaf person.

I did not like the idea of being "fixed" when I feel I am not even damaged in the first place. I was born deaf.

It will take up too much time to learn how to listen.

Hearing aids work just as well, or even better.

In contrast, some respondents commented:

I would like to be able to use the phone again.

It is not appropriate for me at this time. If I were 20 to 25 years younger, I might.

Some respondents also commented on the statements in the survey, such as those listed here.

I think Gallaudet should be more vocal on this cochlear implant issue. We should develop research and disseminate information to students, staff, and faculty. I do not think Gallaudet should take a political side.

I agree with the concept of meeting the needs of students with cochlear implants or providing information about the cochlear implant, but I don't know that we need a special cochlear implant center to accomplish those goals. Existing units and departments are already doing that for individuals.

Implant information should be available to anyone who wants it. Implants do not make a person "normal" but will restore some sense of sound and will aid in the communication process.

It is inhumane to force such an implant on kids under 5 years old because they have no say, and they'll bear this scar of future struggles for the rest of their lives. It is fine with me for the adults to decide to get a cochlear implant. Cochlear implant students at Gallaudet are welcome.

More parents are choosing to have their deaf kids implanted. That is their right to choose. Gallaudet needs to prepare to meet the needs of a more diverse student body if it wants to continue to exist.

I formerly did not support the cochlear implant as I felt it would destroy the deaf community. But now I respect individual choice and feel the cochlear implant is part of deaf culture, anyway. People's perspectives on deaf culture are different now.

Comments like this last one appear to contradict Bonnie Tucker's (1998a) report that cochlear implants are greatly frowned on at Gallaudet, and students are pressured by peers to stop using the implant. Our Gallaudet interviewees tell us that cochlear implant users are increasingly accepted on campus. Nevertheless, even though half of the survey respondents agreed that it is possible to have a cochlear implant and still retain one's identity as a culturally deaf person, the agreement is not as strong for deaf respondents as it is for hearing and hard-of-hearing respondents. This may reflect a transition phase as the deaf community responds to a new reality, specifically that people with cochlear implants are not necessarily rejecting their identity as deaf individuals.

The conflict over pediatric implantation is amply illustrated by the response to the statement about whether children under the age of 5 should be permitted to get an implant after their parents carefully consider the issues. Specifically, over half of the full sample does not accept pediatric implantation. Deaf respondents are far more likely to be opposed in comparison to hearing and hard-of-hearing respondents, supporting Hampton's (1997) findings. This is not surprising in light of the historic deaf community opposition described earlier, as well as concern about long-term implications, which have yet to be determined.

On the other hand, the fact that a clear majority of all respondents agree with the need for Gallaudet to actively recruit students with cochlear implants indicates a realistic understanding of the changing deaf population. Because Gallaudet is often seen as a place where deaf cultural immersion takes place, respondents may see this opportunity as a chance to welcome such students into the deaf community. Support for the need to provide services to students with implants, and information on implants for those requesting it, comes much more from hearing and hard-of-hearing respondents than from deaf respondents. Because the Laurent Clerc National Center on the Gallaudet University campus has added a cochlear implant center as part of its services, it will be interesting to see whether the limited support from deaf respondents changes as they see and experience the emerging reality on campus.

Half of the sample disagree with the suggestion that a sign with voice policy should be encouraged to make Gallaudet "user-friendly" for students who rely more on voice communication. The other half agree or do not know. Additionally, the fact that more deaf respondents disagree, whereas more hearing and hard-of-hearing respondents agree, serves to highlight the sensitive nature of this topic, considering the value of ASL (a language unaccompanied by voice), for those affiliated with deaf culture. It is anticipated that the struggle over the communication issue will continue, at least in the near future, as more students with cochlear implants adjust to the Gallaudet environment.

Although a majority of respondents disagree that the deaf community will eventually disappear, it is surprising to note that proportionately more hearing and hard-of-hearing respondents have faith in the continuing existence of the deaf community in comparison to deaf respondents. When individuals such as Jack Wheeler, formerly of the Deafness Research Foundation, proclaim that deaf babies born each year can become babies who self-identify as hearing kids, this clearly serves to reinforce deaf community perceptions that the goal is for deaf people to become hearing and that cultural genocide is taking place (Manning, 2000). Paradoxically, Wheeler simultaneously confirms the need to preserve deaf culture ("The Death of Deafness?" 2000). Ken Levinson (personal communication, April 3, 2000), a cochlear implant user and member of the Gallaudet University Board of Trustees, predicts that with the eventual improvement of technology, the deaf community will be going through a significant transition for a while, even to the point that its size will diminish. Nonetheless, half of the deaf sample sees the deaf community as strong enough to survive. This is supported by prominent deaf community members such as James Tucker (personal communication, May 31, 2000), superintendent of the Maryland School for the Deaf, and Jay Innes (personal communication, April 28, 2000) of Gallaudet University and the NAD Education Policy and Program Development Center.

Most respondents accurately recognize the appropriateness of the cochlear implant for late-deafened individuals. Interestingly, although most of the hearing respondents support this statement, there was proportionately more support from deaf respondents compared with hard-of-hearing respondents. There continues to be some need for more dissemination of information on the efficacy of the cochlear implant, considering that 26% of the full sample incorrectly agreed with the statement that an implanted person can usually hear as well as a hearing person (or did not know).

The fact that this survey elicited such a variety of responses from the hearing, hard-of-hearing, and deaf subgroups, including a lot of "don't know" responses, for most of the statements supports the need for further education. Jay Innes (personal communication, April 28, 2000) says that the education needed at Gallaudet "includes sensitivity and diversity related educational training. Gallaudet is supposed to serve all deaf individuals who want to be educated at Gallaudet, regardless of communication preference or language.... This will be very challenging for Gallaudet. As biotechnology advances, the challenges will be even greater. Today it is the cochlear implant; tomorrow it will be something else."

Conclusions

As this chapter indicates, the deaf community is facing a new reality. Not only deaf children of hearing parents, but also many signing deaf adults are getting cochlear implants. Some deaf parents are getting their deaf children implanted.

There are deaf people standing on the sidelines, waiting to see how the current proliferation of cochlear implants will impact the deaf community (M. Florsheim, personal communication, April 4, 2000). Like Sharon Applegate (personal communication, April 2, 2000) of the New York Society for the Deaf, many question whether the cochlear implant really means immersion in the hearing world, and whether cochlear implant technology is in fact good enough for 18-month-old children to easily benefit from it. Others see the implant as yet another of the many oppressive threats the deaf community has historically faced. If, as Ben Bahan, chair of Gallaudet University's Department of Deaf Studies, states, cochlear implants are conceptually viewed as devices (similar to hearing aids) that can help make the hearing world more accessible to deaf people rather than changing deaf people into hearing people, and respect for deaf culture and ASL is maintained by educational systems, the deaf community will be more receptive (personal communication, July 15, 2000).

At this point, Jay Innes (personal communication, April 28, 2000) thinks that the deaf community is strong enough and mature enough to tolerate a full range of opinions on the topic of cochlear implants. He sees a "larger, broader, more diverse" deaf community and notes that the worst thing that could happen is for people with cochlear implants not to be welcome into the deaf community. They need the community as much or more than the other deaf people do because they represent a unique aspect of deafness, similar to hard-of-hearing individuals who often feel on the fringe, rooted neither in the hearing nor the deaf world. Therefore, it is time for the deaf community to take down the fence and welcome them.

The deaf community has begun to recognize that individuals with cochlear implants can still be affiliated with the deaf community. They are still deaf. The adolescents and young adults we interviewed confirm this. Information from the Gallaudet survey confirms this. Many of the parents we interviewed recognize this.

More and more, members of the deaf community are considering implants and are beginning to adapt to the reality that children with implants are still perceived as deaf. Their task is to communicate this to parents of deaf children with cochlear implants.

11

Ethics and Choices: Ongoing Dilemma

The question of whether parents have a right to implant a child without the child's consent, or whether they should wait until the child is old enough to decide, hits at the heart of the pediatric implant debate. Experts viewing the same research data often come to diametrically opposed conclusions regarding the ethics of the procedure. Arguments for or against pediatric implantation on ethical principles are played out in various publications and in the public arena. An article in *Silent News,* for example, captures the essence of this dilemma. In reporting on an exchange of opinions during a panel discussion following the showing of the documentary, *Sound and Fury* (Aronson, 1999),[1] Drolsbaugh (2000, p. 7) writes:

> Dr. Harlan Lane, noted author of *Mask of Benevolence* and distinguished professor at Northeastern University, presented a number of research findings opposing the cochlear implant.

---

1. In this film, one deaf brother, Peter Artinian, vehemently rejects the implant for his deaf daughter (after initially considering implantation possibilities), whereas his hearing brother, Chris Artinian, who has married a hearing daughter of signing deaf parents, proceeds to have his deaf twin son implanted.

Immediately afterward, Dr. Pat Chute, a cochlear implant audiologist, challenged Dr. Lane's views with statistics and counterarguments of her own. Watching the two of them slug it out, you could appreciate how difficult it is when hearing parents try to make decisions on how to raise deaf children.

This panel discussion also included members of the Artinian family (featured in the film *Sound and Fury*), who have chosen either one or the other side in the debate. Afterward, the audience was asked to indicate whether the program had changed anyone's mind. Only one person in the audience raised her hand. Granted, many people may not have been willing to publicly acknowledge a change of opinions. Nonetheless, this suggests that people may not change views easily on the issue of pediatric implantation, especially when emotions run high.

Ethics

What do we mean when we talk about ethics? Ethics are moral principles adopted by an individual or group to provide rules for appropriate conduct. Morality in general refers to social conventions about right and wrong (i.e., expectations about human conduct [norms] as shared by a community). This involves an evaluation of actions on the basis of some broader cultural context, value system, or religious standard (e.g., Clark, Cowan, & Dowell, 1997; Corey, Corey, & Callanan, 1993; Jonsen, Siegler, & Winslade, 1998). On this basis, behavior perceived as ethical within one community or culture may be perceived as unethical in another. Pediatric cochlear implantation is clearly a case in point. Those identifying with the culturally deaf community frequently perceive this process as unethical, whereas those who do not identify themselves in this way are more likely to view pediatric implantation as ethical. The situation is complicated by the fact that there are reasons (unrelated to ethics) to question the implantation of children, just as there are reasons to support it (Vernon & Alles, 1994). Therein lies the dilemma for parents, for deaf people, and for professionals working with deaf children.

Use of Technology

The appropriate use of technology lies at the crux of this dilemma. Blume (1993) notes that the medical profession tends to equate "best medical practice" with the use of modern technology; people often want to believe that the use of the latest "cutting edge" technology increases the possibility of amelioration or cure. There is also the implicit assumption that technology will facilitate "normalization" (Stewart-Muirhead, 1998). Whereas ever-improving medical technology certainly has had a positive impact on the lives of many people, including deaf people, varied opinions on the effectiveness of cochlear implants have contributed to the ongoing controversy.

In exploring the potential implications of modern technology on the human condition, George Montgomery (1991) refers to the story of Frankenstein to clarify the fear of what could happen when scientific advances outpace ethical considerations. He feels that cochlear implantation has progressed from the research stage directly to the clinical-commercial stage without what he considers to be an adequate period of evaluation. This is the same argument repeatedly put forth by the National Association of the Deaf (Testimony Before the FDA, 1997). In addition, the position statements of organizations such as Self Help for the Hard of Hearing (1994) and the American Academy of Audiology (1995), which emphasize the benefits of pediatric implantation, acknowledge that the fund of knowledge on the potential auditory and social implications of long-term implant use, as well as the suitability of candidates, is still in its infancy. This is due to the ongoing variability in individual benefits with the implant and the lack of reliable predictors for implant effectiveness. The National Institutes of Health Consensus Development Conference Statement (National Institutes of Health, 1995) concurs that the assessment of psychological impact in implanted children lags behind that for the adult population and recommends further study. Recently, however, there has been general agreement that it is not unreasonable to expect greater cochlear implant success in prelingually deaf children with improved technology and, perhaps, with implantation at a younger age (which, of course, has its own ethical implications). Studies focusing on children implanted at very young ages with more recent state-of-the-art technology are only now appearing in the professional literature (see chapter 9).

Bioethics

The field of medicine, as well as research involving human subjects, is subject to a plethora of bioethical requirements. Bioethics "examines the ethical dimension of problems at both the heart and the cutting edge of technology, medicine, and biology in their application to life" (T. Shannon, 1997, p. 4). Simply put, bioethics deals, in part, with the ethical implications of medical technology, such as the cochlear implant. As part of the evaluative component, medical decisions must take into account the extent to which the expected benefits outweigh the risks, and the extent to which the new technology is an accepted clinical procedure and not primarily a subject of research (Blume, 1994; Clark et al., 1997). These decisions are generally based on the principles of *beneficence, nonmaleficence,* and *respect for autonomy* (Jonsen et al., 1998; T. Shannon, 1997). *Beneficence* essentially means that the duty of physicians is to do good. This duty is closely tied to their ability to fulfill the goals of medicine in conjunction with the patients' preferences about the goals of their lives. It involves judgment about the extent to which individuals believe the technology will be of benefit to them. Corollary to beneficence is the principle of *nonmaleficence,* which is the duty to refrain from causing harm in the interest of maintaining one's well-being. Surgical risks and technology failure need to be considered, as well as psychosocial considerations related to the medical procedure. In medical decision-making, both beneficence and nonmaleficence are essentially judgment calls, which are ultimately based on how degrees of benefit are weighed against degrees of harm. *Respect for autonomy* is based on the principle that individuals must be perceived as capable of deliberating courses of action and making decisions for themselves (T. Shannon, 1997). This process requires informed consent, which is defined as "the willing acceptance of a medical intervention by a patient after adequate disclosure by the physician of the nature of the intervention, its risks, and benefits, as well as of alternatives with their risks and benefits" (Jonsen et al., 1998, p. 55). Informed consent is dependent on the extent to which specific information disclosed to the adult, or to a child's lawful surrogate, is comprehensive, accurate, and intelligible; the value judgment of the person providing the information; and how the recipient of the information (i.e., parent) understands and interprets that information. For these reasons, T. Shannon (1997) considers informed consent to be the most critical problem in bioethics.

Ethical considerations for pediatric implantation are not clear-cut, particularly since both sides of the cochlear implant debate can invoke ethical principles, depending on their viewpoints as to what constitutes "quality of life." Both sides also claim to have the deaf child's best interest at heart. Ultimately, the ethical process becomes an interactive one (Wegener, 1996), as the professionals and families decide what information to pursue, how much value that information contains, and what perspectives are critical in shaping the final decision. We now move to a consideration of how the three principles are interpreted by each side in the debate.

Ethical Perspectives of *Supporters* of Pediatric Implantation

Beneficence

Medical school training focuses on why people do not hear and the methods needed to conquer deafness ("The Death of Deafness?" 2000). For doctors, allied professionals such as audiologists, and the general public, hearing loss is often not seen as a natural occurrence, but as a pathology that adversely affects the individual's quality of life. This easily leads to the social construction of hearing loss as an abnormal condition, handicap, or disability that needs to be corrected or cured to avoid the negative consequences of deafness (Cohen, 1995; Crouch, 1997; Tyler, 1993, p. 498). Creating the ability to hear by providing the child with a cochlear implant is portrayed as an effort to minimize disability, or to "activate a God-given thing," as John Niparko, a cochlear implant surgeon, puts it (Arana-Ward, 1997, p. 1). The principle of beneficence comes into play with the consideration that, by providing communicative value, auditory enjoyment, and enhancing safety, one is "doing good" for the child (Balkany, Hodges, & Goodman, 1996). The hope is that, after implantation, the profoundly deaf child will benefit by mastering a spoken language and interacting more often with hearing peers. This will presumably lead to enhanced opportunities for education, employment, and personal relationships. Based on this perspective, the implanted child will have a chance for an "open future," one that is not necessarily constrained by deafness or by limitations in spoken communication. This open future is generally defined as consisting of infinite possibilities over and above those available when one remains primarily within the deaf community. An ancillary concept is that of freedom of choice. With cochlear implants, the expectation is that children will eventually be able to choose where they want to be, whether among hearing people, part of the deaf community, or straddling both the deaf community and the surrounding hearing society. Because implanted children are usually still perceived and defined as deaf, the "right to be deaf" is not as much of an issue as "the right to choose" when all options theoretically become equally possible.

A related consideration, repeatedly mentioned by the parents we talked with, as well as widely acknowledged in the literature, is that hearing parents would like their children to be "like them" (i.e., part of the hearing mainstream) (Crouch, 1997). On this basis, one can make the argument that enabling the profoundly deaf child to participate in the culture of the parents contributes to the principle of beneficence, or doing good for the child. The alternative possibility is that potential harm could ensue should the child be estranged from the family of origin, or if life possibilities are limited when the child enters the deaf culture/community. This is not to say that those who join the deaf community necessarily become estranged from their family of origin. However, parents do worry about this possibility.

Nonmaleficence

The medical community no longer considers the surgical procedure itself to be experimental. Medical complications occur in a minuscule percentage of patients (Cohen, 1995, 2000a). The Food and Drug Administration approved pediatric implants as being medically safe following years of extensive testing (American Academy of Audiology, 1995), and children were implanted only after extensive work with deaf adults, as based on ethically accepted practices for research (Clark et al., 1997). However, some of the parents we interviewed, as well as parents in the Gallaudet Research Institute (GRI) survey, reported a few surgical problems and some technology failures (see chapter 5). Most technology failures are amenable to correction, with repeat surgery required when the internal components fail. Even if minimal, not only the frequency, but also the severity of technical failure, needs to be considered in the harm versus benefit calculation.

Another factor that needs to be considered in this calculation is the issue of whether the cochlear implant sufficiently facilitates spoken language development and ease of interaction with hearing people to make the procedure a viable option for deaf children. The literature reveals numerous articles that attest to successful outcomes of implantation in children with severe-to-profound hearing loss (e.g., Clark et al., 1997; Niparko, 1998b; Niparko et al., 2000b; R. Shannon, 1998; P. Spencer, this volume [chapter 9]; Waltzman & Shapiro, 1999). Success appears to be narrowly defined as demonstrating improvement in speech perception and production more often than in language development or in social interaction within hearing environments. However, recent studies have noted improvement in expressive and receptive language skills following cochlear implantation, even with maturational changes factored out (e.g., Kelsay & Tyler, 1996; Niparko, 1998b; P. Spencer, this volume [chapter 9]; Waltzman & Shapiro, 1999).

Long-term outcome research covering linguistic, communicative, and psychosocial factors is critical to address further the issue of benefit as compared to risk. Nevertheless, proponents of pediatric implants strongly feel they have sufficient objective outcome research evidence, both medical and speech/language-based, to frame the procedure as an acceptable clinical procedure rather than an innovative and risky one. However, implantation, like any surgery, is an ethically acceptable clinical procedure only with appropriate candidates for whom benefits will potentially outweigh risks (Pollard, 1996). This means that not everyone who comes knocking on the door asking for a cochlear implant is likely to be an acceptable candidate. The ethical principles discussed previously mandate that the selection procedure encompass careful and objective consideration of factors that can impact the outcome. Nevins and Chute (1996) stress the importance of going through what they call the "Children's Implant Profile" as an example of a decision-making checklist that takes into account chronological age, duration of deafness, medical/radiological information, presence of multiple handicapping conditions, functional hearing capacities, speech and language abilities, family structure and support, expectations, educational environment, and availability of support services. Niparko (2000a) outlines assessment procedures that should be followed for the cochlear implant team to provide appropriate expectations matched to implant candidates. In short, to minimize harm, cochlear implant centers ethically must ensure that ideological biases favoring the implant do not interfere with objective evaluation of pediatric candidacy.

Respect for Autonomy

Within the context of pediatric implantation, the third principle, respect for autonomy, essentially means that the patient (or parent in the case of a minor) is accorded respect as a decision-maker and as an agent of self-determination. As stated in Balkany et al. (1996, p. 750), "In exercising autonomy for their children, parents act within the rights of their children, which include freedom of choice, respect for the individual, and free, informed consent to make decisions on behalf of their child" that take the child's best interest into account. The National Institutes of Health Consensus Development Conference Statement (National Institutes of Health, 1995) is explicit in supporting parental responsibility for decision-making. The parents we talked with also strongly endorsed this principle while their children are young (as discussed later in this chapter).

To empower parents in making informed decisions, cochlear implant center staff must inform parents that cochlear implants do not restore normal hearing, outcomes are highly variable, and long-term commitment to rehabilitation is required. Unbiased information covering advantages, disadvantages, reasonable expectations, risks, and alternatives to implantation must be provided (Nevins & Chute, 1996; Tyler, 1993). Professionals are responsible for presenting the information in ways that are easily comprehended by parents. This can include written materials, language translations of these materials, repeated explanations, and whatever else it takes to ensure truly informed consent. This entire process must take place in an atmosphere free of coercion that psychologically allows parents freedom of choice. In short, "professionals who work with deaf children must remain advocates of the children, neither of a technology nor of a culture" (Balkany et al., 1998, p. 313).

Most of the parents in our interview sample report they did not feel pressured by the cochlear implant center to decide in favor of the implant. Parents generally felt they were well-informed consumers who were actively involved in the decision-making process. As indicated in chapter 5, most parents also report having been informed about alternative approaches, benefits, and risk factors. However, the GRI data (table 4.2) indicates that, before implantation, parents are more aware of the potential medical risks than they are of potential social or psychological problems, and are more likely to be aware of the potential benefits, in general, than of the potential risks. How much can be attributed to the way information has been conveyed to parents and how much to parent fallibilities in remembering this information is not clear. However, as a father of a 4-year-old boy implanted at age 2 compellingly stated: *It took me a bit longer to make up my mind only because the people involved that are pro-implant, of course, always talk about the positive end of it and never talk about any possible negatives. And, of course I know that with just about everything else there is going to be downsides too, so I wanted to learn as much as I could about it.* This father also said: *As far as the decision-making, the doctors did leave it up to us. They told us what they suggested or what they think would work well, and they told us about successes and failure rates, but they totally left the decision up to us and that was nice.*

Practically all of the parents we interviewed acknowledged being informed of the possibility that awareness of environmental sounds might be all their child could achieve. Although implant centers try to assess parent expectations to ensure they are realistic (e.g., Nevins & Chute, 1996; Niparko, 1998a), it is common knowledge that parents consciously or unconsciously harbor high expectations for oral communication skills (Kampfe et al., 1993; Kelsay & Tyler, 1996). Mary Koch (personal communication, April 25, 2000), who used to be on the cochlear implant team at The Listening Center at Johns Hopkins University, observes that parents will tell you their hopes (which tend to be relatively realistic), but not their dreams. And Dale Atkins (personal communication, March 30, 2000), a New York City psychologist, adds that, when children are under the age of 2, parents may see the cochlear implant as a magic cure to fully restore the child's hearing, even if they say they understand their child may only hear some environmental sounds.

To minimize the danger of unrealistic expectations, Pollard (1996) recommends that professionals not only focus on informed consent at a technical level (meaning knowledge about the technology, the surgery, and postsurgical aspects, including habilitation) but also on informed consent at a phenomenological level (meaning that one has an unbiased understanding of what life with hearing loss is really like, with or without an implant). Parents should understand that their deaf children can have satisfying lives with or without the implant, as Peters (2000) indicates in his exploration of the pros and cons of implanting his daughter before deciding against the procedure.

In addition, an independent person should ask simple questions of the parent and child (if old enough) to assess expectations and minimize the effect of intangible pressure from those who would benefit from parental decisions to proceed (Clark et al., 1997).

Right of Privacy

A corollary to the principle of autonomy is the right of privacy. During the decision-making phase and afterward, there should be no undue pressure imposed on parents regarding their decision. Balkany et al. (1996) criticize deaf activists for trampling on privacy rights by confronting parents in extremely negative encounters. Some of the parents in our interview sample clearly felt their privacy was violated at times. Understandably, many parents did not appreciate the criticism they received from some deaf people when they were considering an implant for their child. On the other hand, a few parents in our interview sample reported feeling implicit pressure to choose the implant, but were aware enough to recognize it.

Ethical Perspectives of *Opponents* of Pediatric Implants

For opponents of pediatric cochlear implants, the principles of beneficence and nonmaleficence are interpreted in very different ways. The overriding perception is that benefits are not really all that beneficent and harm is being done to deaf children. Additionally, the principle of autonomy is violated by the biased nature of information being provided to parents by those professionals with a vested interest in cochlear implants.

Beneficence and Nonmaleficence

To understand this opposition, it is necessary to refer to the previous chapter, which describes the existence of a large group of culturally deaf people who have adapted to life in self-enhancing ways (Crouch, 1997; Lane & Bahan, 1998a; Stewart-Muirhead, 1998). These people do not see themselves as condemned to an inferior world of silence. Instead, they describe their lives as rich and fulfilling as part of a deaf world that is a vibrant cultural and linguistic community. From their perspective, opening the child up to deaf community membership will facilitate access to a signed language such as American Sign Language (ASL). As some researchers have found, despite misperceptions to the contrary, ASL can provide a link to the written language of the hearing society (Erting, Thumann-Prezioso, & Benedict, 2000; Lane et al., 1996; Marschark, 1998). Thus, this is seen as a form of beneficence. Lane and Bahan (1998a) describe prelingually deaf children as visual, and thereby part of deaf culture, even if their parents are part of the majority hearing society. In this conceptualization, the medical construction of deafness as a disability to be overcome is jettisoned for a social construction of deafness as a characteristic way of life. Also, in this conceptualization, cochlear implant surgery means that the focus is on the disability and not on the child as a deaf person. The surgery forces the child away from a "natural" means of communication (i.e., ASL) into an artificial hearing status that will still not guarantee full acceptance by the hearing community. On the other hand, allowing the deaf child "the right to be deaf" does not necessarily jeopardize connections with the hearing community. Supporting this perspective, the executive director of the National Association of the Deaf writes about the reality of many deaf children and adults functioning in both the deaf and hearing communities (Bloch, 1999).

To opponents of pediatric implants, depriving a deaf child of these opportunities by promoting implants as the prime avenue to accessing hearing society, when there are alternative options that do not require surgery, means that harm is being done. On this basis, the child is denied access to a visual language, the right to be deaf, or to be part of the deaf community.

In addition, many members of the deaf community do not uniformly endorse the perception that pediatric cochlear implant surgery poses minimal risk. Although the increased safety of the surgical procedure is acknowledged, the procedure is still seen as unduly invasive, considering the person being operated on is usually healthy (Lane, Hoffmeister, & Bahan, 1996). Also, there is the risk of technology failure, as discussed earlier. What is at issue is the value of the surgery itself when its major goal is to increase optimal interaction with hearing society through spoken language. Lane and Bahan (1998a, 1998b) contend that surgery continues to be innovative and unproven, given their review of the very same outcome studies relied on by cochlear implant proponents to prove benefit. They arrive at diametrically opposing conclusions, namely that these outcome studies do not show sufficient improvement in spoken language to justify the presence of beneficence. In the studies demonstrating advantages for children with cochlear implants that they review, they suggest that experimenter bias (in the interest of positive research results), as well as greater focus on spoken language therapy for implanted children, may have influenced the results. Based on their evaluation, not a single case has been reported of a child acquiring language because of an implant. In a follow-up to this dialogue, Balkany et al. (1998) indicate total disagreement by referring to additional studies, which they see as providing clear evidence that children with cochlear implants are developing language.

In view of the wide variation in speech and language acquisition among implanted children (see chapter 9), those who question the procedure emphasize that the ethical question of whether the children benefit enough from the cochlear implant to make much difference in their lives demands careful scrutiny (Blume, 1994; Crouch, 1997). Their lives are already impacted by the fact that the path to oral language development is often arduous, with no guarantee of fluency or ease of function in hearing society. Although this is a point repeatedly made by cochlear implant centers, opponents see the pressure to perform as ignoring the potential benefits of being a part of the deaf community. Within the community, being validated as a deaf person able to learn, work, and play, rather than participating in an ongoing struggle to be part of the hearing community, is seen as being of benefit. The right of the child to be a child free of "force" or "undue pressure" to perform is stressed.

There is solid agreement among both proponents and opponents of pediatric implantation that definitive language, educational, psychosocial, and vocational outcomes await further study. Clearly, the current disagreement on outcome studies outlined here and elsewhere will be resolved only with ongoing longitudinal studies supported by researchers from a variety of backgrounds, considering that much of the research reported in the literature has been done by professionals affiliated with cochlear implant centers (Vernon & Alles, 1994). Most of them definitely are ethical researchers, but experimenter bias nonetheless is still a factor. In the meantime, due to the absence of guarantees for success, parents will continue to make a "leap of faith" that the technology will result in better spoken communication and better opportunities for their child (Brauer, 1993;

Simmons, 1985), taking into consideration the extensive speech and language work required for success.

The ethics of candidate selection mandate the careful evaluation of factors that may increase success in pediatric implantation to prove benefit. Success is measured in part by continued use of the implant (M. Koch, personal communication, April 25, 2000). It is noteworthy that although there are ongoing reports of increasing numbers of adults and children being implanted, there are virtually no statistics regarding perceptions of the effectiveness of implants by random samples of prelingually deaf persons who have been implanted since childhood. Currently, the number of people implanted is regularly updated, but not the number of individuals who are no longer using the implant. In one study, Rose, Vernon, and Pool (1996) sent out a brief survey questionnaire to public and private residential and day schools for the deaf in the United States with more than 100 students. With a 70% response rate, 151 children who had been implanted were identified, of whom 71 (47%) were no longer using the implant. However, the *Annual Survey of Deaf and Hard of Hearing Children & Youth* in its 1997 survey identified the percentage of children in the types of schools covered by the Rose et al. (1996) study who have discontinued the implant to be less than 15% (Holden-Pitt, 1998). Holden-Pitt attributes this discrepancy in part to methodological inadequacies in the Rose et al. survey. She notes that, although the definition of success remains open to question, the influence of age at time of implantation (older) and instructional communication (signing environment) within educational settings appear to be critical factors for discontinuation. Now that the average age for pediatric implantation has dropped and visually oriented educational settings are increasingly incorporating auditory input for children with cochlear implants, the circumstances surrounding implant discontinuation will have to be revisited in future research studies.

In the meantime, deaf community activists like Branton Stewart (personal communication, April 3, 2000) express concern that when children with cochlear implants do not respond according to parent expectations and hopes, and eventually stop using the implant, they may end up feeling like failures and could suffer negative psychological consequences. Dale Atkins (personal communication, March 30, 2000) notes that when children grow up orally and subsequently express the desire to learn sign language, parents may frame it as a reflection of failure "to make it in the hearing world." Atkins has to ask the parents what is so awful about learning to sign. However, in our interviews and in the GRI study, parents for the most part were comfortable with the idea of using signs and frequently encouraged their children to associate with deaf peers. There are some implanted children who have transferred from the mainstream to, for example, the Maryland School for the Deaf. According to James Tucker (personal communication, May 31, 2000), superintendent, they have had to struggle with identity issues but are not rejected by their peers. Clearly, we need more research on psychosocial adjustment to the implant.

Based on current information and personal observations on the continuity of use, opponents of pediatric implantation feel justified in continuing to claim that the principle of nonmaleficence has not been adhered to. In other words, the presence of potential harm is a serious consideration, taking into account the fact that deaf children without the implant can and do achieve psychological health, independence, and happiness in adulthood. It is important to clarify that current pediatric implantees represent the first and second generations of children with cochlear implants, as Noel Cohen (2000a, 2000b), a cochlear implant surgeon, and Rebecca Kooper (personal communication, March 31, 2000), a New York audiologist, observe. The third generation of children with cochlear implants represents mostly children implanted with the latest technology prior to the age of 3, and the information that is currently available may not necessarily apply to this new generation.

Respect for Autonomy

Revisiting the issue of respect for parental autonomy, the reader is reminded that this respect involves recognition of a parent's right to decide based on unbiased information. Pediatric implant opponents wonder how alternatives to cochlear implants are presented to parents by cochlear implant teams (Carver, 1990). The National Association of the Deaf continues to question whether parents do receive balanced and unbiased information (Bloch, 1999). Deaf adults who can clarify the implications of all options are rarely represented on cochlear implant teams.[2] As noted in the previous chap-

---

2. One of the authors (Irene W. Leigh) served on a cochlear implant team in the early 1990s.

ter, a study by Bienenstock (1998/1999) reports that the deaf community was not considered a significant factor by implant teams. The parents we interviewed generally acknowledged receiving information about deaf community viewpoints from implant centers, but rarely if at all were they exposed to deaf people who could present such viewpoints as part of the routine screening. Part of the reason may be attributed to the perceptions of a deaf community entrenched in irrational opposition to the implant.

Pollard (1996) feels the medical community could even play a powerful role in providing unbiased information that discounts negative myths about deafness and deaf people. This rarely happens, given the typical medical perception that deaf persons are deprived of the ability to lead positive lives due to lack of hearing. Consequently, opponents of pediatric implantation see informed consent procedures as being rendered suspect by the biases inherent in presenting implants as a means of minimizing the isolation of deafness. Parents therefore psychologically may not have true freedom of choice, contrary to what proponents of cochlear implants believe.

Implant opponents have questioned the parents' ability to make decisions about implantation because of ignorance about the fulfilling lives of many deaf people who do not have cochlear implants. However, according to Bloch (1999), the NAD has consistently maintained the expectation that parents are the decision-making agents for their children, just as proponents of implantation do. The ability to make informed decisions has been confused with the parents' right to make decisions, although extremists on both sides have been guilty of reinforcing the confusion. In the second edition of *The Mask of Benevolence* (Lane, 1999), care is taken to make it clear that the issue is not that of pre-empting parental decision-making, but rather the abrogation of responsibility by government and professional organizations that approved the procedure without sufficient consideration of research evidence, and without sufficiently weighing the broader ethical implications for society.

Ethics and Deaf Community Survival

Currently, there is much talk in the deaf community about its future, not only because of cochlear implants, but also because of the implications of genetic research for correcting hereditary deafness. The latter is beyond the scope of this book, but the possibility of cultural genocide spurred by technology and genetics falls under the rubric of ethics. Although cultural genocide does not directly enter into the parental decision-making process, Lane and Bahan (1998a) ask how the survival of the "Deaf World" can be ensured in a way that does not abrogate the authority of the parents. They conclude that this is up to medical and allied associations, as well as government public health branches—all of which shape public health policy related to pediatric cochlear implants. These bodies have approved pediatric cochlear implantation as having more benefits than risks. Even though the deaf community is currently in no imminent danger of disappearing, Lane and Bahan (1998a) note that the preservation of minority cultures is "good ethics" insofar as it reflects the healthy diversity of humankind. No one is seriously suggesting that surgeons are deliberately setting out to destroy the deaf community, but ultimately this technology has the potential to diminish the size of the deaf community, at least in those countries where implantation is generally available. On that basis, Lane and Bahan question the ethics of the procedure.

Bonnie Tucker, a deaf lawyer, acknowledges that society has moral and ethical obligations to those who are deaf (B. Tucker, 1998a, 1998b). She also states that people who are deaf also have moral and ethical obligations to society. Specifically, people who are deaf should support, rather than reject, research to ameliorate or eliminate deafness, and should agree to accept full responsibility for the ramifications of "chosen" deafness. In other words, Tucker suggests that when deafness becomes increasingly correctable, those who do not choose to correct their hearing loss will lack the moral right to demand that society pay for the costly accommodations needed to compensate for the lack of hearing. She foresees that courts will likely hold that the law does not require that an individual with a physical impairment be provided with accommodations that would not be necessary if the individual obtained reasonable medical treatment that eliminated the need for such accommodations.

Although these two perspectives on the preservation of deafness and deaf culture clearly collide, a "reality check" will help to clarify the current situation. First of all, at this point in time, many people in the deaf community welcome individuals with cochlear implants. We do not see this as changing. Rather, it is likely that even more people in the deaf community will welcome cochlear implant users in the future. Moreover, many implanted children are attending specialized schools for the deaf. Many young adults in the mainstream, at least in our interview sample, are actively searching for or maintaining connections with the deaf community. Implantees from the mainstream continue to attend specialized postsecondary programs that serve deaf students, including Gallaudet University and the National Technical Institute for the Deaf. Most deaf community members who decide to get a cochlear implant remain members of the community, even if they continue to use it (not all do). As noted, many parents are signing with children who have the implant. Many parents also say their children with cochlear implants are still deaf, continue to require an assortment of services even in mainstreamed classrooms, and would benefit from associating with deaf peers. This current chain of events only serves to further Balkany et al.'s (1996) observation that "Welcoming deaf children who are 'different' (because they can use the CI to help them communicate) to be part of their community may actually enlarge and strengthen Deaf society" (p. 753). As members of a cochlear implant team, they clearly do not see themselves as immediately diminishing the deaf community, nor do they see themselves as breaking the ethical imperative to respect the right of a minority culture to exist.

The Principle of Justice

Of equally pressing concern is the fact that technology, including cochlear implants, is not equally available to all deaf persons, as Oscar Cohen (personal communication, April 3 and May 30, 2000) notes. This violates the ethical principle of justice, which deals with the allocation of resources according to "a just standard" (T. Shannon, 1997, p. 27). Deaf children who are poor, including many deaf children of color, do not have the access to technology that more affluent, often white, deaf children do. Even though minorities comprise over 40% of the Gallaudet annual survey of deaf and hard-of-hearing children (Holden-Pitt & Diaz, 1998), the GRI study reveals that approximately 85% of the parents responding to the cochlear implant survey were white. In our interview sample, only one set of parents was from an ethnic minority group. Data from the Allen, Rawlings, and Remington (1993) report on preliminary findings in Texas indicate that 90% of their pediatric implantee sample was white.

Although films such as *Dreams Spoken Here* (Oberkotter Foundation Film Project, 1998) demonstrate sensitivity to multiculturalism by including implanted children from diverse ethnic backgrounds, the reality is that the underrepresentation of racial and ethnic groups is a serious ethical concern. If there is increasing documentation of improved academic performance for deaf children with cochlear implants, the education and development of a growing number of children without access to implants will be threatened. Oscar Cohen accuses many of being silent about this issue and its implications (we return to this issue again in Concluding Thoughts).

The Rights of Children

At what age are children sufficiently competent to participate in the decision-making process? How is the information packaged and presented to the child or adolescent? How vulnerable is the deaf child to pressure from parents and professionals, whether overt or subtle? How seriously is the child's discomfort with the idea of surgery or of wearing the implant paraphernalia addressed? These are all ethical questions that require thoughtful consideration.

The role of children and adolescents in the decision-making process is a sensitive one, especially since the process requires that they undergo surgery and the intensive postsurgical habilitation required to effectively learn how to comprehend and use speech. Legally a child or adolescent need not play a role in decision-making or formally consent to treatment. Ethically, most professionals believe children should be allowed to express preferences, and their assent to treatment should be obtained whenever possible (Deaton, 1996). For this reason, children and adolescents, insofar as possible, should be afforded the principle of autonomy. That is, they should be given the right to participate in the decision-making process, and to share in the informed consent process, with their parents. However, the extent to which young children can collaborate in such decisions is a complex issue.

In their evaluation of factors that need to be considered for implant surgery, Nevins and Chute (1996) note that the population of school-aged children between the ages of 6 and 12 who become candidates for the implant is shrinking because more children are being implanted at younger ages. The 3-year-old child is now "middle-aged" as far as the cochlear implant is concerned (Cohen, 2000a)! Therefore, the right to choose is becoming less of an issue for the school-aged population.

The age group that causes great concern consists of children who are implanted between the ages of 11 and 18, because a large number of them eventually become nonusers or poor performers (Nevins & Chute, 1996). In this age group, self-image, identity, and cosmetic issues are very salient, and adolescents may have unrealistic expectations of what the implant can do for them. At times, well-intentioned parents bring their adolescent to the evaluation process with little or no explanation of its purpose (P. Brice, personal communication, March 28, 2000). According to Clark et al. (1997), the older the child, the more responsibility he or she needs to be given in deciding whether to have a cochlear implant. Pre-implant information sharing and counseling as part of the evaluation process is critical. If the child is age-appropriate, Kelsay and Tyler (1996) recommend that the child be interviewed by cochlear implant staff independently from the rest of the family, thereby allowing the child to openly discuss feelings about the process.

The literature indicates that many parents believe that cochlear implants provide the most flexible option, because the possibility of rejecting it later in life in favor of sign language always exists (B. Tucker, 1998a; Yaffe, 1999). On the other hand, the possibility of learning to speak and hear after being implanted later in life appears to be more remote. On that basis, the parents we interviewed feel they are considering the rights of their child by providing choices. In contrast, implant opponents argue that the implant violates the right and integrity of children, who should be able to make these choices as they grow up (Carver, 1990; Owens, 1999; B. Stewart, personal communication, April 3, 2000). We turn now to the parent interviews to see what parents had to say about the issue of choice.

Parent Perspectives on Choice

Of the 56 parent interviews we conducted, a majority (42 or 75%) indicated that their child was too young to be involved in the decision-making process. The ages of these children ranged from approximately 19 months up to 8 years of age. Many of these parents based their decision on the assumption that there would be more options in the future for their child with an implant than without. Moreover, as noted in chapter 4, parents wanted to maximize the window of opportunity for the development of spoken language. Many parents also acknowledged their child's right to choose not to use the implant as the child matured, but also hoped not to be disappointed in this regard.

The rest of the parents (14 or 25%), who had children ranging from 5 to 17 years of age, said their child either had suggested getting the implant, participated in the decision-making process, or made the decision. It appears that no parents of children under 5 years of age reported giving their child the option. Children between 5 and 8 years of age participated in the decision-making process if the parents felt it was appropriate based on individual readiness. The following comments are representative of the parents' responses:

Well, it's my child, and it's our job to do the best we can for our child, so I believe that until they are mature, that we have to do the best that we can for them, just like you do with other things. Parents don't let their children go do other irresponsible things, either.

Father of a 6-year-old girl implanted at age 2 and
a 4-year-old boy implanted at age 2

My child herself made the suggestion that she would like a cochlear implant. This is what prompted us to consider the matter very seriously.

Father of a 12-year-old girl implanted at age 9

We did not want to make the decision. We wanted her [the 11-year-old] to make this decision because she's old enough.

Mother of a girl recently implanted at age 11 and
an 8-year-old girl implanted at 4

We felt like he was old enough to kind of give us some feedback [about] what he wanted to do. We explained that you were going to get cut and he ... wanted to do it. And he had seen pictures we made of him with a bandage on his head and all that stuff. And you know, he asked, Mmmm, cutting hurt, same as picture? And he said, he wanted ... to hear. ... And he wanted to do it.

Parent of a 9-year-old boy facing a third
surgery due to implant failure

But some parents do acknowledge their child might see them as having pushed for implantation. One parent said:

> For us he was completely involved. It was completely his decision. He would not have been forced to have the implant, not as a teenager, certainly. [A famous audiologist] even said, If it ain't broke, don't fix it. He's happy and . . . so no one was saying, You should do this, but we were just exposing him to it. . . . And he might say that we were pushing it, but I can tell you honestly, we weren't.
>
> *Mother of an 18-year-old young man implanted at age 16*

Some parents were concerned about the implications of waiting for the child to be old enough to choose.

> How old does a child have to be before he can make an informed decision. . . . If [my son] is 6, 7, 8, 9 years old, I think I can very well influence what he feels he wants to do. Because what does a 7-year-old say if daddy is saying, You want an implant, don't you? He'll go, Yeah. Now, is that considered informed consent?
>
> *Father of a 2-year-old boy implanted at 19 months*

> I feel like by the time a child is old enough to make a decision for him or herself, their opportunities to really use the implant effectively has diminished [based on brain research], so I felt like we needed to make the decision now and not wait till our children were old enough to think they might want it.
>
> *Mother of a 6-year-old girl implanted at age 2 and*
> *a 4-year-old boy implanted at age 2*

> At first, one of our opinions was that this is kind of an intrusive operation and I think this opinion was formed from people in the deaf community. I think we bought into that for a while, that she should make this decision on her own—it's her body—but as we thought about it and talked about it, and came around to it, we as parents want her to have every opportunity to be able to have these things available to her, and it's part of our duty as a parent to find this information out, to evaluate it, and give her the opportunity. . . . We prayed for a miracle. And to us there is

nothing wrong with deafness. There is nothing wrong with hearing. They're both the same. It's just that in this hearing world, my child seemed to not be getting full advantage like everyone else. So our prayer for a miracle was that she would be able to hear in this hearing world so that she could live fully.

Father of a 6-year-old girl implanted at age 5

We were told, if we didn't make the decision and waited until he was 18 to make the decision, we were actually making the decision [not to implant] because it would be too late.

Father of a 5-year-old boy implanted at age 2

What most parents had to say should their child later reject the implant is captured by this sentiment:

But no matter what she chooses or decides to do, we'll always be there to back her up.

Mother of a 6-year-old girl implanted at 19 months

A parent who chose not to implant had this to say: *If we gave him the implant, when he grew up he could say, Why did you do that to me? So it could go either way.... I think that's why we felt that we had to document our research so that we could say to him, This is why. And, you know ... I still feel confident that we made the right decision.*

All the parents we interviewed did not make the decision to implant lightly. As two parents stated:

As a parent, you want nothing but the best for your children. And as a parent you are going to be constantly faced with choices for your children that you have to make and all you can do is gather the information you can, try to make the most informed decision you can, and then hope you did it right.

Father of an 11-year-old boy implanted at age 8

I had days where I was convinced we'd done the right thing, and I had days where I was convinced we did the wrong thing. And I don't have days anymore where I think we did the wrong thing.

Mother of a 5-year-old boy implanted at age 2

Young Adult Perspectives on Choice Issues

For the young adults we interviewed, ages of implantation ranged from 4 to 20. This clearly impacts on the extent to which they had input into the decision to implant. First, we report on the perspectives of the 13 nonusers and then on those of the 14 continuing users (see chapter 10 for a description of the sample).

Three of the nonusers reported they were too young to understand much about the surgery, having been implanted at ages 4, 5, and 7, respectively. Another nonuser, implanted at age 7, reports that her mother did not ask her how she felt about the cochlear implant: *I was scared and said nothing.* She had to undergo a second surgery at age 11 because of technical difficulties with the first implant, and claims that if her mother had asked her, she would have said no.

A female implanted at age 13 reported that her parents did not ask her if she wanted the cochlear implant. She was taken to the hospital without explanations or any interpreting of what was going on. When she woke up, she had an implant. The other female who was implanted at age 13 said, *My parents asked me. It was my decision if I wanted this cochlear implant thing. I ... said yes, fine, but my main reason was to please my parents. They seemed to be so excited over this new thing that can help me hear....I mean, I was 13 years old, and I had a hard time with the whole concept of not wanting to be shown that I'm deaf.... A lot of conflicting feelings, but as time went on I was ready for it.* People were honest with her, but the problem was that she really wanted to be normal. However, she said she *freaked out* when shown by the doctor what the surgery would be like and started crying en route to surgery, wishing the procedure would stop. Three males, implanted at ages 7, 8, and 13, also reported not really having a choice and acceding to parent wishes.

Two young adults said that they expressed desire for a cochlear implant. One of them, implanted at age 6, badly wanted sound back, having lost her hearing at age 3, whereas the other had seen a classmate with an implant and wanted it as well.

Finally, one female decided to get implanted at the age of 20 because, she said: *There was a lot of debate and I wanted to go ahead and prove that it didn't work on me.* She was disappointed that it worked to the extent that she could identify environmental sounds (voices were more difficult)!

The issue of choice includes not only the decision to start, but also the decision to stop using the implant. The 20-year-old female just described decided that, after one year of use, she had had enough and went back to what she called *quiet time*. Additionally, hearing people would not gesture to her or recognize that she was still deaf, which made it difficult for her considering her identity as a deaf person. The 12 other nonusers stopped using the cochlear implant during adolescence. They said it either did not work, it was too noisy, discriminating sound was too difficult, they got headaches, or there was no real change in communication. For them, the benefits were not worth the effort to use the implant. Some of them also mentioned identity issues, peer pressure, and the desire to be connected with deaf culture.

One person said: *It was a frustrating experience and they* [peers in a Total Communication program to which the interviewee had transferred as a teenager] *made fun of me. On top of all that I had this wire hanging down from my head. It was all cosmetic, but it's part of teenage peer pressure. When I stopped using the cochlear implant, I explained to my parents the issue of identity, the lack of improvement in hearing, and the fact that I could still speak.... They felt that by removing the implant, I was removing the options. They couldn't understand why I couldn't be deaf, use sign language, and have an implant.... Later, I realized my initial intentions were wrong* [in light of increasing acceptance of cochlear implants in the deaf community] *but the overall results were good because the implant was not helping me.*

Another interviewee said: *In high school it was the worst time for me with the cochlear implant because I was really trying to find my identity with the cochlear implant.... I never accepted my deafness. And the cochlear implant in some ways showed me that no matter what, the moment I take it off, I'm deaf. I'll never be hearing 24 hours.*

While at Gallaudet, this young adult was exposed to deaf people who were not embarrassed about their deafness in public. Then, as she states, she started to let her deafness be part of her.

No nonuser expressed intense anger at parents for having chosen an implant. As a matter of fact, three appreciated having had the chance to use the implant, to know what hearing was like, even though one of them blamed her father for wanting her to be implanted. A fourth person, who had been implanted at age 13, felt *half and half* about having had the chance to be exposed to hearing stimuli, but wished that her parents had asked her if she wanted an implant.

Two of the interviewees who were asked about implanting young deaf children responded that parents should wait until these children were old enough to make their own choices, preferably in late adolescence. *I never wanted to put a child through the emotions and mental stuff that I went through. The kid would feel confused, angry, and ask why did the parent do that to him.*

A third suggested age 10 as a reasonable age when the child could participate in the decision-making process. Two were equivocal:

If you want to have all the benefits of the implant and everything that it is designed to do, medically speaking, it is better to implant a child. But ethically, you'd be taking away an individual's right to freedom. If they implant and sign, or do not implant and sign, I'd be happy, but if they do implant and not sign, I am upset.

I believe that children should have the cochlear implant, but expose them to deaf culture. This person has two deaf children and has decided against the implant for them.

Regarding the phenomenon of nonuse, Mary Koch (personal communication, April 25, 2000), auditory education consultant, believes it parallels that of taking off hearing aids as part of identity exploration rather than having anything to do with the cochlear implant itself. She feels that many will return to hearing aids or cochlear implants when interacting more with hearing people. Indeed, some of the nonusers we talked with mentioned the possibility they might return to use of the implant when in hearing-oriented environments, although some were concerned about symptoms like headaches. According to Koch, such symptoms should not occur if the mapping is done well and appropriately within the framework of good rehabilitation programs.

Moving on to the group of 14 adolescent and young adult users, six clearly indicated they chose the implants for themselves. Their ages at the time of surgery ranged from 13 to 17. One 16-year-old reported that her mother even asked her if she was really sure she wanted the implant because she did so well with hearing aids. Her response was that she felt she could do even better with the implant: *I always wanted to have the best hearing that I could, so I said, Why not give it a chance?* A 15-year-old female said: *I want the implant to make me able to listen and be able to understand hearing people because, you know, later on in life I will be working with hearing people.*

One 18-year-old female initially expressed skepticism about the effectiveness of the implant over hearing aids. Additionally, she hated doctors, but decided to pursue implantation at the age of 15 after seeing her implanted friends surpass her in oral communication skills. Her parents were the reluctant ones!

The Gallaudet University female who continues to use her implant initially resisted implantation when her mother and audiologist suggested it at age 14 because, as she said, *I was afraid of having something in my head.* When she turned 17, she became curious about whether she could hear more with it than with her hearing aid, and makes it clear she decided for herself. She feels she would not have wanted it as a young child.

Five of the users reported having been too young to participate in the decision-making process since all were under the age of 4 when they had the surgery. Currently, they all indicate continuing satisfaction with the implant. Another interviewee expressed the desire to hear at age 6, and one 14-year-old female described parental pressure when she was 13: *To be honest, I never wanted the cochlear in the first place.... The main reason I didn't want the cochlear was because I was comfortable with my hearing aid, and now I have to get used to something else.... I didn't decide to do it. My parents wanted me to do it. ...I just gave up in the end.... Now I just don't care.* She acknowledges that now she can carry on phone conversations without too much trouble. Finally, one 18-year-old male implanted at age 12 said: *Honestly, I don't think I made the decision, Okay, go for it. I think I trusted my parents.* He also adds: *What right does the deaf community have to say I violated my personal integrity? I might have been 12 years old, but I was a 12-year-old that grew up with hearing aids* [and then lost the remainder of his residual hearing].

One of the six users, when asked about young children being implanted, indicated opposition:

> Parents are wasting their money trying to force their kids
> to have an implant, and then later, because kids are kids,
> they are going to be hating it, they are going to grab it,
> throw it, break it.
>
> *Female age 18, implanted at age 16*

The rest, who had been implanted during early childhood or as adolescents, were supportive to varying degrees:

> If the hearing aids were not helping them, if they had a profound loss, I would probably give them the implant. At the same time, I would influence them about deaf culture and the deaf community when they were young, you know. . . . I mean, I want to give them choices when they are young, so they can grow older and consider which side they would like.

> If I had deaf kids, which I probably won't, I would probably choose for the kid . . . at the early stages of life. . . . I just don't think they would be mature enough to think for themselves.

> At first I would let my kids start out with hearing aids, and then when they got old enough to understand the difference between cochlear implants and hearing aids, then I could tell them my [experiences] and they could take their own risks and choices in deciding whether or not they want cochlear implants.

Clearly, those implanted young people we interviewed, both users and nonusers, do not take choice issues lightly. Nor do the respondents in the Gallaudet University survey. Half of the full sample felt parents should not be permitted to choose the implant for children under the age of 5, even after careful research (see chapter 10).

How strongly do young deaf adults agree with the decision their parents made to implant them when they were children? The interviews reported here indicate variability in agreement, with a good number of users and nonusers both expressing concern about very young children being implanted. Consequently, parents need to take their children's opinions and feelings into account if possible. Whether the children participate or not, parents need to carefully weigh potential risks and benefits in terms of successive stages of development. This involves not only exploring the literature and talking to a wide spectrum of professionals, but also meeting members of the deaf community—both those who have grown up with implants and those who have not. When they have done all these things, their final decision to proceed or not will have been fully informed. Parents owe that to their children, who live with the consequences of that decision.

Concluding Thoughts

"I think one of the reasons I really wanted to do this study is because I'm really happy that you're trying to get a cross-section, and to understand. I think people need to know there's a lot of confused information out there. So if you guys can help straighten that out a little, it'll be great."

Mother of an 18-year-old young man
implanted at age 16

One of our goals in writing this book was to try and straighten out that confusion, especially for new parents. These parents often have to search far and wide to get the information that will help them understand the choices they are making for their deaf child. To aid them in their search for understanding, we wanted to get a cross-section of parents and report on their experiences and their perspectives. Even though our interview sample was weighted toward parents of children and youth who continue to use the implant, we believe we did get a spectrum of perspectives on the issues parents face as they navigate the pathways to implantation and beyond.

Although the cochlear implant has clearly been a boon for some, the variability in results makes it difficult to successfully predict how well children will do with the implant. This is true for the children in our interview sample, as well as children included in the research reported in chapter 9. Consequently, the extent to which the cochlear implant does make a significant difference in their lives is still being determined. As discussed earlier, factors such as level of intellectual functioning, the presence of cognitive impairment, age at implantation, educational placement, systematic exposure to language, and the ability to absorb spoken language, among others, will factor into the ultimate usefulness of pediatric cochlear implants. Our parent interviews clearly indicate that most parents are aware there is no guarantee that their child will sufficiently benefit from having a cochlear implant to make the surgery worth doing. Indeed, many cochlear implant centers typically stress this point. Even those children who do well with the implant continue to need support services such as note-taking, captioning, and speech, auditory, and language therapy. Moreover, cochlear implants do not typically enable the user to overcome communication difficulties caused by group situations and noisy backgrounds. All these reasons reinforce perceptions of most of the parents we talked with that implanted children, including their own, are still children who are deaf. Most of the parents realize that the implant is not a miracle cure, contrary to media headlines and statements by some implant advocates proclaiming that it is.[1] Most parents, however, do see the implant as enhancing their child's quality of life.

The new National Association of the Deaf (NAD) position statement (NAD, 2000b) strongly emphasizes that quality of life can be good even without the implant. On the other hand, many parents note positive post-implant differences, such as enhanced family communication, among other things. This difference of opinion can be explained by the fact that quality of life means different things to different people who frame life situations differently, based on their own cultural experiences.

Presenting available options to parents without creating the impression of bias is no easy task. In "Does God Have a Cochlear Implant?" Michael Harvey (2001) writes a fascinating description of

---

1. For example, in a letter to the editor in response to a lengthy article about cochlear implants in the *The Washington Post* (Colburn, 2000), the writer, Elizabeth Foster, the director of the National Campaign for Hearing Health, found a way to use the word "miracle" to describe implants three times in her short letter (Foster, 2000).

the struggle to examine his own biases as a professional who works with people on both sides of the cochlear implant debate. His major struggle has been to try to reconcile the perspective of cochlear implant technology, which promises increased accessibility and a more equal playing field, with the perspective of oralism (in the guise of cochlear implants) as an evil behemoth trampling on the rights of deaf persons. Harvey himself has seen devastating failures, as well as amazing successes subsequent to cochlear implantation. Consequently, he says, *"You need to have and understand all the relevant information.* And that's easier said than done" (p. 78; italics in original).

In addressing the question of what professionals and cochlear implant centers can do to enhance collaboration with parents, we note that parents are very sensitive to the various factions that tout their own philosophy about what they believe is best for deaf children. A number of parents in our interview sample had difficulties dealing with professionals who strongly advocated for their particular approaches. In fact, as one parent said: *People have their own feelings, and their own biases, and their own needs to validate their choices, and their own strongly held beliefs, and it was very difficult to sort of discover that, and then filter through what people were telling us, and try to separate fact from emotion and the whole bit.*

Most parents felt comfortable with professionals and cochlear implant staff members who tried to explain what the various communication and technology options were and who did not try to push the parents in a specific direction. They respected professionals who respected them and their struggles. In order for professionals to get to that point and increase their awareness of their biases, one mother suggested that they: *Break down some of the walls between auditory-verbal, sign language,* [and] *cochlear implant groups. My child is an example of someone who has thoroughly benefited by our conscientious integrating of different modalities, giving him pieces of each of them to suit his temperament. And that seems to not be very easy for individuals, professionals, to really be able to do that, because they're kind of territorial, it seems like.* Another mother asked of professionals: *If you haven't walked in my shoes, don't judge me. And the professionals hadn't walked in my shoes. They chose deafness, I didn't.*

From our interviews and from the Gallaudet Research Insititute (GRI) survey, it appears that parents generally felt they were provided with a fairly comprehensive picture of what to expect and what their child's life might be like with the implant. Generally, the focus appears to have been on positive aspects related to the procedure at the expense of potentially negative consequences. Even if unintentional, that in and of itself can be related not only to what parents want to or are able to remember, but also to how the relevant information is packaged and delivered to them. For this reason, some health care professionals need to critically evaluate how they deliver information to parents.

Another sensitive area that involves professionals and their biases is the issue of how they present opinions expressed by deaf people who question the implant's effectiveness. Parents are much more likely to meet professionals and cochlear implant center staff members than deaf people themselves. Consequently, these parents will typically be getting "deaf community perspectives" about the cochlear implant from audiologists, physicians, education specialists, and other professionals who are not part of the deaf community. Parents, most of who have rarely, if ever, even met a deaf person before, are largely unaware of the nature of this community and how deaf people interact within this community. As one parent remarked: *I think it scares the parents even more sometimes when they ... hear or read things from the deaf community that, to them, sound so foreign to what they're used to. It solidifies their decision to do everything they can to keep their child from becoming one of them.*

The new NAD position paper on cochlear implants, which emphasizes the diversity of deaf people, with or without implants, will likely improve the way parents perceive the deaf community (assuming, of course, that parents become aware of the position paper). In the same vein, professionals need to ask themselves whether they can honestly convey to parents what their child's life in the deaf community could be like if they decide against implantation. Are health care professionals able to accurately describe opportunities for in-depth socialization and interaction with people in the deaf community, or is the deaf community negatively depicted as a limiting influence that stands in the way of interacting with hearing peers? Is it absolutely true that becoming part of the deaf community severs connections with hearing peers? Since that typically is not the case, careful consideration of the ethics involved in this debate (as discussed in chapter 11) will enhance the ability of professionals to think about all aspects of this issue and impart information to parents in a way that facilitates truly aware informed consent regarding implantation, whatever the parents finally decide.

It seems to us that the walls between those who support pediatric implantation and those who oppose the procedure are, if not crumbling, at least beginning to show some noticeable cracks. Both parties are more willing to pay attention to the other side of the argument, even though they may not necessarily agree (see, e.g., Balkany et al., 1998; Lane & Bahan, 1998a, 1998b; R. Shannon, 1998). As we wrote in the Introduction, another goal in writing this book was to elicit some common ground. Many of the parents and young people we interviewed clearly crave this common ground. They are not interested in "either-or" thinking, whether it be oralism or manualism, implants or signing; they support a move to a more inclusive approach that is tolerant of diversity. Parents who continue to sign to their children after implantation are a prime example of this; most of the parents in both our sample and the GRI survey have not stopped signing to their implanted children, nor do they think that signing necessarily hinders the development of spoken language. This flies in the face of the pervasive myth that children with implants are no longer allowed to sign once they get the implant. Whether children sign or not depends, of course, on the educational program philosophy that the parents or the children themselves choose. Many of the parents in our sample appear to have chosen programs that encourage signs to maintain communication, as needed, while continuing to focus on audition. As noted in chapter 9, new research on language development supports this approach. There is no question that, for children with implants, the emphasis on post-implant auditory training continues to be critically important, even with signs. But many young people who are the products of various regimens are nevertheless interested in reaching out to the deaf community while simultaneously maintaining ties to hearing peers. They want to embrace diversity and not be boxed in by the constraints of only one community.

By the same token, there are increasing numbers of deaf community members who welcome cochlear implant users. It used to be that deaf people who functioned easily in a speaking environment were viewed as suspect, as being "too hearing," even if they continued to interact with signing members of the deaf community. In fact, in American Sign Language, there is even a derogatory sign for deaf people who are perceived as being too close to hearing people, who "think hearing." In the same vein, children, youth, and adults with cochlear implants were seen as individuals trying to be "hearing," and for this reason were often ostracized by many if not most deaf community signers. Today, the tide has clearly begun to change. Our interviewees, both users and nonusers of the implant, increasingly tell us that young people with cochlear implants are a part of an inclusive deaf community, that they are still deaf. This is based on the recognition that cochlear implants do not automatically entail a repudiation of deaf community values. Additionally, this process is a reflection of the deaf community's move from the cultural to the bicultural, as Carol Padden (1996), a deaf scholar and a member of Gallaudet University's Board of Trustees, describes it. Deaf people have recognized the need to not withdraw from, but rather to deal with hearing-deaf tensions in positive, bridge-building ways as they negotiate boundaries with hearing peers. Confronting and adapting to the cochlear implant issue are manifestations of how these tensions are being handled.

One wall that still needs to be broken down is that between hearing parents of deaf children and deaf adults, particularly those that could serve as role models for children with cochlear implants who are in the mainstream and rarely see deaf adults. Although some parents gravitate easily toward interacting with deaf people, most find it difficult, whether due to communication issues, feelings about the deaf community, or discomfort about the condition of deafness as a disability. What some of these parents may forget is that, in more ways than one, *deaf adults are their children grown up.* Deaf adults who sign, as well as those who do not, have experienced what life is like as a deaf person, and they have advice and wisdom to pass on to parents and children. Increasingly, there will be deaf adults who have grown up with cochlear implants who can also serve as mentors for parents, as well as their deaf children. If deaf adults, particularly those who consider themselves part of the deaf community, are willing to listen to what parents have to say about cochlear implants and their deaf child, parents are likely to be more willing to start a dialogue with them and create a process of mutual understanding and learning about what might be best for their deaf child. As one mother says, *I still think nobody knows their child like a parent.* Another parent said: *I've never understood why a deaf person would be unkind to someone who functions well in the hearing world. Are you supposed to hold yourself back because others don't want to cross over? I don't understand.* Deaf adults need to respect that feeling on the part of parents. Our research indicates they have begun this process as they see the increasing numbers of children and peers with implants. Hopefully, greater respect and understanding on all sides will lead to a reduction of the "either-or" thinking reflected in this mother's lament.

As a means of encouraging interaction between parents and deaf adults, one parent we talked with recommends that: *It probably would be better, instead of giving somebody a stack of papers and organizations, . . . if, in the initial stages of finding out if a child is deaf, to have a deaf counselor assigned to people, or something.* Another parent adds that: *Maybe there should be a network of deaf people that audiologists can recommend to hearing parents of deaf children, maybe some sort of mentor program.* This might go a long way toward enhancing the perception of deaf people as valuable resources for parents and, in turn, for professionals working within cochlear implant programs.

As we discussed in chapter 8, most parents said that if they had to start over again, they would consider implanting their child earlier. They were encouraged by their perceptions of success or improvement in contrast to their child's pre-implant performance. The definition of success, and of failure, however, is not clear-cut. Success can be defined by criteria ranging from recognition of environmental sounds to facility in the use of spoken language. Failure can be defined by lack of auditory comprehension in noisy situations, or by the inability to move beyond the recognition of environmental sounds. The reasons for failure are still subject to conjecture (Kluwin & Stewart, 2000). We come to the conclusion that success and failure dimensions are very subjective. Objective criteria for different levels of success, including measures of psychological and psychosocial wellness (Lane & Bahan, 1998a; R. Shannon, 1998) need to be developed. The meaning of failure needs specification as well.

In addition to figuring out what constitutes failure, we need to consider the implications of failure. Failure, especially defined in terms of permanently discontinuing implant use, affects parents, the child, and other members of the family. Considering that recruiting parents of children and youth who no longer use the implant for research purposes is no easy task, we can also assume the presence of emotional factors that need to be dealt with. Are parents' unconscious hopes for their child's facility in spoken communication dashed? Do parents struggle with guilt about "not doing enough" or "doing the wrong thing" for their child? How does the child or adolescent deal with the disappointment of the parents? How does this process of rejecting the implant affect the child's self-esteem? In studies reporting speech and language results for implanted children, what are the psychosocial and emotional consequences for children who do not perform well? Do families go for counseling to help them deal with the feelings of failure or of "wasted effort"? We would possibly know more about minimizing future problems if implant centers could follow children who discontinue the implant. This becomes difficult when families move and are then lost to follow-up, or when they do not respond to research requests.

Additional issues are emerging on the educational front. One of us (Irene W. Leigh) grew up in the era of oral education that involved lipreading training, which is very visual, and auditory training classes a couple of times a week to hone listening skills with old-fashioned headsets connected to auditory units. The need to accent both vision and audition is still salient, especially in the case of schools that currently embrace sign language-based programs and visual avenues for enhancing the education of deaf children. Many of these institutions, especially residential schools, are beginning to grapple with strategies for integrating auditory education to accommodate children with cochlear implants. The Laurent Clerc National Deaf Education Center at Gallaudet University is a case in point. Gallaudet's new cochlear implant center is unique in that it will "develop and evaluate programming for children with implants with an educational framework that integrates American Sign Language" (Fernandes, 2000a). Such programming will emphasize the development of both spoken and visual language skills. At the same time, oral-based schools are becoming more aurally oriented in response to this new influx of deaf children. These new demands of specialized schools heighten the need to search for the most effective educational interventions for this specialized population. Due to the variability in results that currently exists, we are still light years away from doing away with schools for the deaf, cost-effectiveness studies of pediatric implantation (e.g., Niparko et al., 2000a) notwithstanding.

Whereas the establishment of a cochlear implant center at Gallaudet is undoubtedly surprising to some, so far it has not provoked any visible opposition from students or others on campus or, as far as we know, from any other subgroups within the deaf community. It obviously takes a good amount of time to change attitudes, particularly about something as controversial and challenging as cochlear implants. But our findings indicate that attitudes on campus are changing. The fact that cochlear implant forums take place on campus without overt protest is powerful testimony to the effect that a new reality exists.

Regarding mainstream education, the most typical expectation is that cochlear implantation will facilitate entry into mainstream educational programs, which range from self-contained classrooms in which deaf children spend most of their time to partial and full-time mainstreaming, most often with support services. In numerous cases, parents have to fight hard to get quality support services for their deaf children. In the high school years, some children do gravitate from mainstream programs to schools for the deaf, and vice versa. That was true for some of the families in this study. The education of deaf children has always been a complex undertaking, dependent on what these children need at various stages of development and what local areas have to offer. At this point in time, the implant by itself does not consistently provide complete, full access to a spoken language system for every young child with a cochlear implant, intensive speech and listening therapy notwithstanding. Mainstream educational programs must acknowledge the special needs of deaf children with cochlear implants. Ignorance and cost considerations must be put aside in the interest of providing an appropriate education for each child.

The science of predicting which young child will benefit from the cochlear implant is still in its infancy. In this regard, as far as children whose deafness is caused by genetic factors is concerned, Hedi Rehm (personal communication, July 20, 2000), of the Department of Neurobiology at Harvard Medical School, has told us that the genetic basis of the deafness, and therefore the exact pathology present in the cochlea, may have the potential to influence how well a given child does with implants.

No one has yet done a study of an exact genetic condition that correlates it to the outcome of the cochlear implant. A recently developed genetic test for deafness is one that detects mutations in the connexin 26 gene. Now that connexin 26 testing is increasingly common, researchers are beginning to look at this specific genetic group and examine cochlear implant performance. As tests develop for additional genes for deafness, we can anticipate further study in this area. However, it remains clear that factors extraneous to the genetic basis for deafness, such as individual variability and environmental input, will continue to play a critical factor in predicting cochlear implant success. Hence, the possibility of predicting implant success for infants younger than 12 months is unlikely to increase drastically in the near future. We ask whether it is possible and advisable to determine whether or not a child under 12 months of age has a moderate to severe hearing loss, and therefore could benefit from using hearing aids, before implantation is considered? (There are exceptions such as in the case of meningitis, which, of course, does not have a genetic etiology, although susceptibility for hearing loss due to meningitis may have a genetic component [Collins, 2001].)

Research on whether and how hair cell regeneration can be artificially stimulated in mammals has begun (Contanche, 2000). Scientists hope to identify pathways for inducing functional regeneration of hair cells in cochleas. Another future possibility includes the development of a "biological cochlear implant," where sensory hair cells could be implanted into the inner ear. This area of research is still in its infancy, and it will be years before anyone can capitalize on biological and gene-based interventions.

Currently, there are many advances on the technology front. For example, Advanced Bionics, the manufacturer of the Clarion cochlear implant, has developed electrodes that are capable of selectively stimulating targeted groups of hearing nerve fibers. Implantable hearing aids are now available (R. Shannon, 2000). Efforts to miniaturize cochlear implant components are bearing fruit, with the new behind-the-ear device now available. The technology for a fully implantable cochlear implant exists today, and this instrument will be ready for marketing sooner rather than later (R. Shannon, 2000). Clearly, science and technology are collaborating in the effort to create improved access to hearing.

However, with all the technology advances, we need to pause and consider what the potential problems might be. It will be some time before we have adults who have had implants for 25 years or more. Questions about the long-term effects of having a magnet in one's head have not yet been answered. What about reimplantation as technology improves, or to counteract unanticipated problems? Is this process going to become a viable, easily accomplished procedure? Will insurance companies be willing to subsidize reimplantation, considering the present difficulties in getting a number of insurance companies to even approve cochlear implant surgery in the first place?

Ultimately, the final word about the usefulness of cochlear implants will come from the cochlear implant users themselves. The adolescents and young people we interviewed provided a variety of perspectives that was refreshing. However, a good number of the ongoing users expressed concern about very young children being implanted and how they might eventually feel about this process. The fact that most of our interviewees were not implanted before the age of 3 may have been a factor in their responses. Yet, considering what these young people said, and in view of the fact that the average age of pediatric implantation continues to drop, it behooves us to look very closely at how this population is adjusting to life with the implant. As scholars on opposing sides of this debate have suggested, it is time to stop looking solely at speech and language results, or at cost-effectiveness numbers, and to start looking also at important psychosocial issues. Are these children making friends? Do they communicate in comfortable ways with the world around them? How do they explain the implant to themselves and to others? Are they participating in classroom situations, whether in the mainstream or in specialized schools? Are they ostracized or accepted as children or teenagers who happen to use an implant? When they grow up, with whom do they socialize? Do they cherish both deaf and hearing friends? Whom do they choose as life partners? What kinds of jobs do they get? Do they continue to use the implant on a consistent basis? These are questions about "life" for which the answers are sorely lacking. We look forward to seeing how the future evolves as cochlear implant users and the deaf community work to create new pathways toward coexistence.

One issue that needs to be addressed by the cochlear implant community is the unequal distribution of implants among various racial, ethnic, and socioeconomic groups in the United States. In the 1999 GRI survey, for example, more than 85% of the respondents were white, about 4% were African-American, and 6% were Latino (5% other). According to the U.S. Census Bureau (1999), about 72% of the population is white, 12% is African-American, and slightly more than 11% is Latino.[2] Whites are overrepresented in the GRI study just as they are in the pediatric cochlear implant population at large. In addition, in the GRI study, slightly more than 57% of the families reported an annual income of more than $50,000. Again, this is far from a typical cross-section of the American population. In 1998, slightly less than 47% of the white population reported an annual family income above $50,000, whereas only about 26% of African-American families reported a family income above this figure (U.S. Census Bureau, 1999). Perhaps because affluent families are more likely to have health insurance that pays for implantation as well as other resources (including an awareness of how the health care system functions and what it frequently takes to get a response from insurance companies and health care professionals), they are more likely to be successful in their effort to secure an implant for their child. Moreover, in general, affluent people are more likely to be better educated, and consequently perhaps more likely to be aware that implants are even an option, than their less affluent neighbors. One challenge facing everyone concerned about the future of deaf children is the need to try to avoid a situation where affluent white youngsters have access to the latest technology, while less affluent young people, especially young people of color, are left with residual resources. Therefore it behooves any professional this latter group may encounter to facilitate access to the best services possible, including Medicaid and other public services, when appropriate.

2. As reported in *The Economist*, the 2000 U.S. Census found that 69.1% of the population is white, 12.1% is African-American, and 12.5% is Latino ("Primary Colours," 2001).

Another issue involving implantation centers around the question of the extent to which those who are theoretically eligible for a cochlear implant are, in fact, considering one or even aware that they might benefit from using one. As noted earlier, both adults and children who are considered candidates for an implant must have, among other things, a severe to profound sensorineural hearing loss and should receive little or no benefit from a hearing aid.

In an effort to determine how many people there are who might be eligible for a cochlear implant, in 1999 the Project HOPE Center for Health Affairs investigated the severely to profoundly deaf population in the United States. After reviewing several studies (Project HOPE did not conduct the original research itself), the authors of the report (Blanchfield, Dunbar, Feldman, & Gardner, 1999) estimated that there are approximately 464,000 to 738,000 severely to profoundly deaf people in the United States. (This is approximately .17% to .27% of the total United States population.) About 8%, or somewhere between 37,000 and 60,000 severely to profoundly deaf people, are children under the age of 18.

At the present time there are more than 35,000 people in the entire world who have cochlear implants. About half of these are children and half are adults, and the vast majority reside in one of the "First World" nations (especially the United States, Australia, Japan, and countries in Western Europe). It is not known how many of these people are still using their implant. At the current rate of growth, approximately 4,000 to 6,000 people, half of them children under 18, are implanted annually around the world.

Project HOPE concludes, "implantation of the device is extremely low among those who could benefit [in the United States]" (Blanchfield et al., 1999, p. iv). Given the numbers above, that conclusion is certainly not surprising, and it obviously means that there is a great deal of potential growth for implantation in the future, among both children and adults. The report also found, however, that "most of the severely to profoundly hearing-impaired population are, on average, poorer than other Americans" (p. iii) and are less likely to have comprehensive private insurance coverage than more affluent Americans. Thus, although there is clearly a market for implants in the United States, there are a number of factors that might make it difficult for the implanted population to diversify beyond the fairly homogeneous racial and socioeconomic categories discussed above.

And this, of course, says nothing about cochlear implantation in the Third World where the vast majority of the severely to profoundly deaf population in the world lives. The Population Reference Bureau (2000) estimates that the world's population is currently about 6,067,000,000 and is increasing (births minus deaths) at the rate of more than 200,000 people per *day.* Approximately 97% of this increase is in the Third World (Warrick, 1998). Although deafness prevalence rates undoubtedly vary among countries (Schein, 1989), if one uses the .17% to .27% figure noted above for the United States as a rough estimate and applies that rate to the entire world population, it is apparent that there are approximately 10,000,000 to 16,000,000 severely to profoundly deaf people in the world today. In addition, perhaps 360 babies are born in the world each day with severe hearing problems (if a prevalence rate of one of every 1,000 live births, a commonly suggested figure, is applied on a worldwide scale where there are now approximately 360,000 births each day).

One way to look at this exercise is to say that the market for cochlear implants is not likely to ever be saturated and the growth potential is unlimited. Although this is undoubtedly true, it is also somewhat pointless, given the current inequitable distribution of medical resources around the world. There is simply no way countries in sub-Saharan Africa, for example, which may have one doctor for every 20,000 people and a per capita income of $500 per year or less, could even begin to consider implantation on a wide scale for the deaf children and adults who live there.

In the final analysis, it appears that cochlear implantation is unlikely to ever reach more than a relatively small proportion of those who could theoretically benefit from the device. This is likely to be true for a large number of severely and profoundly deaf people in countries like the United States, and it is certainly true in less industrialized nations. This conclusion is at odds with some observers who apparently feel that it is only a matter of time before pediatric implantation becomes almost routine, at least in the United States (e.g., "The Death of Deafness?" 2000). Even if universal infant screening for hearing loss is instituted in all states (something we strongly endorse), it remains to be seen whether there will be sufficient numbers of implant surgeons and centers, audiologists trained in cochlear implant mapping procedures, speech and language therapists, particularly in public schools, willing parents, insurance carriers willing to pay for the procedure, and so on. It seems more reasonable to predict that pediatric implantation will continue to grow, but that significant structural barriers, as well as individual choices, will likely lead to something less than a fully implanted population of deaf children.

In summary, although it is conceivable that in the years ahead the cost of implantation could be drastically reduced, or emerging technologies or procedures could even make the implant obsolete, at the present time the implant's impact and availability are likely to be more limited than some people expect. This means that there will still be millions of deaf people around the world who will need other services and products, who will continue to form sign language-based deaf communities in the countries where they live, and who will continue to need basic educational opportunities that are unevenly available. In the rush to embrace modern technology, we cannot ignore the needs of those whose access to this technology is, and will continue to be, severely constrained.

We hope that the perspectives of the parents, the deaf implant users and nonusers that we interviewed, and the Gallaudet University survey respondents will help facilitate movement toward the common ground that we were looking for as we embarked on the research for this book. Cochlear implant centers and allied professionals working with pediatric implantees can benefit from what the parents and young people have to say about the process. The NAD, in its new position paper, has taken a giant step in building a bridge to parents. This is a message for the deaf community to follow suit so that parents can build on their feelings of comfort about entrusting their child to both the deaf community and the hearing world.

One strong message coming out of this research is that of teamwork. Parents, deaf people, and professionals, both deaf and hearing, need to build on collaborative efforts to benefit any deaf child, including a child with a cochlear implant, as we await the results of ongoing research. It is hoped that this forthcoming research will indicate the extent to which the potential benefits of cochlear implants are available to all children whose parents select this option.

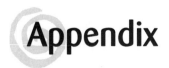

Appendix

Cochlear Implant Companies

Product: Clarion
Advanced Bionics Corporation
12740 San Fernando Road
Sylmar, CA 91342
818-362-7588
800-678-2575
http://www.cochlearimplant.com/
info@advancedbionics.com

Product: Nucleus
Cochlear Corporation
61 Inverness Drive East
Suite 200
Englewood, CO 80112
303-790-9010
800-523-5798
http://www.cochlear.com/

Product: Combi
Med-El Corporation
2222 East NC Highway 54, Suite B-180
Durham, NC 27713
919-572-2222
http://www.medel.com/
implants@medelus.com

References

Aiello, P., & Aiello, M. (2000, July). *Misconceptions of cochlear implants in the deaf community.* Symposium conducted at the National Association of the Deaf 45th Biennial Conference, Norfolk, VA.

Albinhac, D. (1978). Les implantes cochleaires. In *Contribution a l'histoire de l'experimentation humane.* Rennes: Thesis, Ecole Nationale de la Sante Publiques (as cited in Blume, 1999).

Allen, A. (2000, May 24). Sound and fury. *Salon* [On-line]. Available: http://www.salon.com/health/feature/2000/05/24/cochlear/index.html

Allen, T., Rawlings, B., & Remington, E. (1993). Demographic and audiological profiles of deaf children in Texas with cochlear implants. *American Annals of the Deaf, 138,* 260-266.

American Academy of Audiology. (1995). A position statement: Cochlear implants in children. *Audiology Today, 7* (3), 14-15.

Anderson, E. (1999). *Code of the street: Decency, violence, and the moral life of the inner city.* New York: Norton.

Andersson, Y. (1994). Do we want cochlear implants? *WFD News, 1,* 3-4.

Apicella, R. (1993, April/May). A parent's right. *Hearing Health,* 18-23.

Arana-Ward, M. (1997, May 11). As technology advances, a bitter debate divides the deaf. *The Washington Post,* p. A1.

Aronson, J. (Producer & Director). (1999). *Sound and Fury* [Film]. (Available from Aronson Films & Public Policy Productions, 35 E. 20th St., New York, NY 10003.)

Aschendorff, A., Marangos, N., & Laszig, R. (2000). Surgical technique for implantation of the CI24M. In S. B. Waltzman & N. L. Cohen (Eds.), *Cochlear implants* (pp. 157-158). New York: Thieme.

Balkany, T., Hodges, A., & Goodman, K. (1996). Ethics of cochlear implantation in young children. *Otolaryngology-Head and Neck Surgery, 114,* 748-755.

———. (1998). Additional comments. *Otolaryngology-Head and Neck Surgery, 119,* 312-313.

Balkany, T. J., Cohen, N. L., & Gantz, B. J. (1999). Clinical results with the Clarion multi-strategy cochlear implant. *Annals of Otology, Rhinology and Laryngology, 108* (Suppl. 177), 27-30.

Barker, E., Daniels, T., Dowell, R., Dettman, S., Brown, P. M., Remine, M., Psarros, C., Dornan, D., & Cowan, R. (2000, June). *Long term speech production outcomes in children who received cochlear implants before and after 2 years of age.* Symposium conducted at the Fifth European Symposium on Pediatric Cochlear Implantation. Antwerp, Belgium.

Barringer, F. (1993, May 16). Pride in a soundless world: Deaf oppose a hearing aid. *The New York Times,* pp. A1, A22.

Bat-Chava, Y., & Deignan, E. (2001). Peer relationships of children with a cochlear implant. *Journal of Deaf Studies and Deaf Education, 6,* 186-199.

Battmer, R. D., Haake, P., Zilberman, Y., & Lenarz, T. (1999). Simultaneous analog stimulation (SAS)—Continuous interleaved sampler (CIS) pilot comparison study in Europe. *Annals of Otology, Rhinology and Laryngology, 108* (Suppl. 177), 69-73.

Baumgartner, W., Youssefzadeh, S., Franz, P., Steurer, M., & Gstoettner, W. (2000). First results of magnetic resonance imaging in Combi 40 cochlear implant patients. In S. B. Waltzman & N. L. Cohen (Eds.), *Cochlear implants* (pp. 108-110). New York: Thieme.

Beiter, A. L., & Shallop, J. K. (1998). Cochlear implants: Past, present, and future. In W. Estabrooks (Ed.), *Cochlear implants for kids* (pp. 3-29). Washington, DC: Alexander Graham Bell Association for the Deaf.

Biderman, B. (1998). *Wired for sound: A journey into hearing.* Toronto, Canada: Trifolium.

Bienenstock, M. (1998/1999). The cochlear implant: Issues and controversies. *A Deaf American Monograph, 48,* 13-15.

Bilger, R. C., & Black, F. O. (1977). Auditory protheses in perspective. *Annals of Otology, Rhinology and Laryngology, 86* (Suppl. 38), 3-10.

————, Black, F. O., Hopkinson, N. T., Myers, E. N., Payne, J. L., Stenson, N. R., Vega, A., & Wolf, R. V. (1977). Evaluation of subjects presently fitted with implanted auditory prostheses. *Annals of Otology, Rhinology and Laryngology, 86* (Suppl. 38), 3-20.

Blamey, P. (1995, May). Factors affecting auditory performance of postlinguistically deaf adults using cochlear implants: Etiology, age, and duration of deafness. *Cochlear implants in adults and children* (pp. 15-20). Bethesda, MD: NIH Consensus Development Conference.

————, Sarant, J., Paatsch, L., Barry, J., Bow, C., Wales, R., Wright, M., Psarros, C., Rattigan, K., & Tooher, R. (2001). Relationships among speech perception, production, language, hearing loss, and age in children with impaired hearing. *Journal of Speech, Language, and Hearing Research, 44* (2), 264-285.

————, Sarant, J., Serry, T., Wales, R., James, C., Barry, J., Clark, G., Wright, M., Tooher, R., Psarros, C., Godwin, G., Rennie, M., & Meskin, T. (1998, November-December). Speech perception and spoken language in children with impaired hearing. *Fifth International Conference on Spoken Language Processing* (Vol. 6, pp. 2615-2618). Sydney, Australia.

Blanchfield, B., Dunbar, J., Feldman, J., & Gardner, E. (1999). *The severely to profoundly hearing impaired population in the United States: prevalence and demographics.* Available: http://www. projhope.org

Bloch, N. (1999). Update: The NAD and childhood cochlear implants. *The NAD Broadcaster, 21*(5), 5.

Blume, S. (1993, January). *Cochlear implantation.* Paper presented at the meeting of the Association GESTES, Paris, France.

——. (1994). *Making the deaf hear: The cochlear implant as promise and as threat.* Unpublished manuscript.

——. (1999). Histories of cochlear implantation. *Social Science & Medicine (49),* 1257–1268.

Bollard, P., Popp, A., Chute, P., & Parisier, S. (1999). Specific language growth in young children using the Clarion cochlear implant. *Annals of Otology, Rhinology and Laryngology, 108,* 119–123.

Bornstein, H., & Saulnier, K. (1981). Signed English: A brief follow-up to the first evaluation. *American Annals of the Deaf, 126* (1), 69–72.

——, Saulnier, K., & Hamilton, L. (1980). Signed English: A first evaluation. *American Annals of the Deaf, 125* (4), 467–481.

Brauer, B. (1993, June/July). Leap of faith. *Hearing Health,* 1-4.

Bravin, P. (2000). *Cochlear implants: Covering the basics* [Film]. (Available from DawnSign Press, 6130 Nancy Ridge Drive, San Diego, CA 92121-3223.)

Brown, C., & Yaremko, R. (1991). Special considerations of cochlear implants in children. *Australian Journal of Human Communication Disorders, 19* (2), 25–30.

Brueggemann, B. J. (1999). *Lend me your ear: Rhetorical constructions of deafness.* Washington, DC: Gallaudet University Press.

Bykowski, M. (2000, Summer). Allows enrollment at mainstream schools. *Soundwaves, 33,* 6.

Byrd, T. (1999, Fall). Cochlear implants: Where do you stand? *Gallaudet Today,* 16-24.

Carver, R. (1990, March 31). Cochlear implants in prelingual deaf children: A deaf perspective. *Cochlear implant forum.* Available: http://www.deafworldweb.org/pub/c/rc/cicarver.html

Cheng, A., Grant, G., & Niparko, J. K. (1999). Meta-analysis of pediatric cochlear implant literature. *Annals of Otology, Rhinology and Laryngology, 108* (4), 124–128.

——, Haya, K., Rubin, R., Powe N. R., Mellon, N. K., Francis, H.W., & Niparko, J. K. (2000, August 16). Cost-utility analysis of the cochlear implant in children. *Journal of the American Medical Association, 284,* 850–856.

Chouard, C. H. (1978). *Entendre sans Oreilles.* Paris: Robert Laffont (as cited in Blume, 1999).

Christiansen, J. (1999, February). Panel of cochlear implant users. Distinguished Faculty Presentation. Gallaudet University: Washington, DC.

————, & Barnartt, S. (1995). *Deaf president now! The 1988 revolution at Gallaudet University.* Washington, DC: Gallaudet University Press.

Clark, G. M. (1997). Historical perspectives. In G. M. Clark, R. S. C. Cowan, & R.C. Dowell (Eds.), *Cochlear implantation for infants and children: Advances* (pp. 9-27). San Diego: Singular Publishing Group, Inc.

————. (1999, October/November). Interviews with Patricia Spencer. Bionic Ear Institute, University of Melbourne, Australia.

————, Cowan, R., & Dowell, R. (1997). Ethical issues. In G. M. Clark, R. S. C. Cowan, & R. C. Dowell (Eds.), *Cochlear implantation for infants and children: Advances* (pp. 241-249). San Diego: Singular Publishing Group, Inc.

Clay, R. (1997). Do hearing devices impair deaf children? *APA Monitor, 28,* 1, 29-30.

Cochlear implants in children. (1991, March). *The NAD Broadcaster, 13 (3),* 1.

Cohen, N. (1995). The ethics of cochlear implants in young children. In A. Uziel & M. Mondain (Eds.), *Cochlear implants in children: 2nd European Symposium on Paediatric Cochlear Implantation* (pp. 1-3). Basel, Switzerland: Karger.

————. (2000a, April 2). *Cochlear implant forum.* Panel presented at the cochlear implant forum, New York University School of Medicine, New York City.

————. (2000b). Surgical techniques for cochlear implants. In S. B. Waltzman & N. L. Cohen (Eds.), *Cochlear implants* (pp. 151-156). New York: Thieme.

Colburn, D. (2000, October 3). Wired for sound. *The Washington Post Health Magazine,* 12-18.

Collins, F. (2001, July). The human genome project: Health care implications. Presentation at The Human Genome Project and Hearing Loss Conference, Bethesda, MD.

Connor, C., Hieber, S., Arts, A., & Zwolan, T. (2000). Speech, vocabulary, and the education of children using cochlear implants: Oral or total communication? *Journal of Speech, Language, and Hearing Research, 43 (5),* 1185-1204.

Contanche, D. (2000). Hair cell regeneration and the development of a biological cochlear implant. *Biotechnology and the cochlea* (pp. 4-6). Washington, DC: A. G. Bell Association of the Deaf.

Copmann, K. S. (1996). The audiological assessment. In S. Schwartz (Ed.), *Choices in deafness* (2nd Ed., pp. 17-38). Bethesda, MD: Woodbine House.

Corey, G., Corey, M., & Callanan, P. (1993). *Issues and ethics in the helping professions* (4th Ed.). Pacific Grove, CA: Brooks/Cole.

Corker, M. (1994). *Counseling: The deaf challenge.* London: Jessica Kingsley.

Crouch, R. (1997). Letting the deaf be deaf: Reconsidering the use of cochlear implants in prelingually deaf children. *Hastings Center Report, 27,* 14-21.

Davis, J., Elfenbein, J., Schum, R., & Bentler, R. (1986). Effects of mild and moderate hearing impairments on language, educational, and psychological behavior of children. *Journal of Speech and Hearing Disorders, 51* (1), 53-62.

Davis, L. (1995). *Enforcing normalcy: Disability, deafness, and the body.* London: Versace.

The death of deafness? The heart of the matter. (2000, March/April). *Hearing Health, 16* (2), 25-39.

Deaton, A. (1996). Ethical issues in pediatric rehabilitation: Exploring an uneven terrain. *Rehabilitation Psychology, 41,* 33-52.

Debate continues: FDA approves new cochlear implant device (1997). *The NAD Broadcaster, 19* (6), 1.

Demonstrations against childhood implants. (1994, April). *WFD News, 1,* 4.

Dorman, M. F. (1998). An overview of cochlear implants. In B. P. Tucker (Ed.), *Cochlear implants: A handbook* (pp. 5-28). Jefferson, NC: McFarland and Co.

Dowell, R., Blamey, & Clark, G. M. (1997, March). Factors affecting outcomes in children with cochlear implants. *Proceedings, XVI World Congress of Otorhinolaryngology-Head and Neck Surgery* (pp. 297-303). Sydney, Australia.

Drolsbaugh, M. (2000, June). Sound and fury: Choices, choices. *Silent News, 32,* 1, 7-8.

Ear implants are found to aid profound deafness. (1999, March 24). *The Boston Globe,* p. A9.

Easterbrooks, S., & Mordica, J. (2000). Teachers' ratings of functional communication in students with cochlear implants. *American Annals of the Deaf, 145* (1), 54-59.

Eilers, R., Cobo-Lewis, A., Vergara, K., & Oller, D. K. (1997). Longitudinal speech perception performance of young children with cochlear implants and tactile aids plus hearing aids. *Scandinavian Audiology, 26* (Suppl. 47), 50-54.

————, Cobo-Lewis, A., Vergara, K., Oller, D., & Dolan-Ash, M. (1995). A cohort study of children using multichannel tactile aids and cochlear implants. *Seminars in Hearing, 16* (4), 382-392.

Epstein, J. (1989). *The story of the bionic ear.* Melbourne, Australia: Hyland House.

Erting, C., Thumann-Prezioso, C., & Benedict, B. (2000). Bilingualism in a deaf family: Fingerspelling in early childhood. In P. Spencer, C. Erting, & M. Marschark (Eds.), *The deaf child in the family and at school* (pp. 41-54). Mahwah, NJ: Lawrence Erlbaum.

Ertmer, D. K., Kirk, K., Sehgal, S., Riley, A., & Osberger, M. (1997). A comparison of vowel production by children with multichannel cochlear implants or tactile aids: Perceptual evidence. *Ear & Hearing, 18,* 307–315.

Estabrooks, W. (1996). The auditory-verbal approach. In S. Schwartz (Ed.), *Choices in deafness* (2nd Ed., pp. 53–87). Bethesda, MD: Woodbine House.

Fernandes, J. (2000a, June 28). *Cochlear implant center opening.* E-mail distribution to the Gallaudet University community.

———. (2000b, Winter). Integrating cochlear implant technology. *Odyssey: New Directions in Deaf Education,* 17–19.

Fishman, A. J., & Holliday, R. A. (2000). Principles of cochlear implant imaging. In S. B. Waltzman & N. L. Cohen (Eds.), *Cochlear implants* (pp. 79–107). New York: Thieme.

Fleischer, L. (1993, April/May). Whose child is this? *Hearing Health,* 18–23.

Foster, E. (2000, October 10). Cochlear implants: Thousands unserved. *The Washington Post Health Magazine, 16* (4), 4.

Francis, H. W., Koch, M. E., Wyatt, J. R., & Niparko, J. K. (1999). Trends in educational placement and cost-benefit considerations in children with cochlear implants. *Otolaryngology-Head and Neck Surgery, 125,* 499–505.

Gallaudet Research Institute. (1999). *Regional and national summary report of data from the 1998-99 annual survey of deaf and hard of hearing children & youth.* Washington, DC: Gallaudet University.

Gannon, J. (1989). *The week the world heard Gallaudet.* Washington, DC: Gallaudet University Press.

Gary, L., & Hughes, C. (2000, February). *A second look at "tweeners." Candidacy considerations for 8 to 14.* Paper presented at the meeting of the Sixth International Cochlear Implant Conference, Miami, FL.

Gatty, J. (1996). The oral approach: A professional point of view. In S. Schwartz (Ed.), *Choices in deafness* (2nd Ed., pp. 163–171). Bethesda, MD: Woodbine House.

Geers, A., Brenner, C., & Davidson, L. (2000a). Speech perception changes in children switching from MPEAK to SPEAK coding strategy. In S. B. Waltzman & N. L. Cohen (Eds.), *Cochlear implants* (pp. 211–212). New York: Thieme.

———, & Moog, J. (1994). Speech perception results: Audition and lipreading enhancement. *Volta Review, 96,* 97–108.

———, Nicholas, J., Tye-Murray, N., Uchanski, R., Brenner, C., Crosson, J., Davidson, L., Spehar, B., Terteria, G., Tobey, E., Sedey, A., & Scrube, M. (2000b). *Cochlear implants and education of the deaf child: Second-year results.* Available: http://www.cid.wustl.edu/research

———, & Tobey, E. (1992). Effects of cochlear implants and tactile aids on the development of speech production skills in children with profound hearing impairment. *Volta Review, 94,* 135–163.

Gibson, W. (1991, August). Opposition from deaf groups to the cochlear implant. *Medical Journal of Australia* (as cited in Blume, 1993).

Hampton, J. (1997). *A survey of the current perspectives on cochlear implants.* Unpublished manuscript, Gallaudet University, Washington, DC.

Harvey, M. (2001). Does God have a cochlear implant? *Journal of Deaf Studies and Deaf Education, 6* (1), 70–81.

Heward, W. L. (1996). *Exceptional children: An introduction to special education* (5th Ed.). Englewood Cliffs, NJ: Prentice-Hall.

Hill, K. (1999, July). Letter to the editor: Confessions of a burned-out deafie. *Silent News,* pp. 4–5.

Hodges, A., Ash, M., Balkany, T., Schloffman, J., & Butts, S. (1999). Speech perception results in children with cochlear implants: Contributing factors. *Otolaryngology-Head and Neck Surgery, 121,* 31–34.

Holden-Pitt, L. (1998). *Discontinuation of cochlear implant use among prelingually-deaf children.* Unpublished manuscript, Gallaudet University, Washington, DC.

——, & Diaz, J. (1998). Thirty years of the annual survey of deaf and hard-of-hearing children and youth: A glance over the decades. *American Annals of the Deaf, 143,* 72–76.

House, W. F. (1995). *Cochlear implants: My perspective.* Available: http://www.marshall.edu/commdis/audiology/house/implants.html

——, & Berliner, K. (1991). Cochlear implants: From idea to clinical practice. In H. Cooper (Ed.), *Cochlear implants: A practical guide* (pp. 9–33). London: Whurr Publishers.

Humphries, T. (1993). Of deaf mutes, the strange, and the modern deaf self. In N. Glickman & M. Harvey (Eds.), *Culturally affirmative psychotherapy with deaf persons* (pp. 99–114). Mahwah, NJ: Lawrence Erlbaum.

Johnson, J., & Newport, E. (1989). Critical period effects in second-language learning: The influence of maturational state on the acquisition of English as a second-language. *Cognitive Psychology, 21,* 60–99.

Jonsen, A., Siegler, M., & Winslade, W. (1998). *Clinical ethics* (4th Ed.). New York: McGraw-Hill.

Kampfe, C., Harrison, M., Oettinger, T., Ludington, J., McDonald-Bell, C., & Pillsbury, H. (1993). Parental expectations as a factor in evaluating children for the multichannel cochlear implant. *American Annals of the Deaf, 138,* 297–303.

Kelsay, D., & Tyler, R. (1996). Children and cochlear implants. In F. Martin & J. Clark (Eds.), *Hearing care for children* (pp. 249–262). Boston: Allyn & Bacon.

Kluwin, T., & Stewart, D. (2000). Cochlear implants for younger children: A preliminary description of the parental decision process and outcomes. *American Annals of the Deaf, 145* (1), 26–32.

Lane, H. (1993, February/March). Cochlear implants: Boon for some— bane for others. *Hearing Health,* 19–23.

————. (1999). *The mask of benevolence: Disabling the deaf community.* (2nd Ed.). San Diego, CA: DawnSign Press.

————, & Bahan, B. (1998a). Ethics of cochlear implantation in young children: A review and reply from a deaf-world perspective. *Otolaryngology-Head and Neck Surgery, 119,* 297–307.

————, & Bahan, B. (1998b). Reply to the review. *Otolaryngology-Head and Neck Surgery, 119,* 309–312.

————, Hoffmeister, R., & Bahan, B. (1996). *A journey into the deaf-world.* San Diego, CA: DawnSign Press.

Leigh, I. W. (Ed.). (1999). *Psychotherapy with deaf clients from diverse groups.* Washington, DC: Gallaudet University Press.

————, & Lewis, J. W. (1999). Deaf therapists and the deaf community. In I. W. Leigh (Ed.), *Psychotherapy with deaf clients from diverse groups* (pp. 45–65). Washington, DC: Gallaudet University Press.

————, Sullivan, V. J., Graham-Kelly, M. P., & Aiello, P. (1998, July). *Cochlear implants and deaf adults: Implications for the deaf community from within.* Panel presentation at the National Association of the Deaf 44th Biennial Conference, San Antonio, TX.

Lomax, M. (2001, July). Hair cell regeneration. The potential for gene-based approaches. Presentation at The Human Genome Project and Hearing Loss Conference, Bethesda, MD.

Luxford, W. (2000, February). *Evaluation of the 12-18 month old cochlear implant candidate.* Paper presented at the meeting of the 6th International Cochlear Implant Conference, Miami, FL.

Mahshie, J. & Nussbaum, D. (2000, April 26). Campus forum shares information on cochlear implants. *On the Green* (4), 1.

Manning, A. (2000, May 2). *The changing deaf culture: Improved implants bring concern for a beautiful language.* Available: http://www.usatoday.com/usatonline/20000502/2217736s.htm

Markon, J. (1998, November 30). A gain or a loss. *Newsday,* pp. A5, A7.

Marschark, M. (1998). *Raising and educating a deaf child.* New York: Oxford University Press.

Mecklenburg, D., & Lehnhardt, E. (1991). The development of cochlear implants in Europe, Asia and Australia. In H. Cooper (Ed.), *Cochlear implants: A practical guide* (pp. 34–57). London: Whurr Publishers.

Meyer, T., Svirsky, M., Kirk, K., & Miyamoto, R. (1998). Improvements in speech perception by children with profound prelingual hearing loss: Effects of device, communication mode, and chronological age. *Journal of Speech and Hearing Research, 41* (4), 846–858.

Montgomery, G. (1991). Bionic miracle or megabuck acupuncture? The need for a broader context in the evaluation of cochlear implants. *Perspectives on Deafness: A Deaf American Monograph, 41,* 97–106.

Moores, D. F. (1996). *Educating the deaf* (4th Ed.). Boston: Houghton Mifflin.

Morford, J., & Mayberry, R. (2000). A reexamination of "early exposure" and its implications for language acquisition by eye. In C.

Chamberlain, J. Morford, & R. Mayberry (Eds.), *Language acquisition by eye* (pp. 111-127). Mahwah, NJ: Lawrence Erlbaum.

National Association of the Deaf (NAD). (1991). Report of the task force on childhood cochlear implants. *The NAD Broadcaster, 13,* 1-2, 6-7.

———. (2000a, April). NAD participates in XV WFD General Assembly. *The NAD Broadcaster, 22,* 27.

———. (2000b, October). *NAD position statement on cochlear implants.* Available: http://www.nad.org/infocenter/newsroom/papers/CochlearImplants.html

National Institute on Deafness and Other Communication Disorders. (1996). National strategic research plan. Bethesda, MD: National Institutes of Health (as cited in Niparko, 2000c).

National Institutes of Health. (1988, May 4). *Consensus development conference statement: Cochlear implants* (Vol. 7). Bethesda, MD: Author.

———. (1995). *Cochlear implants in adults and children: NIH consensus development conference statement, May 15-17, 1995.* Available: http://text.nlm.nih.gov/nih/cdc/www/100txt.html

Nevins, M. E., & Chute, P. M. (1996). *Children with cochlear implants in educational settings.* San Diego, CA: Singular Publishing Group.

Nikolopoulos, T., O'Donoghue, G., & Archbold, S. (1999). Age at implantation: Its importance in pediatric cochlear implantation. *The Laryngoscope, 109,* 595-599.

Niparko, J. K. (1998a, September/October). An update on cochlear implants, Part II: Implant candidacy: Would a cochlear implant be right for me? *Hearing Loss,* 20-22.

———. (1998b, November/December). An update on cochlear implants, Part III: Results and rehabilitation. *Hearing Loss,* 19-23.

———. (1999, March 7). *Cochlear implants.* Presented at the meeting of the Cochlear Implant Support Group Forum, Gallaudet University, Washington, DC.

———. (2000a). Assessment of cochlear implant candidacy. In J. K. Niparko, K. I. Kirk, N. K. Mellon, A. M. Robbins, D. L. Tucci, B. S. Wilson (Eds.), *Cochlear implants: Principles and practices* (pp. 173-177). Philadelphia, PA: Lippincott Williams & Wilkins.

———. (2000b). Culture and cochlear implants. In J. K. Niparko, K. Kirk, N. Mellon, A. Robbins, D. Tucci, D., & B. Wilson (Eds.), *Cochlear implants: Principles and practices* (pp. 371-379). Philadelphia, PA: Lippincott Williams & Wilkins.

———. (2000c). The epidemiology of hearing loss: How prevalent is hearing loss? In J. K. Niparko, K. Kirk, N. Mellon, A. Robbins, D. Tucci, D., & B. Wilson (Eds.), *Cochlear implants: Principles and practices* (pp. 88-92). Philadelphia, PA: Lippincott Williams & Wilkins.

———, Cheng, A. K., & Francis, H. W. (2000a). Outcomes of cochlear implantation: Assessment of quality of life implant and economic evaluation of the benefits of the cochlear implant in relation to costs. In J. K. Niparko, K. Kirk, N. Mellon, A. Robbins, D. Tucci, D., & B. Wilson (Eds.), *Cochlear implants: Principles and practices* (pp. 269–288). Philadelphia, PA: Lippincott Williams & Wilkins.

———, Kirk, K., Mellon, N., Robbins, A., Tucci, D. & Wilson, B. (2000b). *Cochlear implants: Principles and practices.* Philadelphia, PA: Lippincott Williams & Wilkins.

———, & Wilson, B. S. (2000). History of cochlear implants. In J. K. Niparko, K. I. Kirk, N. K. Mellon, A. M. Robbins, D. L. Tucci, & B. S. Wilson (Eds.), *Cochlear implants: Principles and practices* (pp. 103–107). Philadelphia, PA: Lippincott, Williams & Wilkins.

Oberkotter Foundation Film Project (Sponsor). (1998). *Dreams spoken here* [Film]. (Available from Oberkotter Foundation Film Project, P.O. Box 50215, Palo Alto, CA 94303-9465.)

O'Donoghue, G., Nikolopoulos, T., Archbold, S., & Tait, M. (1999). Cochlear implants in young children: The relationship between speech perception and speech intelligibility. *Ear & Hearing, 20* (5), 419–425.

Olkin, R. (1999). *What psychotherapists should know about disability.* New York: Guilford.

Osberger, M., & Fisher, L. (1999). SAS-CIS preference study in postlingually deafened adults implanted with the Clarion cochlear implant. *Annals of Otology, Rhinology and Laryngology, 108* (Suppl. 177), 74–79.

———, Fisher, L., Zimmerman-Phillips, L., Geier, L., & Barker, M. (1998). Speech recognition performance of older children with cochlear implants. *The American Journal of Otology, 19*, 152–175.

———, Robbins, A., Todd, S., & Riley, A. (1994). Speech intelligibility of children with cochlear implants [Monograph]. *Volta Review, 96* (5), 169–180.

———, Robbins, A. M., Todd, S. L., Riley, A., Kirk, K. I., & Carney, A. E. (1996). Cochlear implants and tactile aids for children with profound hearing impairment. In F. H. Bess, J. S. Gravel, & A. M. Tharpe (Eds.), *Amplification for children with auditory deficits* (pp. 283–310). Nashville, TN: Bill Wilkerson Center Press.

Otto, S. R., Ebinger, K., & Staller, S. J. (2000). Clinical trials with the auditory brainstem implant. In S. B. Waltzman & N. L. Cohen (Eds.), *Cochlear implants* (pp. 357–366). New York: Thieme.

Owens, D. (1999, January 15). Breaking the silence: Cochlear implants give the profoundly deaf a new hope of hearing, but not everyone is impressed. *The Orlando Sentinel,* p. E1.

Padden, C. (1980). The deaf community and the culture of deaf people. In C. Baker & R. Battison (Eds.), *Sign language and the deaf community* (pp. 89–103). Washington, DC: National Association of the Deaf.

———. (1996). From the cultural to the bicultural. In I. Parasnis (Ed.), *Cultural and language diversity and the deaf experience* (pp. 79–98). New York: Cambridge University Press.

————, & Humphries, T. (1988). *Deaf in America: Voices from a culture.* Cambridge, MA: Harvard University Press.

————, & Rayman, J. (2000). *The future of American Sign Language.* Unpublished manuscript, University of California, San Diego.

Patkowski, M. (1980). The sensitive period for the acquisition of syntax in a second language. *Language Learning, 30,* 449-472.

Peters, E. (2000). Our decision on a cochlear implant. *American Annals of the Deaf, 145,* 263-267.

Pisoni, D. (2000). Cognitive factors and cochlear implants: Some thoughts on perception, learning, and memory in speech perception. *Ear & Hearing, 21* (1), 70-78.

Pollard, R. (1996). Conceptualizing and conducting preoperative psychological assessments of cochlear implant candidates. *Journal of Deaf Studies and Deaf Education, 1,* 16-28.

Ponton, C., Moore, J., & Eggermont, J. (1999). Prolonged deafness limits auditory system developmental plasticity: Evidence from an evoked potentials study in children with cochlear implants. *Scandinavian Audiology, 28* (Suppl. 51), 13-22.

Population Reference Bureau. (2000). *2000 world population data sheet.* Washington, DC: Author.

Preisler, G., Ahlstrom, M., & Tvingstedt, A. (1997). The development of communication and language in deaf preschool children with cochlear implants. *International Journal of Pediatric Otorhinolaryngology, 41,* 263-271.

Primary colours. (2001, March 17). *The Economist,* 27-28.

Pyman, B., Blamey, P., Lacy, P., Clark, G. M., & Dowell, R. (2000). Development of speech perception in children using cochlear implants: Effects of etiology and delayed milestones. *American Journal of Otology, 21,* 57-61.

Quigley, S., & Paul, P. (1990). *Language and deafness.* San Diego, CA: Singular Publishing Group.

Rose, D., Vernon, M., & Pool, A. (1996). Cochlear implants in prelingually deaf children. *American Annals of the Deaf, 141,* 258-262.

Rosen, R. (1986). Deafness: A social perspective. In D. M. Luterman (Ed.), *Deafness in perspective* (pp. 345-355). San Diego, CA: College Hill Press.

————. (1992, December). President Rosen on cochlear implants. *NAD Broadcaster, 14,* 6.

Sacks, O. (1989). *Seeing voices: A journey into the land of the deaf.* Berkeley, CA: University of California Press.

Schein, J. (1989). *At home among strangers.* Washington, DC: Gallaudet University Press.

Schick, B., & Moeller, M. P. (1992). What is learnable in manually coded English sign systems? *Applied Psycholinguistics, 13* (3), 313-340.

Schindler, R. A. (1999). Personal reflections on cochlear implants. *Annals of Otology, Rhinology and Laryngology, 108* (Suppl. 177), 4–7.

Schwartz, S. (1996). *Choices in deafness* (2nd Ed.). Bethesda, MD: Woodbine House.

Self Help for the Hard of Hearing (1994, January/February). Position on cochlear implants. *SHHH Journal, 15,* 32–33.

Shannon, R. (1998). Review. *Otolaryngology-Head and Neck Surgery, 119,* 308–309.

———. (2000, March 4). Cochlear implant workshop technical discussion. *HOH-LD News, 2.* Available: HOH-LD-News-owner@onelist.com

Shannon, T. (1997). *An introduction to bioethics* (3rd Ed.). New York: Paulist Press.

Shapiro, W. H. (2000). Device programming. In S. B. Waltzman & N. L. Cohen (Eds.), *Cochlear implants* (pp. 185–193). New York: Thieme.

Simmons, F. B. (1985). Cochlear implants in young children: Some dilemmas. *Ear & Hearing, 6,* 61–63.

Solomon, A. (1994, August 28). Defiantly deaf. *The New York Times Magazine,* 38–45, 62, 65-68.

Spencer, L., Tye-Murray, N., & Tomblin, J. B. (1998). The production of English inflectional morphology, speech production and listening performance in children with cochlear implants. *Ear & Hearing, 19* (4), 310–318.

Spencer, P. (2000a). Every opportunity: A case study of hearing parents and their deaf child. In P. Spencer, C. Erting, & M. Marschark (Eds.), *The deaf child in the family and at school* (pp. 111–132). Hillsdale, NJ: Erlbaum.

———. (2000b, October). *She's still deaf, but now she can talk.* Paper presented at the meeting of the 15th Annual Conference on Issues in Language and Deafness, Boys Town National Research Hospital, Omaha, NE.

———. (2000c, November). *Factors contributing to English language development after early cochlear implantation.* Conference of American Speech, Language, and Hearing Association, Washington, DC.

Stewart, L. (1992). Debunking the bilingual/bicultural snow job in the American deaf community. In M. Garretson (Ed.), *Viewpoints on Deafness: A Deaf American Monograph, 42,* 129–142.

Stewart-Muirhead, E. (1998, Aug.). "Fixing" deafness: Ethical issues in cochlear implantation. *Bioethics Bulletin, 6* (4). Available: http://www.ualberta. ca/~ethics/bb6-4fix.htm

Svirsky, M., & Meyer, T. (1999). Comparison of speech perception in pediatric Clarion cochlear implant and hearing aid users. *Annals of Otology, Rhinology and Laryngology, 108* (4), 104–109.

————, Robbins, A., Kirk, K., Pisoni, D., & Miyamoto, R. (2000). Language development in profoundly deaf children with cochlear implants. *Psychological Science, 11* (2), 1-6.

Swidler, A. (1986, April). Culture in action. *American Sociological Review, 51,* 273-286.

Synopsis of the 6th International Cochlear Implant Conference. (2000). Miami, FL: Advanced Bionics. Available: http://www.cochlearimplant. com/CI2000Summ1.html

Tait, M., Lutman, M., & Robinson, K. (2000). Preliminary measures of preverbal communicative behavior as predictors of cochlear implant outcomes in children. *Ear & Hearing, 21* (1), 18-24.

Teissl, C., Kremser, K., Hochmair, E. S., & Hochmair-Desoyer, I. J. (2000). Magnetic resonance imaging compatibility of a cochlear implant. In S. B. Waltzman & N. L. Cohen (Eds.), *Cochlear implants* (pp. 112-115). New York: Thieme.

Testimony Before the FDA. (1997, June). *The NAD Broadcaster, 19* (6), 2, 6-7.

Tomblin, J. B., Spencer, L., Flock, S., Tyler, R., & Gantz, B. (1999). A comparison of language achievement in children with cochlear implants and children using hearing aids. *Journal of Speech, Language, and Hearing Research, 42,* 497-511.

Tucci, D. L., & Niparko, J. K. (2000). Medical and surgical aspects of cochlear implantation. In J. K. Niparko, K. I. Kirk, N. K. Mellon, A. M. Robbins, D. L. Tucci, & B. S. Wilson (Eds.), *Cochlear implants: Principles and practices* (pp. 189-224). Philadelphia, PA: Lippincott Williams & Wilkins.

Tucker, B. (1998a). *Cochlear implants: A handbook.* Jefferson, NC: McFarland & Company, Inc.

————. (1998b). Deaf culture, cochlear implants, and elective disability. *Hastings Center Report, 28,* 6-14.

Tucker, J. (1996, Spring). Questions, questions, and questions. . . . *The Maryland Bulletin,* 10.

————. (1999, Spring-Summer). An open letter to editors of newspapers, magazines, and electronic newsletters. *MDAD News, 39* (2-3), 8-9.

Tye-Murray, N., Spencer, L., & Woodworth, G. (1995). Acquisition of speech by children who have prolonged cochlear implant experience. *Journal of Speech and Hearing Research, 38,* 327-337.

Tyler, R. (1993, March). Cochlear implants and the deaf culture. *American Journal of Audiology,* 26-32.

U.S. Census Bureau. (1999). *Statistical abstract of the United States.* Washington, DC: U.S. Government Printing Office.

Vernon, M., & Alles, C. (1994). Issues in the use of cochlear implants with prelingually deaf children. *American Annals of the Deaf, 139,* 485–492.

Vincent, C., LeJeune, J., & Vaneecloo, F. (2000). The Digisonic auditory brain stem implant: Report of the first three cases. In S. B. Waltzman & N. L. Cohen (Eds.), *Cochlear implants* (pp. 369–371). New York: Thieme.

Waltzman, S. B., & Cohen, N. L. (1998). Cochlear implants in children younger than 2 years old. *American Journal of Otology, 19,* 158–162.

———, & Shapiro, W. (1999). Cochlear implants in children. *Trends in Amplification, 4,* 143–162.

Warrick, J. (1998, October 28). AIDS's shadow cools global population forecast. *The Washington Post,* p. 3E.

Weber, B. P., Neuburger, J., Dillo, W., Battmer, R., & Lenarz, T. (2000). New magneticless cochlear implant: Concept and clinical results. In S. B. Waltzman & N. L. Cohen (Eds.), *Cochlear implants* (pp. 115–116). New York: Thieme.

———, Neuburger, J., Goldring, J. E., Santogrossi, T., Eng, B., Koestler, H., Battmer, R. D., & Lenarz, T. (1999). Clinical results of the Clarion magnetless cochlear implant. *Annals of Otology, Rhinology and Laryngology, 108* (Suppl. 177), 22–26.

Wegener, S. (1996). The rehabilitation ethic and ethics. *Rehabilitation Psychology, 41,* 5–17.

Williams, J. M. (2000, May 5). Do health-care providers have to pay for assistive tech? *Business Week.* Available: http://www.businessweek.com/bwdaily/dnflash/may2000/nf00505c.htm

Wrigley, O. (1996). *The politics of deafness.* Washington, DC: Gallaudet University Press.

Yaffe, S. (1999, March). To hear or not to hear. *Toronto Sun* (Canada). Available: http://www.deafworldweb.org/pub/c/ci.march99.html

Young, N. M., Grohne, K. M., Carrasco, V. N., & Brown, C. (1999). Speech perception in young children using Nucleus 22-channel or Clarion cochlear implants. *Annals of Otology, Rhinology and Laryngology, 108* (Suppl. 177), 99–103.

Zimmerman-Phillips, S., & Murad, C. (1999). Programming features of the Clarion multi-strategy cochlear implant. *Annals of Otology, Rhinology and Laryngology, 108* (Suppl. 177), 17–21.

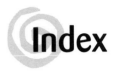# Index

Please note: Page references in *italics* indicate figures; page references in **boldface** indicate tables.

DATE DUE